Public Health
LEADERSHIP &
MANAGEMENT

The cover artwork by Gustav Klimt (1862-1912) is Hygeia—the Greek goddess of health. It is part of a larger work titled *Medicine* that was painted between 1900 and 1907 and destroyed by fire in 1945. Images of Hygeia are frequently used to represent the profession of public health. For example, in 1970 a marble bust of Hygeia was installed outside the main entrance of the Centers for Disease Control and Prevention (CDC) in Atlanta, Georgia. Klimt, in his extraordinary painting, portrays the Greek goddess with her traditional cup and snake—symbols that represent the waxing and waning of life and death. Born in Austria, Klimt became the foremost exponent of art nouveau in Vienna. His greatest works were portraits and landscapes of exotic sensibility, with symbolic themes and extravagent rhythms. Klimt was significantly influenced by the vibrant colors of Byzantine mosaics, clearly evident in his Hygeia.

Public Health
LEADERSHIP&
MANAGEMENT
Cases and Context

Stuart A. Capper
University of Alabama at Birmingham

Peter M. Ginter
University of Alabama at Birmingham

Linda E. Swayne
University of North Carolina at Charlotte

Sage Publications
International Educational and Professional Publisher
Thousand Oaks ■ London ■ New Delhi

For information:

Sage Publications, Inc.
2455 Teller Road
Thousand Oaks, California 91320
E-mail: order@sagepub.com

Sage Publications Ltd.
6 Bonhill Street
London EC2A 4PU
United Kingdom

Sage Publications India Pvt. Ltd.
M-32 Market
Greater Kailash I
New Delhi 110 048 India

Printed in the United States of America

Library of Congress Cataloging-in-Publication Data

Capper, Stuart A.
    Public health leadership and management : cases and context / by
Stuart A. Capper, Peter M. Ginter, and Linda E. Swayne.
        p. cm.
    Includes bibliographical references and index.
    ISBN 0-7619-2318-7
    1. Public health administration—Case studies.   I. Ginter, Peter M.
II. Swayne, Linda E. III. Title.
    RA425 .C34 2001
    362.1'068—dc21   2001003380

This book is printed on acid-free paper.

                     06   7   6   5   4   3   2

Acquisition Editor:	Marquita Flemming
Editorial Assistant:	MaryAnn Vail
Production Editor:	Sanford Robinson
Editorial Assistant:	Cindy Bear
Typesetter:	Tina Hill
Indexer:	Molly Hall
Cover Designer:	Michelle Lee

Contents

FOREWORD   ix

      William L. Roper, MD, MPH

PREFACE   xi

PART I: Improving Public Health Leadership and Management   1

CHAPTER 1. ANALYZING PUBLIC HEALTH CASES   3

      Stuart A. Capper, Peter M. Ginter,
      Linda E. Swayne, and W. Jack Duncan

CHAPTER 2. INFORMATION SOURCES FOR PUBLIC HEALTH LEADERS   21

      Arthur P. Liang and Sherrill Snuggs

CHAPTER 3. ORAL PRESENTATIONS IN PUBLIC HEALTH SETTINGS   35

      Gary F. Kohut and Carol M. Baxter

CHAPTER 4. FINANCIAL ANALYSIS FOR HEALTH CARE ORGANIZATIONS   55

      Mahmud Hassan

PART II: Public Health—Context   83

INDUSTRY NOTE 1: THE U.S. HEALTH CARE SYSTEM   85

      Stuart A. Capper

INDUSTRY NOTE 2: THE U.S. PUBLIC HEALTH SYSTEM   109
Ray M. Nicola

PART III: Public Health—Cases   131

**CASE 1—CDC AND THE MANTOOKAN BLOOD SUPPLY:
A TOUGH MANAGEMENT DECISION**   133
Terrie C. Reeves, Stuart A. Capper, Arthur P. Liang,
and Gail W. McGee

CASE 2—AIDSCAP NEPAL   155
Ven Sriram and Franklyn Manu

**CASE 3—THE INDIANA STATE DEPARTMENT OF
HEALTH: MANAGING STRATEGICALLY**   173
Peter M. Ginter, Linda E. Swayne, and W. Jack Duncan

**CASE 4—COOPER GREEN HOSPITAL AND THE
COMMUNITY CARE PLAN**   199
Alice M. Adams, Peter M. Ginter, and Linda E. Swayne

**CASE 5—INTERMARK: DESIGNING UNICEF'S ORAL
REHYDRATION PROGRAM IN ZAMBIA**   221
Ronald Stiff

**CASE 6—THE NEW YORK STATE WEST NILE VIRUS
OUTBREAK: WHAT SHOULD BE NASSAU
COUNTY'S RESPONSE?**   237
Written by Amy Dreibelbis, Jason Farley,
William Lovett, and Stephanie Waldrop under the
supervision of Susan L. Davies, Peter M. Ginter,
Robert R. Jacobs, Donna J. Petersen, and Dale O. Williams;
revised by Stuart A. Capper, Peter M. Ginter, and
Linda E. Swayne

**CASE 7—INDIAN HEALTH SERVICE:
CREATING A CLIMATE FOR CHANGE**   265
Robert Tusatto, Terrie C. Reeves, W. Jack Duncan,
and Peter M. Ginter

CASE 8—THREE VEXING CASES IN HEALTH CARE ETHICS   285
John M. Lincourt

CASE 9—DEKALB COUNTY BOARD OF HEALTH (A):
   SELECTING A NEW DIRECTOR   289

CASE 9—DEKALB COUNTY BOARD OF HEALTH (B):
   REDEFINING THE PARADIGM OF SUCCESS   295
   Jane C. Nelson and Thomas C. Neil

CASE 10—RED TIDE AND RED INK IN
   ESCAMBIA COUNTY, FLORIDA   299
   Written by Tina Cummings, Willie Lipato,
   Mustafa Mohd, and Alan Rowan under the
   supervision of Susan L. Davies, Peter M. Ginter,
   Robert Jacobs, Donna J. Petersen, and Dale O. Williams;
   revised by Stuart A. Capper, Peter M. Ginter, and
   Linda E. Swayne

CASE 11—THE NEW MEXICO
   MENINGOCOCCAL OUTBREAK   307
   Gary Simpson, Maria Goldstein, Patricia Barnett,
   Paul Ettestad, Judith Candelaria, and Stuart Capper

CASE 12—C. W. WILLIAMS COMMUNITY HEALTH CENTER   319
   Linda E. Swayne and Peter M. Ginter

CASE 13—BUILDING FOR THE FUTURE OF
   PUBLIC HEALTH IN ALABAMA   339
   Rueben E. Davidson, Stuart A. Capper, and
   Mahmud Hassan

CASE 14—POSSIBLE BIOTERRORISM IN NEW HAMPSHIRE:
   A PUBLIC HEALTH RESPONSE   369
   Stuart A. Capper

CASE 15—¡DESPIERTA! A PHYSICIAN'S STARK ENCOUNTER
   WITH THE GRIM HUMAN TOLL OF A
   PREVENTABLE PUBLIC HEALTH PROBLEM   379
   Daniel J. Derksen

INDEX   383

ABOUT THE AUTHORS   393

Foreword

During my career, I have been fortunate to work in a variety of senior positions with local, state, federal, and private health organizations. As I think back on my experiences, I recognize that there was little in my formal education that prepared me for the breadth and complexity of the leadership and management judgments I was called on to make.

Throughout my medical education, with the guidance of faculty, I studied case after case and refined my ability to help individual patients through difficult clinical judgments. However, during my public health education, there was little if any opportunity to practice applying the powerful science I was learning to real world public health judgments. This book aids significantly the important process of filling a void in public health leadership and management education by providing cases that allow students a classroom experience somewhat akin to real life public health decision-making.

The fifteen case studies in this book place the reader in a wide variety of real public health leadership situations, ranging—as one reviewer commented—from babies to bioterrorism. Each situation is presented to the student with the swirl of communications, conflicts, and conundrums that I have found accompany any difficult public health leadership judgement. The diversity of the organizational settings is quite wide. Students will find themselves grappling with issues from local, state, and federal public health agencies as well as private organizations that have substantial public health missions. The setting for these organizations is within many different geographic regions, both domestic and international.

As I have moved around this country to assume various health leadership positions, I have been struck by the influence that local and organizational contexts can have on the decisions that are made. The case writers have done a very good job of placing the student in public health decisional situations that, to me, feel like the reality of my own professional life.

As Professors Capper, Ginter, and Swayne mention in their preface for this book, the cases are not presented to illustrate correct or incorrect decision making. I believe this is as it should be. My experience suggests that few of the difficult decisions our public health leaders face in the future will have a clearly right answer. Instead, they will be called upon to make difficult judgments and to be ready and willing to explain and be accountable for the decisions they have made. Participating in discussions of the timely and complex cases in this book will give future, as well as current, leaders the opportunity to practice the essence of our profession.

Having been a public health practitioner and now, as a public health academic, I am especially pleased to see the extensive collaboration that occurred between these two groups. The realism, relevance, and quality of this book are not because of either public health practice or public health academics. Rather, it is the collaboration that created the success.

This book is both good education and a good read. It is my hope that it will substantially aid the research, writing, and teaching by the case method that needs to be established within the profession of public health.

William L. Roper, MD, MPH
Dean, School of Public Health
The University of North Carolina at Chapel Hill

Preface

Noted educators and business writers Warren Bennis and Burt Nanus stated, "Managers are people who do things right, and leaders are people who do the right thing." This statement suggests that management is more about efficiency, whereas leadership is more about effectiveness. The often cited Institute of Medicine (IOM) study *The Future of Public Health* called for public health education to increase its emphasis on both managerial and leadership skills. The implications of the IOM study were that public health institutions need to be more effective in carrying out their mission and use their available resources much more efficiently.

Over the past fourteen years, a variety of public health organizations have sought ways to respond. Federal agencies such as the Centers for Disease Control and Prevention (CDC) and the Health Resources and Services Administration (HRSA) have funded and worked within public health to develop management and leadership institutes at the national and regional levels. Many state and local public health systems have established public health leadership training programs within their jurisdictions. Schools of public health have worked with federal and foundation funding partners in addition to state and local public health agencies to establish and conduct leadership training through continuing education and certificate programs as well as degree-granting programs. It is our belief that case studies are a valuable tool to develop the management and leadership skills envisioned by the Institute of Medicine and that these skills will, in turn, make public health institutions more effective and efficient. Learning to apply independent critical analysis in the making of difficult public health judgments is the essence of professional public health practice. The dilemma is how to develop the ability to make good public health decisions without undo risk to the public's health. As educators, we believe it is important to incorporate these difficult decisions in the classroom for students to practice and develop the skills with full, frank, and critical discussion of the students' recommendations.

Definitive answers to tomorrow's public health problems will not be found in the public health leadership programs of today. The complexity of national and international public health practice and the rapid changes in the context for public health leadership mean that there will be few situations where rote learning will provide solutions. Public health professionals must learn to apply an independent critical analysis and to make judgments that balance conflicting and completing interests, interests that may or may not accept the best public health science that, in a rapidly evolving situation, may or may not provide clear guidance.

For more than 100 years professionals in medicine, law, and management have relied on case studies as a didactic method for education. Case studies are an ideal pedagogy to practice professional decision-making and leadership skills because they place the student in real situations—situations that actually were encountered by professionals—with all the information, conflicts, and confusions inherent in the difficult decisions that were faced. Cases do not reveal to the student what the professional decided or how the decision was made. The cases do provide students with the situation and opportunity to practice making tough professional judgments. The ensuing discussion offers a chance to present and defend the logic of a particular recommendation and listen to others who have different views. Thinking is the method of intelligent learning, and case studies help teach discussion participants how to think.

This book is designed to overcome the lack of public health practice case studies. Each case provides a wide variety of public health leadership challenges based on actual events in public health practice. The cases were not written to illustrate correct or incorrect decision making; rather, the cases give students the chance, in a protected and collegial environment, to develop their public health management and leadership skills.

Organization of the Book

This book is divided into three parts. Part I contains four chapters that provide methods to improve public health management and leadership through case analysis and decision making. Chapter 1 includes a framework for case analysis, Chapter 2 presents a valuable list of sources for public health information, Chapter 3 provides guidance for making effective oral presentations, and Chapter 4 presents a brief primer on health care finance.

Part II of the book provides descriptive information about the U.S. health care system and the U.S. public health system to provide the context for public health decision making. Although public health leaders have some control over the organizations they manage, they have little control over the forces outside their agencies that influence public health practice. The "rules" for successful public health leadership are defined outside public health organizations.

Part III contains fifteen public health case studies that present a wide array of challenging and complex public health issues. The cases are based on field research conducted in a variety of public health agencies. Many have been coauthored by public health practitioners. The cases encompass all the core public health disciplines and engage the student in integrating these disciplines into management and leadership practice.

Acknowledgments

Many people helped and encouraged us as we worked on this book. First, we would like to thank all the authors of the cases. Case writing is a difficult art requiring many hours of library research, personal interviews, and detailed analyses. The case contributors in this text represent some of the finest researchers anywhere. They have greatly enhanced the important body of public health case literature. In addition, we want to pay a special tribute to the authors of the chapters in this text. It has been a wonderful experience to work with each of them.

We would like to provide special recognition to all the state and local public health leaders who have assisted us, including Don Williamson, Carole Samuelson, Max Michael, Clyde Barganier, Kathy Vincent, and Frances Kennamer of Alabama; Pat Cleaveland, Barak Wolff, Norty Kalishman, and Alex Valdez of New Mexico; Joe Hunt of Indiana; Jesse Greenblatt of New Hampshire; Joe Kimbrell of Louisiana; Gail Gannaway and Lewis Leslie of Arkansas; and Paul Wiesner of Georgia. At the federal level, we are indebted to Earl Fox and Ron Merrill of HRSA as well as Stephen Thacker, Andrew Dannenberg, and Edward Baker of CDC.

Within the academic community, we have many outstanding colleagues who have contributed to our work in a variety of ways. They include Dean Eli Capilouto and Associate Dean Donna Petersen of UAB, Dean Ann Anderson of Tulane, and Dean Claude Lilly of UNC Charlotte as well as Professors Jack Duncan and Michael Maetz. We offer special thanks to Bill Roper for writing the forward to this book. Dr. Roper has been an important leader in public health and has always been supportive of our projects.

Thanks to our collaborators at Sage Publications—Marquita Flemming, our editor, with whom we have had an enjoyable and productive relationship, and Rolf Janke, whose unfailing enthusiasm for our work is always motivational.

We deeply appreciate the support and comradeship of all the individuals who have influenced and encouraged us. Most important, we want to recognize the patience, love, and support of our families. After all, they are what it is all about.

Stuart A. Capper
Peter M. Ginter
Linda E. Swayne

PART I

Improving Public Health Leadership and Management

P art I contains four chapters that provide tools for decision making and case analysis. The first chapter presents a process for addressing and solving public health case studies. It provides a broad template for thinking through and making decisions in complex public health situations. Chapter 2 presents a valuable list of sources for public health information including abstracts, electronic information sources, dictionaries, directories, handbooks and guides, journals, and Internet public health resources. These information sources are essential for the public health practitioner addressing actual public health issues and for the case analyst searching for additional case information. Chapter 3 provides recommendations for making effective oral presentations. These presentation suggestions are appropriate for both classroom presentations and presentations required in public health practice. The last chapter presents a brief primer on health care finance. The primer is designed to provide a broad view of health care finance that may be applied to a variety of health care and public health situations.

CHAPTER 1

Analyzing Public Health Cases

Public health management and leadership roles often call for far-reaching decisions that will affect the health of a community. Decisions must be made despite conflicting data, divergent opinions, and competing political agendas. Therefore, public health management and leadership require an understanding of current and emerging community health issues as well as the agency's resources and capabilities. In addition, in making these decisions, public health managers and leaders must understand public health practice and science. Public health management and leadership decisions typically require simultaneously balancing community issues, organizational issues, and public health science. In this complex decision environment, there are many competing issues, and public health science informs the judgment—it does not make the decision.

How does a leader and manager learn to make decisions in public health organizations? The most valuable way is to practice making decisions. The public's health may suffer until a leader develops his or her skills by on-the-job trial and error. Another way to acquire experience is to observe the decision making of others. Unfortunately, learning by observing others is not practical in most rapidly changing environments, nor is it practical in the often unique situations that public health leaders face.

Even if trial-and-error learning or learning by observation were feasible, it would be very risky; therefore, public health organizations, hospitals, and other health providers would trust important decision making only to the most "seasoned managers." As a result, case studies have been used successfully to provide aspiring leaders with the opportunity to practice making decisions without "betting the organization" and the public's health on the outcome. In other words, case studies offer an opportunity to deal with real decisions in a low-risk environment.

This chapter was written by Stuart A. Capper, Peter M. Ginter, Linda E. Swayne, and W. Jack Duncan.

The case studies presented in this book contain situations actually faced by managers and leaders in public health organizations and are documented in a way that makes them useful in educating decision makers. The decisions required to solve these cases represent a wide range of complexity, so that no two cases are addressed in exactly the same manner. In the following discussion, one method of case analysis is presented. This approach is useful because it is a logical method of decision making. Exhibit 1.1 offers a process or way of thinking about cases rather than prescribing the only way to analyze them.

First, it is important to gather information and identify the issues. Often, there will be many issues in a case that eventually will lead to defining the problem or identifying an opportunity. Identifying as many of the issues as possible is critical to understanding the problem clearly. Ultimately, the decision maker may not be able to deal with every issue. However, knowing the issues and being able to prioritize them is fundamental to defining the problem and crafting a decision. Information in the case may or may not be useful. Part of the process of identifying issues is to evaluate the information and differentiate between factual information, inferential information, speculations, and assumptions.

Second, it is important to understand the decision context or external forces that may affect public health—the political/legal, economic, social/cultural, technological, competitive, and health issues that public health leaders face. These forces represent the *context* that frames the decision. At this point, relating the capabilities of the organization to the decision context becomes important. To do this, a thorough and objective analysis of the organization's internal strengths and weaknesses is required. One of the most useful ways to look introspectively at a public health organization is to examine its resource base and the capabilities possessed by its professional and nonprofessional employees. In addition, it is necessary to understand the unique culture of the organization, including its mission and goals.

Once the situation analysis is complete—examining the decision context, the organization, and the organization's mission and goals—the problem or opportunity should be identified and alternatives generated as possible solutions. At least some thought must be given to the outcomes likely to result from the different choices. The effectiveness of the various alternatives must be evaluated. Then one of the alternatives needs to be chosen to become the recommendation and its method of implementation considered.

Although the approach outlined here is logical, it is important to remember that a case should be approached and appreciated as a unique opportunity for problem solving. The organization, context, and decision make each case different.

Cases: Real and Hypothetical

Many different types of cases are used for public health leadership and management education. Sometimes cases are invented to illustrate a specific point. Usually these appear as "ABC Public Health Department" or some similar name. Other cases are real but disguised. A writer may, for example, have information from an organiza-

Exhibit 1.1. Process of Analysis for Public Health Cases

Steps of the Process	*Processes*
■ Gather information and identify preliminary issues	□ Read the case □ List key issues □ Use the administrative disciplines and core public health disciplines to cue and screen issues □ Reread the case and take notes on evidence (documentation) of issues □ Evaluate evidence as facts, inferences, assumptions, and judgments □ Obtain additional information on issues not presented in the case (if required)
■ Analyze the present situation	□ Evaluate the decision context specifying the relevant economic, regulatory, demographic, technological, health care, service area, and service category issues/forces □ Identify the organization's strengths and weaknesses including culture, marketing, organization, human resources, finance, and information systems □ Evaluate the importance of the strengths and weaknesses in light of the decision context (SWOT analysis) □ Evaluate the mission of the organization □ Evaluate the goals of the organization
■ Finalize issue identification	□ Eliminate symptoms and identify causes □ Finalize "core" issues (problems/opportunities) □ Prioritize core problems/opportunities □ State the issues
■ Analysis	□ Develop a theoretical perspective □ Generate alternative solutions or actions □ Evaluate alternatives using administrative and core public health discipline theory and methods
■ Make recommendation	□ Select alternatives □ Present theoretical underpinning □ Illustrate how the recommendation addresses the problem/opportunity
■ Develop action plan	□ Specify the activities necessary to achieve the selected alternative □ Group activities and suggest persons responsible for achieving the activities □ Specify timeline for accomplishing activities
■ Finalize report	□ Prepare written report □ Prepare oral report

tion such as the Veterans Administration or Medicaid in Illinois but for some reason have been asked not to use the name of the organization.

The best cases, like those in this book, are real and undisguised. Cases such as "CDC and the Mantookan Blood Supply" and "The Indiana State Department of

Public Health" are obviously about real organizations. The cases in this book have been selected because of the important issues they present for public health leaders. Sometimes the issues presented are not even problems. Often the greatest challenge facing an organization is recognizing and acting on an opportunity rather than solving a problem.

Cases that have obvious solutions that everyone agrees with are not good for practicing decision making. Leaders in public health organizations rarely face decisions where the solution is obvious to everyone. Real life is quite complex, and so are most cases. For example, public health science may be in conflict with political realities, economic issues may be at odds with social issues or priorities, and optimal alternatives may not be feasible. Although there is seldom a single correct answer in case analysis, some recommendations clearly are better than are others. The evaluation of a case analysis is often based more on the approach and logic employed than the precise recommendation offered. This often mirrors the way a choice by a public health decision maker will be evaluated in the practice setting. Because difficult judgments are often required, and because there will be no absolutely correct or incorrect decision, constituents may evaluate the decision of the public health leader based on his or her logic and approach rather than the specific decision. As long as the decision is rational in the context of the community, the logic and approach used by the public health leader to reach the decision often will form the foundation of the leader's credibility and the basis for the community's acceptance of the decision.

Cases, Management, and Public Health

Cases offer practice in decision making that is impossible to achieve through other means. Cases rarely give us all the information we need; decision makers in public health organizations rarely have all the information they want or need when they face decisions. Risks must be taken in real-life decision making, and a good case analysis will involve similar types of risks. A poor case analysis may be embarrassing for the student, but it will not result in unnecessary health risks, poor policy decisions, misinterpretation of science, or declining health status for a community. At the same time, the lessons learned by analyzing cases and participating in discussions will build problem-solving skills.

Many future public health decision makers are not familiar with how to analyze cases. For this reason, this chapter has been included—not to prescribe how all cases should be solved but to offer some initial direction on how to "surface" the real issues presented in the cases and carry out logical analysis.

Solving Case Problems

Solving a case is much like solving any problem. First, the issues are defined, information is gathered, and alternatives are generated, evaluated, recommended, and implemented. Although the person solving one of the cases from this book seldom has the opportunity to implement a decision, he or she should always keep in mind that recommendations must be tempered by the limitations imposed on the organization in terms of its human and nonhuman resources. As the likely success or failure of the recommendation is analyzed and discussed, lessons are learned that can be applied to future decision making.

Alternative Perspectives: Passion or Objectivity

Public health management and leadership cases have to do with people in organizations trying to make decisions in the face of uncertainty. Therefore, the key decision maker and the organization must be identified. Public health is an organized effort to create healthy people in healthy communities, and it is through our organizations and their leadership that public health makes a difference. It is thus important to identify a decision-making role (as case analyst) in the case.

Different hypothetical roles can be assumed when analyzing cases. Some students prefer to assume the organization leader's position in order to become a passionate advocate of a particular course of action. Others prefer to observe the case from the detached objectivity of a consultant who has been employed by the organization to solve a problem.

Either perspective can be useful, but the first offers some unique advantages. Because there are no absolutely correct or incorrect answers to complex cases, the most important lesson to learn is why managers and leaders behave as they do, why they select one alternative in preference to others, and why they pursue specific alternatives under the conditions presented in the case. When students think about or discuss a case with others in terms of "we," as in "we don't have the manpower to vaccinate all children in the community" or "we don't have the time to go through normal channels for approval," the case analysts have "internalized" the case, creating a decision-making opportunity that is their own.

The consultant's perspective allows the student to step back, look at decision makers who are engaging in strategies that may be radically different from those of their counterparts in the same service area, and objectively assess the likely outcomes of their actions. The consultant can more easily play the devil's advocate and point out how actions are at odds with current theory. Although the fun and excitement of case analysis is enhanced by assuming the decision maker's role, the options can often be expanded through the more objective and detached outlook of the consultant.

Feel the excitement and fear of doing new and innovative things in a dynamic and complex public health environment. Defend recommendations and challenge others to defend what they have recommended. Through this discussion, a better recommendation may emerge. The goal of case analysis discussion is to try to surface all possibilities and attempt to make the best recommendation for the community and the organization—whether the passionate role of the leader or the objective role of the consultant is taken.

Preparation:
An Essential Aspect of Case Analysis

Effective case analysis begins with the first reading of the case. If a student skims the case several days before beginning the analysis, "free" thinking can be obtained. Often problems presented in cases are complex and require considerable thought. Thinking through the issues may take some time and consideration of multiple issues. Therefore, it is helpful if the initial reading is done several days ahead of the assignment's due date. Often a case has to be read a number of times. Rarely can anyone absorb enough information from the first reading of a comprehensive case to adequately solve it. Therefore, collect information and make notes about details as the case unfolds—try to develop a preliminary list of issues.

Gathering Information

The information required to solve a case successfully comes in a number of forms. The first type of information is given as part of the case and may includes things such as the history of the public health department, community health center, or federal agency; its organization; its leadership; and its financial situation (administrative information). In addition, public health data and science may be presented—epidemiological, health behavior, environmental health, biostatistical, or health policy data, theory, and applications (core public health disciplines). Students will have to assess the accuracy and relevancy of the data, methodology, and interpretation of such information. Some cases will include extensive information about the decision context, but others will not.

"Obtainable" information is not provided in the case or by the instructor but is available from secondary sources in the library or from the Internet. Examples of sources of obtainable public health information are given in Chapter 2. If the case does not include extensive information, the instructor may expect students to do some research before proceeding. Be sure to understand whether your instructor expects class members to work within the information—and time frame of the case— or whether class members are expected to search for additional—and perhaps more current—information.

Not all information is "fact" or information that can be verified. The case analyst often will have to make "inferences" from the information in the case. In other words, the case analyst has to make judgments on the basis of the evidence in the case. When some information is outright lacking in a case, the analyst will sometimes have to use his or her own experience or knowledge at the time of the case and make assumptions. Assumptions used should be clearly stated, and they must be reasonable. It is not fair to assume, for example, that "there will be no changes in health services legislation over the next five years." The uncertainty of the decision context is one of the most difficult aspects of being a leader in public health.

Identifying Public Health Issues

From the very first reading of the case, start to list the issues (threats and opportunities) facing the organization. When identifying relevant management and leadership issues, students can use both the administrative disciplines (finance, marketing, human resources, and so on) and the core public health disciplines (epidemiology, biostatistics, health behavior, environmental health sciences, and health policy) to cue and screen actual and potential threats or opportunities.

When a threat or opportunity is discovered, mark it for more detailed examination. Are the threats to the community as a whole or to a specific group? Is the budget expected to be cut? Do the primary issues appear to be those of human resources? Perhaps there are few, if any, apparent threats. The strategic issue facing the organization may be an opportunity to be exploited or at least investigated: "Teenage pregnancies are down this year compared with last year. What can we do to further decrease the pregnancy rate among teenagers?"

Analysis of the Present Situation

After pinpointing the initial impressions of the major issues in the case, the next step is to understand what is going on with the organization, the decision context, and the decision makers at the time a decision is needed. This is called *situational analysis*. The objective of this stage of the case analysis is to obtain a clear picture of the forces external to the organization that will have an influence on the key issues and to profile the organization that must deal with the issues.

Situational analysis is one of the most important steps in analyzing a case. The list below highlights some of the important areas that could be included in this stage of case analysis.

The Decision Context

Every decision is made within a context that includes the situation surrounding it. A number of questions are suggested to spur the analysis.

Decision Context Factors

- What are the prevailing economic conditions, regulatory philosophies, lifestyle and demographic factors, technological factors, and health care forces that are likely to influence decision making in public health?
- How many other organizations offer similar services?
- Is the number increasing or decreasing?

- What is the nature of other organizations that are competing for the same budget money?
- If we don't provide this service, what other organizations are available to provide it?

Service Area

- Is the market for the organization's services geographically concentrated?
- Who are the organization's primary customers—children, elderly residents of long-term-care facilities, the homebound ill?
- To what extent are the clients or customers loyal to the organization's services?
- Is waiting time a major determinant in the clients' decision to use our services?
- Will clients travel and be otherwise inconvenienced to obtain the organization's services?

Services (Service Categories)

- Does the organization offer a full range of public health services?
- Is the present service mix complementary, or does the organization compete with itself in some areas?
- Could the overall level of benefit to the community be significantly increased if selected new services were added?

The Organization

There is another decision context within the organization that is more internally focused. Questions posed may have very straightforward answers or may raise important issues.

Mission

- Does the organization have a clear sense of mission? Is there a mission statement? Is it communicated to those responsible for accomplishing it?
- Are there well-developed and well-communicated long- and short-range goals?
- Does the organization have the human and nonhuman resources necessary to accomplish its mission?

Culture

- What do we know about the culture of the organization?

- Will the culture allow innovation, or are management and employees bound to familiar ways of doing things?

Marketing Strategies

- How sophisticated is the organization in terms of its marketing?
- Is any education carried out in the media?
- Has serious thought been given to a health communications strategy?
- Has the appropriate channel of distribution been identified and utilized?
- How flexible are the organization's marketing policies?
- When was the last time management tried something innovative in the area of marketing?
- More important, perhaps, has the organization ever done any serious marketing of its services and programs?

Finance

- Are the financial resources needed to deliver an appropriate level of service available, or is the organization underfunded?
- How do the finances of this organization compare with others that provide similar services?
- Does the organization do meaningful financial planning, and are all leaders and managers aware of the financial consequences of their decisions?

Information Systems

- Are the information systems providing information that is used by decision makers?
- Can data on outcomes be generated so that the organization can make informed judgments?

Strengths, Weaknesses, Opportunities, and Threats (SWOT) Analysis

Once the situational analysis has been reviewed, a better evaluation of the opportunities and threats facing the organization can be made. Ask, "How can we take advantage of the opportunities and avoid the dangers (threats) in the decision context?" An effective way of summarizing the results is through the use of a simple two-by-two chart listing strengths, weaknesses, opportunities, and threats.

To illustrate how to relate strengths, weaknesses, opportunities, and threats, assume a leadership role in a large county public health department that has received numerous complaints from citizens about a company that recycles lead batteries. The employees of the battery recycling company and local public officials believe that the county health department is unfairly accusing the company of producing harmful pollutants and will not cooperate with efforts to test and determine how much exposure employees have received. Employees and public officials are concerned that jobs will be lost (the company employs 105 people in the small town where it operates). Despite repeated attempts to gain the company's compliance with air pollution rules and regulations, no changes have been made.

Strengths in the situation might be the carefully crafted and well-defined air pollution standards for the county. The judge assigned to the case has a chemical engineering background and understands the technical problems of lead exposure. Recycling of lead batteries is better for the environment than having them in landfills. Weaknesses may include the inability to gain cooperation of employees to be screened for lead exposure so that actual test results could be introduced into the legal case. Threats include significant health problems among employees and residents of the area as well as the Environmental Protection Agency (EPA) coming down hard on the county health department because of noncompliance. Opportunities may include a better-educated public that wanted a cleaner environment and new technology in battery manufacturing. Exhibit 1.2 illustrates how this SWOT analysis might be summarized and aid in the situational analysis.

Purpose or Mission of the Organization

Well-known management philosopher Peter Drucker says that anyone who wants to "know" a business must start with understanding its purpose or mission. The same is true for a public health organization. If a mission statement is included in the case, does it serve the purpose of communicating to the public why the organization exists? Does it provide employees with a genuine statement of what the organization is all about?

Mission statements provide valuable information, but they may leave much to be inferred and even imagined. Missions are broad, general statements outlining what makes the organization unique. When the mission is understood, a number of things are known that will help in arriving at a good solution to the case. When you read the assigned case, ask if you know enough about the organization's mission to confidently speculate about the following:

1. Who are the customers/clients? The customers may be children, older adults, women, or individuals with an STD. The group or groups must be identified before any serious analysis of the organization can be initiated.

2. What are the organization's principal services? Does the organization have unique experience and expertise in home health care, sanitation, HIV/AIDS, or some other area of specialization?

Exhibit 1.2. SWOT Analysis

Strengths	*Weaknesses*
■ Well-crafted set of air pollution standards ■ Judge who is an engineer by training ■ Support of upper management ■ Lead recycling is better than lead in landfills ■ Dedication of the county air pollution engineers	■ Lack of cooperation from employees, "Mill town" effect ■ Lack of OSHA involvement ■ Only lead smelting operation in the state ■ No lead information in the state
Opportunities	*Threats*
■ Media interest in pollution from lead ■ New technology in battery manufacturing ■ Public education about environmental concerns ■ A better-educated public wants a cleaner environment	■ Health problems of employees and citizens ■ Unfavorable media coverage ■ Negative economic impact for the city ■ Loss of federal funding because of non-compliance with EPA guidelines

3. Where does the organization compete? Is the case about a small public health department that serves only one local market, or is it a national agency expected to deliver services to a population that is nationwide?

4. Who are the competitors? Is the case about a county health department that has to battle for its fair share of the budget with police, schools, and so on? In other words, how much competition is actually present in the market where the organization competes or intends to compete?

5. What is the preference of the organization with regard to its public image? If a home health care organization wants to be perceived in certain ways, it may have to limit its options when defining and solving strategic issues. Is it, for example, important to the organization's leadership that it be regarded as a uniquely caring or affordable "citizen" of the community, or is the mere fact that it creates a large number of jobs sufficient?

6. What does the organization want to be like in the future? Does the information in the case indicate that the organization wants to continue to operate as it does at the present time, or does it wish to expand the programs and the services it offers or even change its own basic operating philosophy?

If a formal mission statement is not presented in a case, it is important to attempt to construct one from the information provided.

Goals: More Specific Directions

Mission statements are broad and provide general direction. Goals should be specific and explicitly point to where the organization wants to be at a particular time in the future. Sometimes the case will indicate what the public health organization plans to achieve in the next year, or where it hopes to be in three years, or even in five years. As with mission statements, if the goals are not explicitly stated, there is a need to speculate about them, because they will be the standards against which the success or failure of a particular strategy will be evaluated.

When constructing or modifying a public health agency's or other health care organization's goals, be sure they are as measurable as possible. This is important so that decision makers can use them as a reflection of organizational priorities and as a way to determine their own personal and professional priorities. Make sure that the objectives are motivational and inspirational, yet feasible and attainable. Moreover, because goals are futuristic and no one can predict the future with complete accuracy, goals should always be adaptable to the changing conditions of the organization and the area. Sometimes an organization will have to face a major strategic problem simply because it was unwilling to alter its goals in light of changing conditions in the environment.

As a test of your understanding of the case and the organization under examination and before attacking problems, reflect on what an initial reading of the case reveals about the mission and goals of the organization:

1. Identify two or three of the primary values of the organization and speculate about the type of goals that it would like to accomplish. How important, for example, is the quality as well as the quantity of clinic services delivered by the organization?
2. Speculate about the indicators that should be used to judge whether or not the values are being realized and goals are being accomplished. Is there an adequate means of professional review and evaluation to ensure outcomes are actually being achieved and that the basic values are not simply given lip service?
3. Are the aspirations of the organization's leaders realistic in view of the competition and the organization's strengths and weaknesses?
4. Are the goals being pursued consistent with what you understand to be the mission of the organization?

If the questions raised cannot be easily answered, reread the case yet again.

Finalizing Identification of Issues

Situation analysis is designed to further surface present and potential public health issues. In case analysis, problems include not only the usual idea of a "problem" but also situations where things may be working well but improvements are possible. As noted previously, the "problem" may not be negative, but rather may be a situation that can be capitalized on by the organization if it acts consciously and decisively.

When issues are analyzed carefully, patterns can be detected, and discrepancies between what actually is and what ought to be become more apparent. In other words, fundamental issues, not mere symptoms, begin to emerge.

Looking for Causes, Not Symptoms

It is important to realize that the things observed in an organization and reported in a case may not be the "real" or essential problems and opportunities. Often symptoms are observed, rather than the more serious core problems. For example, tropospheric ozone measurements that are much higher than EPA guidelines are not a problem but the symptom of a problem. The problem may be the geographic terrain of a community (not likely to be changed) or the number of polluters in the environment (a problem that can be tackled). In organizations as complex as public health systems, problems may have more than a single cause, so do not be overly confident when a single, simple reason is isolated. In fact, the suggestion of a simple solution should increase rather than decrease skepticism.

Uncovering core problems requires that information be examined and analyzed carefully. Further application of the administrative disciplines and the core public health disciplines will flesh out core problems. For example, information from biostatistical, epidemiological, or financial theory or analysis may be useful in identifying core problems in an organization.

In arriving at the ultimate determination of core problems, try not to suffer from "paralysis by analysis" and waste more time than is necessary on identifying problems. At the same time, don't make premature judgments about problem areas because the "real" issues may be missed.

Always review the obtainable sources of data before moving to the next step. One general guideline is that when research and analysis cease to generate surprises, the analyst can feel relatively, though not absolutely, sure that adequate research has been conducted and the core problems have been identified.

The threat and opportunity discovery process should not become myopic. There may be a tendency on the part of individuals interested and experienced in public health policy to see all problems in terms of policy. A physician/epidemiologist approaching the same case will likely focus on the clinical and epidemiological implications. A health educator might see only the behavioral implications. Each of these represents too limited a view for effective decision makers. Successful case analysis requires managers and leaders to transcend a single function and attempt to develop recommendations that solve problems. Insistence on approaching case analysis exclusively from the viewpoint of one's own expertise and training is not likely to produce an accurate overall picture of the situation facing the organization, nor is this approach likely to improve the organization's performance.

Never accept information, either given or obtained, at face value. The statistics on a state's STDs may look strange, but are they? Before jumping to such a conclusion, look at the data in a historical perspective and think about the population from which the data are obtained. Determine case facts and differentiate carefully between facts, inferences, speculations, and assumptions.

Stating the Issues

Once the problems are identified, they must be stated precisely and their selection defended. The best defense for the selection of the core problem is the data set used to guide the problem discovery process. The reasons for selection of the problems and issues should be briefly and specifically summarized, along with the supportive information on which your judgments have been based. It is often useful to state the problem in the form of a question. Later, when alternatives are being developed, each one should be a possible answer to the question. If the alternatives that are generated do not answer the question, it may be that the question is not really the correct problem (or the alternatives might not be right if the question is still considered to address the right issue).

The problem statement stage is not the time for solutions. Focusing on solutions at this point will reduce the impact of the problem statement. If you assume the role of consultant, the problem statement you present must be convincing, precise, and logical to the client organization, or your credibility will be reduced. If you select the role of the decision maker, you must be equally convincing and precise as a case analyst. The decision maker should be as sure as possible that the correct problems have been identified in order to pursue the appropriate alternatives. After all, the leader will be the one responsible for ensuring that the recommendations are implemented.

The statement of the problem should relate only to those areas where actions have a chance of producing results. The results may be either increasing gains or cutting potential losses. Long- and short-range aspects of problems should be identified and stated. It is important to keep in mind that most decision makers can deal with only a limited number of issues at a single time; therefore, it is vital to identify key result areas that will have the greatest positive impact on organizational performance.

Analysis

After the problem is satisfactorily defined, decision context analyzed, and organizational resources and capabilities evaluated, the decision must be analyzed and framed. This involves (1) developing a theoretical perspective, (2) generating alternative solutions or actions, and (3) evaluating the alternatives.

Developing a Theoretical Perspective

One of the most serious mistakes made in case analysis is to attempt analysis inside a "theoretical vacuum." It is important that the problems are defined and opportunities are evaluated according to some consistent theoretical perspective. Both the administrative and core public health disciplines have theoretical underpinning and analysis methods.

Students must decide which of the disciplines to apply to case issues. For example, are the problems the kind that biostatistical analysis can assist in solving? Are the issues facing the organization problems of leadership, organization, or control? It might be that problems concerning lack of revenue growth are really problems of not responding adequately to client needs—the lack of a marketing orientation. Many revenue shortfalls could be resolved with the use of the relatively simple marketing philosophy. A proper theoretical perspective, for example, might suggest that clients are less concerned with the location of a public health office than they are with how they are treated when they arrive.

Alternative Actions and Solutions

If the job of obtaining and organizing information has been done well, the generation of alternatives will be a challenging yet attainable task. To investigate options, the given and obtained information must be matched with what is known about epidemiology, biostatistics, health behavior, environmental health science, health policy, financial analysis, marketing, human resources management, and so on, so that actions that are promising, feasible, and consistent with the mission can be generated.

Good alternatives possess specific characteristics. The alternatives should be grounded in theory and be practical or no one will seriously consider them. However, alternative courses of action that are too theoretical or abstract to be understood by those who have to accomplish them are not useful. Alternatives should be stated carefully, with a brief justification as to why they could be used to solve at least one of the core problems in the case.

Alternatives should be specific. Relate each alternative to the core problem it is intended to address. This is a good check on the analyst's thinking. If the alternatives generated do not directly address core problems, ask how important they are to the case analysis.

Finally, alternatives should be usable. A usable alternative is one that can be reasonably accomplished within the constraints of the human and nonhuman resources available to the organization. Alternatives should be able to be placed into action in a relatively short period of time. If it takes too long to implement a proposed solution, it is likely that the momentum of the recommended action will be lost. Of course, implementation should always take place in light of potential long-range effects of shorter-term decisions.

After the alternatives have been generated and listed, each one must be (1) evaluated in terms of the core problems and key result areas isolated in the prior analysis,

(2) evaluated in terms of its relative advantage or disadvantage compared to other possible solutions to core problems, and (3) justified as a potentially valuable way of addressing the issues found in the case.

Evaluating Alternatives

Alternatives should be evaluated according to both quantitative and qualitative criteria. Analysis methods of each of the administrative and core public health disciplines may be required. For instance, financial analysis provides one basis for examining the impact of different courses of action. However, a good alternative course of action is more than merely the one with the highest payoff. It may be that the culture of the organization cannot accommodate some of the more financially promising alternative courses of action.

For example, an established policy and practice in the state may tolerate no more than a certain percentage of debt financing. Although the financial analysis illustrates that additional debt is a low-cost way to finance expansion, top state government officials can be expected to reject the level of debt required, which will make other options necessary. On the more qualitative side, a state public health system with a reputation for avoiding layoffs at all costs could be expected to reject any strategic alternative that involves closing a program and reducing staff.

Once the alternatives have been evaluated, one must be selected. At this point, it is essential to completely understand the criteria upon which the selection is being made and the justification for the criteria. Sometimes the key to identifying the criteria is in the case itself. The chief executive officer may have clearly stated the basis on which decisions are to be made. At other times it is necessary to look outside to what is going on in the public health sector. Is competition for new state dollars so fierce that decisions to expand programs are likely to radically affect the organization's ability to compete? If so, should the health department intentionally postpone short-term actions to ensure that sufficient resources are dedicated to the modernization of facilities and the purchase of up-to-date technologies to improve the chances of long-range growth and development?

Making Recommendations

Making good recommendations is a critical aspect of successful case analysis. If recommendations are theoretically sound and justifiable, people will pay attention to them. If they are not, little is likely to result from all the work.

One effective method for presenting recommendations is to relate each one to issues in the decision context and to organizational strengths. If necessary, a recommendation can instead illustrate how it assists in avoiding known weaknesses. If the organization has sufficient financial strength, the recommendations should highlight how each alternative will capitalize on the strong financial condition. If, on the other hand, resources are limited, it will be important to avoid recommendations that rely on resources that are not available.

It will be particularly useful to ask the following questions when making recommendations:

1. Is the public health science underlying the decision sound?
2. Does the public health organization have the financial resources needed to make the recommendation work?
3. Does the organization have the personnel to accomplish what will be required by each recommendation?
4. Does the organization have the controls needed to monitor whether or not the recommendations are being accomplished?
5. Is the timing right to implement each recommendation? If not, when will the timing be right? Can the organization afford to wait?

Developing a Plan of Action

Once the alternative has been selected, an action plan is required. Action planning moves the decision maker from the realm of strategy to operations. Now the question becomes, "How do we get all this done in the most effective and efficient way possible?"

The task of case analysis does not require that the student implement a decision in a real organization; however, because our alternatives must be "implementable," it is necessary that thought be given to how each alternative actually would be put into action. This is called *action planning*, and it requires three important steps for each recommended alternative. First, the decision maker must decide what activities are needed to accomplish the alternative action. This involves thinking through the process and outlining all the steps that will be required.

Next, the list of required activities should be reviewed carefully, and tasks should be grouped logically. Those that relate to human resources go into one group, service delivery activities go into another, and financial activities go into a third. Each itemized activity must be placed into such a group, and any activities that do not fit neatly into the existing organization should be placed in another category of miscellaneous tasks. (Note that if this "other" list is too long, it may suggest that the structure of the organization needs revision.)

Finally, the responsibility for accomplishing the different groups of tasks must be clearly assigned to the appropriate individuals in the organization. Although this is not always possible in case analysis, it is important that consideration be given to how, in a real organization, the recommendations would be accomplished. If, in the process of thinking about getting the different activities completed, it becomes apparent that the organization lacks the resources or the structure to accomplish the recommendations, other approaches should be proposed.

People must ultimately accomplish all actions; therefore, the action plan for accomplishing recommendations should be assigned to individuals. Who will be responsible for getting each of the recommendations accomplished? Is this individual likely to have the skills required to complete the task? If not, what actions will be necessary before the recommendation can be fully implemented?

The process of action planning should never be neglected. Organizations sometimes spend large amounts of money and resources developing plans only to discover that they are not prepared to implement them.

Finalizing the Report

Presentation is the final part of case analysis. The report can be either written or oral, depending on the preference of the instructor. Although the form is slightly different, the goal is the same—to summarize and communicate in an effective manner what the analysis has uncovered. Ultimately, public health leaders and managers have to persuade others through oral arguments. Chapter 3 deals with oral presentations in greater detail.

Conclusions

Case analysis is an art—there is no one precise way to accomplish the task. Adapt the analysis to the case problem under review. Keep in mind that case analysis is a logical process that involves (1) understanding the organization and the decision context; (2) clearly defining problems and opportunities; (3) generating alternative courses of action; (4) analyzing, evaluating, and recommending the most promising courses of action; and (5) providing at least some consideration of the operational aspects of how and by whom the recommendations will be accomplished.

The work of case analysis is not over until all these stages are completed. Often, a formal written report or oral presentation of the recommendations is required. Case problems provide a unique opportunity to integrate all you have learned about decision making and direct it toward specific problems and opportunities faced by real organizations. They provide an exciting way to gain experience and decision-making skills. Take case analysis seriously and develop systematic, defensible ways of solving problems faced by leaders in public health practice.

CHAPTER 2

Information Sources for Public Health Leaders

Although well-researched case studies have as much information as the decision maker had available at the time, the individuals in the case often have a deeper understanding of the situational context than is practical to provide in a case chapter. In case analysis, it is often useful to perform at least part of the situational analysis by investigating secondary data. In addition, some instructors may want the students to deepen their understanding of the environment for a particular case. This chapter provides an aid in locating information sources that are generally available about both the health care and the public health environments. Resources that typically are available in university libraries or are electronically accessible are listed. Brief descriptions of each resource are provided.

Abstracts

Abstracts of Health Care Management Studies. Ann Arbor: Health Administration Press for the Cooperative Information Center for Health Care Management Studies, School of Public Health, University of Michigan (quarterly).

This publication provides abstracts of materials recently published on public policy, planning, and management. Its primary focus is on the delivery of health care.

Excerpta Medica. Amsterdam: Excerpta (ten issues per year, with semiannual accumulations).

An international abstracting service that covers all aspects of health care, this publication can be used as a general index as well as a specialized resource.

This chapter was written by Arthur P. Liang, National Center for Infectious Diseases, Centers for Disease Control and Prevention, Atlanta, Georgia, and Sherrill Snuggs, School of Public Health, University of Alabama at Birmingham.

Health Planning and Services Research: An Abstract Newsletter. Springfield, VA: National Technical Information Service (weekly).

>This weekly newsletter contains information on health services, facility use, health personnel requirements, health-related costs, and methods of funding.

Medical Care Review. Ann Arbor: Bureau of Public Health Economics, School of Public Health, University of Michigan (monthly).

>This publication reviews the current literature and contains abstracts from articles as well as entire journal articles. A section on federal and state legislation is included.

Standard and Poor's Industry Surveys. New York: Standard and Poor's Corporation (quarterly).

>This source contains extensive information for sixty-nine major domestic industries. Some of the industries included are health care, computer and data processing equipment, leisure time, and liquor.

Bibliographies

Business Information Sources, 3d ed., by Lorna M. Daniells. Berkeley: University of California Press, 1993.

>This guide provides a selected, annotated list of books and reference sources for businesses including the health care industry. This edition contains several new sections covering such topics as competitive intelligence, economic and financial measures, and health care marketing. Handbooks, bibliographies, indexes and abstracts, on-line databases, dictionaries, directories, statistical sources, and periodicals are included.

Federal Information Sources in Health and Medicine: A Selected Annotated Bibliography, by Mary G. Chitty. New York: Greenwood Press, 1988.

>This bibliography annotates government publications and databases from federal agencies, institutes, and information centers. The subject bibliography is divided by publication type. About 1,200 government publications and 100 databases from some 90 federal agencies, institutes, and information centers are described.

Medical Books and Serials in Print: An Index to Literature in the Health Sciences. New York: Bowker (annual).

>This index includes a listing of books and other materials in the medical and allied health sciences fields currently available from publishers.

Public Health Administration: Monographs, 1970–1987, by Mary Vance. Monticello, IL: Vance Bibliographies, 1988.

>This source combines information in the public administration field and the health administration area.

Where to Find Business Information: A Worldwide Guide for Everyone Who Needs the Answers to Business Questions, 2d ed., by David M. Brownstone and Gorton Carruth. New York: John Wiley & Sons, 1982.

>This book contains a descriptive list of more than 5,000 sources of current business information, concentrating on periodic publications and services such as magazines, newsletters, and computerized databases.

Computerized Information Services

A large number of electronic database services is available for subscription, and others can be accessed through various public institutions. A student is able to access a large amount of information on many topics in a short amount of time through the use of these databases; however, it should be noted that information technology is a vast and ever-changing source of information. Only a very few sources, therefore, will be listed here. These sources should be viewed as a starting point in the search for knowledge, not as an all-inclusive list.

ABI/Inform. Ann Arbor, MI: UMI Web site: www.umi.com

> ABI/Inform is the largest and oldest database of bibliographical information. The major health care administration journals are indexed, along with an impressive number of business periodicals. The database includes articles from 1971 to present.

Cumulative Index to Nursing and Allied Health. Glendale, CA: Cinahl Information Systems.

> This database indexes more than 12,000 journals from all disciplines of nursing and allied health, plus pamphlets, dissertations, software, and other items. Indexing begins with 1982. Citations are provided from *Index Medicus* as well as other sources.

Health Planning and Administration. Bethesda, MD: U.S. National Library of Medicine.

> This database contains references to nonclinical literature on health care planning, management, human resources, and licensing and certification. The references are compiled from the *Hospital Literature Index* and *Medline*.

Health Reference Center Database. Foster City, CA: Information Access Company.

> Formerly known as the Health Periodicals Database and the Health & Wellness ASAP Database, this full-text database provides references to journals covering the entire range of health issues in both consumer health and professional medical journals. Topics include health product announcements and reviews, prenatal care, AIDS, and health care administration, as well as clinical descriptions and research findings in layperson's terms. Author and nontechnical abstracts are included. About 35 percent of the file is full text.

Medline. Bethesda, MD: National Library of Medicine.

> This database contains more than 11 million articles published in 4,300 biomedical journals on all aspects of medical and biomedical literature. Most of the articles are written for health professionals.

Dictionaries

Health Services Cyclopedia Dictionary: A Compendium of Health Care and Public Health Terminology, 3d ed., edited by Thomas C. Timmerick. Boston: Jones and Bartlett, 1997.

Miller-Keane Encyclopedia and Dictionary of Medicine, Nursing, and Allied Health, 6th ed., edited by Benjamin F. Miller and Thomas Eoyang. Philadelphia: W. B. Saunders, 1997.

The New American Medical Dictionary and Health Manual, 7th ed., by Robert E. Rothenberg. New York: Penguin USA, 1999.

Directories

American Hospital Association Guide to the Health Care Field. Chicago: American Hospital Association (annually).

>This guide provides information on health care facilities, the AHA, health care organizations, and national hospital statistical data.

Directory of Local Health Departments. Washington, DC: National Association of County and City Health Officials (updated quarterly).

>This directory contains contact information for all local public health agencies in NACCHO's comprehensive database.

Medical and Health Information Directory, 9th ed. Detroit: Gale Research, 1998.

>This directory provides information on the locations of agencies, institutions, associations, and companies involved with health care at the state and national levels.

Handbooks and Guides

Chronic Disease Epidemiology and Control, 2d ed., edited by Ross C. Brownson, Patrick L. Remington, and James R. Davis. Washington, DC: American Public Health Association, 1998.

>A good source on chronic disease epidemiology, prevention, and control, the book is divided into three major sections: public health approaches to chronic disease control, selected lifestyle risk factors, and major chronic diseases.

Control of Communicable Diseases Manual, 17th ed., edited by James E. Chin. Washington, DC: American Public Health Association.

>This book provides information and recommendations for communicable disease prevention.

Critical Condition: Human Health and the Environment: A Report by Physicians for Social Responsibility, edited by Michael McCally, Howard Hu, and Eric Chivian. Cambridge: MIT Press, 1993.

>This report discusses human health consequences of various environmental conditions such as the depleting ozone layer, species extinction, and the loss of biodiversity.

Environmental & Occupational Medicine, 3d ed., by William N. Rom. Philadelphia: Lippincott/ Williams & Wilkins, 1998.

>This comprehensive text covers the fields of epidemiology, toxicology, clinical medicine, and ethics.

Environmental Epidemiology and Risk Assessment, edited by Tim Aldrich, Jack Griffin, and Christopher Cooke. New York: Van Nostrand Reinhold, 1993.

>This book could be used as a reference source. It provides an explanation for conducting epidemiologic studies about disorders caused by environmental factors. Examples of real situations from the past are used to illustrate how the public reacts to these tragedies and the importance of communicating scientific findings when they occur.

Environmental Health: New Directions (Advances in Modern Environmental Toxicology), by J. Shields. Princeton, NJ: Princeton Scientific Publications, 1990.

>A textbook that covers air, water, hazardous waste, pesticides, and foods.

Environmental Management in Healthcare Facilities, edited by Kathryn D. Wagner. Philadelphia: W. B. Saunders, 1998.

> This reference book addresses hazardous and nonhazardous waste treatment alternatives, air quality, chemical hazards, and regulations.

Environmental Toxicants: Human Exposure and Their Health Effects, 2d ed., edited by Morton Lippman. New York: John Wiley & Sons, 1999.

> This reference text is for public health officials, industrial safety managers and hygienists, epidemiologists, and primary health care professionals who make decisions on risk assessment and risk management for individuals and populations. It provides in-depth, critical reviews on chemical, physical, and classes of agents that either have or could have major impacts on the health of the general public. The introductory chapter and the three closing chapters deal with generic issues and concerns, placing the critical review chapters in a larger perspective.

Global Health Statistics: A Compendium of Incidence, Prevalence and Mortality Estimates for over 200 Conditions (Global Burden of Disease and Injury), edited by Alan D. Lopez et al. (World Health Organization) and Christopher J. Murray. Boston: Harvard University Press, 1996.

> The book provides estimates for all major diseases and injuries. More than 100 disease experts analyzed these data, collected from exhaustive searches of registration data and published and unpublished studies. A comprehensive set of tables presents more than 200 causes with estimates of mortality, incidence, prevalence, and duration by age, sex, and region.

Guide to Clinical Preventive Services: Report of the U.S. Preventive Services Task Force, by U.S. Preventive Services Task Force Staff. Washington, DC: U.S. Department of Health and Human Services, 1997.

> This guide summarizes the scientific basis for a number of clinical preventive interventions. It is divided into three sections that cover detailed screening information for various conditions, and counseling patients on lifestyle choices, as well as immunizations and chemoprophylaxis.

Handbook of Immigrant Health, edited by Sana Loue. New York: Plenum, 1998.

> This book contains review articles on the behavioral, social, and cultural issues most important in the consideration of immigrant health and health care.

Health, United States, 2000, With Adolescent Health Chartbook. Hyattsville, MD: National Center for Health Statistics, 2000 (annually).

> The book is from the NCHS series describing national trends in health statistics on such topics as birth and death rates, infant mortality, life expectancy, morbidity and health status, risk factors, use of ambulatory care and inpatient care, health personnel and facilities, financing of health care, health insurance and managed care, and other health topics. The chartbook focuses on the adolescent population (10–19 years of age) and measurements of health status during the transition from childhood to adulthood.

Healthy People 2010, edited by the U.S. Department of Health and Human Services. Washington, DC: Reiter's Scientific & Professional Books, 2000.

> *Healthy People 2010* is a nationwide health promotion and disease prevention agenda that sets specific health objectives for the year 2010. It is designed to improve the health of all Americans, eliminate disparities in health, and improve years and quality of healthy life. This program builds on the goals and initiatives of Healthy People 2000.

How to Manage in the Public Sector, by Gordon Chase. New York: McGraw-Hill Higher Education, 1983.

> This book is an excellent complement to books on management and organizational theory. It provides practical advice on working with political appointments, elected officials, the community, and the media, as well as personnel and financial management offices.

Introduction to Environmental Health, 2d ed., edited by Daniel S. Blumenthal and A. James Ruttenber. New York: Springer, 1995.

> This book is divided into four parts: principles of environmental health, agents of environmental disease, routes of exposure, and environmental health practice. Some of the topics included in the sections are infectious agents, toxic substances, radiation, air and water pollution, and environmental law.

Mandell, Douglas, and Bennett's Principles and Practice of Infectious Diseases, 5th ed., edited by Gerald L. Mandell, John E. Bennett, and Raphael Dolin. Philadelphia: Churchill Livingstone, 2000.

> Written for a medical audience, the book discusses major clinical syndromes, pathologic microbes, and special problems in infectious disease.

Maxcy-Rosenau-Last Public Health and Preventive Medicine, 14th ed., edited by Kenneth Fuller Maxcy, M. J. Rosenau, John M. Last, and Robert B. Wallace. New York: McGraw-Hill Professional Publishing, 1998.

> This book covers most aspects of public health. Research methods, communicable diseases, environmental and occupational health, social and behavioral factors, noncommunicable and chronic disabling conditions, injury and violence, and health care planning, organization, and evaluation are all discussed in detail. An extensive and comprehensive variety of topics is included.

Merck Manual of Diagnosis and Therapy, 17th ed., edited by Mark H. Beers and Robert Berkow. Whitehouse Station, NJ: Merck & Co., 1999.

> This well-known medical text provides information on a vast array of human diseases, disorders, and injuries. It lists the symptoms and recommended therapy for each disease.

The Nation's Health, 5th ed., edited by Philip R. Lee and Carroll L. Estes. Boston: Jones and Bartlett, 1997.

> This is a compendium of articles on factors affecting the health of Americans. Some of the topics covered include tobacco, immunization, HIV/AIDS, managed competition, and the rationing of health care. Preventive care, cost of health care, and the relationship between socioeconomic class and health are included.

Oxford Textbook of Public Health, 3d ed., edited by Roger Detels, Walter Holland, James McEwen, and Gilbert Omenn. Oxford, UK: Oxford University Press, 1997.

> This reference book provides a comprehensive review of the field of public health. This edition has been updated to reflect the challenges faced by public health professionals because of the increasing fiscal and political pressures to reduce government support for a number of community health programs. Discussions on HIV, drug-resistant strains of previously treatable diseases, and new emerging viruses that are a threat to public health have been added.

Principles of Public Health Practice, by F. Douglas Scutchfield and C. William Keck. Albany, NY: Delmar Publishing, 1997.

> This book provides public health practitioners with complete and authoritative information and developmental tools on public health practice. It examines how today's public health system works and includes a look at future trends in public health practice.

Public Health Administration: Principles for Population Based Management, edited by Lloyd F.
  Novick and Glen P. Mays. Gaithersburg, MD: Aspen, 2000.

> This textbook covers the basics of administration, including organizational design, law,
> human resources, budgeting and financing, marketing, and communications. In addi-
> tion, it discusses areas such as health information management, geographic informa-
> tion systems, performance measurement and improvement, ethics, leadership, and
> community partnerships.

Public Health Administration and Practice, 9th ed., by George Pickett and John J Hanlon. New
  York: McGraw-Hill Higher Education, 1989.

> A well-established textbook for students in a variety of health-related fields. Considers
> the historical, biological, psychological, environmental, developmental, management,
> and public policy aspects of public health practice in the United States.

Public Health and Human Ecology, 2d ed., by John M. Last. Stamford, CT: Appleton & Lange,
  1998.

> This book provides descriptions and historical backgrounds of public health problems,
> including ecological viewpoints.

Public Health and Related Journals

American Journal of Health Promotion. Keego Harbor, MI: The American Journal of Health
  Promotion, Inc. (bimonthly).

> Goals of this journal are to provide a credible forum for discussion among the many dis-
> ciplines that promote health and to provide an interface between health promotion re-
> searchers and practitioners. The journal publishes original research, literature reviews,
> editorials, and case studies on a wide variety of health promotion topics.

American Journal of Public Health. Washington, DC: American Public Health Association
  (monthly).

> The official journal of the American Public Health Association, the largest organization
> of public health professionals. The journal publishes a broad range of peer-reviewed
> scientific reports relevant to public health as well as editorials, book reviews, and public
> health practice-oriented reports.

Harvard Journal of Minority Public Health. Boston: Harvard School of Public Health (quarterly).

> The journal considers itself to be a major "venue for dialogue on the health concerns of
> communities of color." It "reports on health services delivery and research technology,
> community intervention projects and health policy and management strategies as they
> affect the health of traditionally underserved populations."

Hazardous Substances and Public Health. Atlanta, GA: ATSDR.

> Newsletter from the Agency for Toxic Substances and Disease Registry. Provides a com-
> plete archive of its issues.

Health and Medical Informatics Digest—HMID. Madison: University of Wisconsin Board of
  Regents.

> This monthly digest examines on-line medical informatics for practitioners, academics,
> and researchers.

Health Management Technology. North Nokomis, FL: Nelson Publishing (monthly).

> Emphasizes feature stories on health care informational technology solutions and is-
> sues, columns and monthly departments that highlight case studies, and a database of
> health care information technology companies.

Health Service Journal. London: Emap Healthcare Ltd, Greater London House (weekly).
   News, opinions, and feature stories as well as book reviews and other resources for
   health care managers, primarily from a British perspective.
Health Services Research Journal. Chicago: Health Research and Educational Trust.
   Covers the latest research in public policy and health-services management.
International Journal of Health Care Quality Assurance. Bradford, UK: MCB University Press Ltd.
   Presents information, comment, and debate on quality assurance issues, trends, and
   developments that affect the health care industry.
Journal of Medical Screening. London: BMJ Publishing Group.
   Journal for professionals that encompasses screening statistics, techniques and proce-
   dures, and public health issues.
Journal of Public Health Management & Practice. Gaithersburg, MD: Aspen.
   Provides practical information applicable to the design and implementation of public
   health programs.
Journal of Public Health Policy. South Burlington, VT: National Association for Public Health
   Policy.
   Covers such subjects as alcohol and illicit drugs; mental, dental, and environmental
   health; and diseases such as cancer.
ODPHP—Prevention Report. Washington, DC: Office of Disease Prevention and Health Pro-
   motion, U.S. Department of Health and Human Services.
   Oriented to preventive medicine, with significant content on the Healthy People initiatives.

On-Line Journals and Publications

Advance Data From Vital and Health Statistics of the CDC NCHS
www.cdc.gov/nchs/products/pubs/pubd/ad/ad.htm
   This Web site provides early release of data from the National Center for Health Statistics' health and demographic surveys. Many of these releases are followed by detailed
   reports in the Vital and Health Statistics series.
American Journal of Epidemiology
www.aje.oupjournals.org
   This page contains information on the *American Journal of Epidemiology* (AJE) as well
   as *Epidemiologic Reviews* and the Society for Epidemiologic Research. The AJE is devoted to the publication of empirical research findings, methodologic developments in
   the field of epidemiologic research, and opinion pieces. It is aimed at both fellow
   epidemiologists and those who use epidemiologic data, including public health workers
   and clinicians.
American Journal of Preventive Medicine (8 times/year)
www.elsevier.com/locate/ajpmonline
   Features searchable tables of contents, abstracts, and selected full-text articles with references linked to MEDLINE abstracts. Some full-text articles link to relevant content
   that does not appear in the print journal.
American Medical Association—Journals of the AMA Archives Journals
pubs.ama-assn.org/archive_home.html
   This site provides a collection of links to AMA journals in a wide range of clinical specialties. Many of the current and past issues of these journals are available through this site.

Annual Review of Public Health

publhealth.annualreviews.org

>   Contains on-line archives of the *Annual Review of Public Health* with full-text articles for the past five years.

Centers for Disease Control and Prevention—Publications

www.cdc.gov/publications.htm

>   This site of the Centers for Disease Control and Prevention in Atlanta, Georgia, provides links to a broad array of publications produced by the various scientific centers and program offices within CDC.

Clinician's Handbook of Preventive Services, 2d ed. Washington, DC: Department of Health and Human Services, 1998.

www.ahcpr.gov/clinic/ppiphand.htm

>   This handbook summarizes recommendations of the U.S. Preventive Services Task Force on screening information for various conditions, counseling patients on lifestyle choices, and immunizations and chemoprophylaxis.

Journal of Community Health

www.wkap.nl/journalhome.htm/0094-5145

>   Publishes original articles on the practice, teaching, and research of community health, on topics such as coverage of preventive medicine, new forms of health manpower, analysis of environmental factors, delivery of health care services, and the study of health maintenance and health insurance programs.

Journal of Epidemiology and Community Health

www.jech.com

>   An international journal on all the aspects of epidemiology and public health. It publishes original papers, leading articles, reviews, and short papers concerned with the study and improvement of communities worldwide.

MMWR—Morbidity and Mortality Weekly Report

www2.cdc.gov/mmwr/

>   The *MMWR* series is prepared by the Centers for Disease Control and Prevention. The data in the weekly *MMWR* are provisional, based on weekly reports to CDC by state health departments.

New England Journal of Medicine

www.nejm.com

>   This site provides abstracts for articles in current and past issues of this journal. Full-text articles are available only by paid subscription.

Pediatric and Perinatal Epidemiology

www.sper.org/links.htm

>   Affiliated with the Society for Paediatric and Perinatal Epidemiologic Research, the journal links the epidemiologist and the pediatrician, obstetrician, or child specialist with the intent of ensuring that important pediatric and perinatal studies reach them.

Preventive Medicine

www.academicpress.com/pm

>   This site provides access to abstracts of current and past issues of this journal. Full-text articles are available only by paid subscription.

Public Health Reports

www.phr/oupjournals.org

>   *Public Health Reports* is the journal of the U.S. Public Health Service and is published bi-monthly in collaboration with the Association of Schools of Public Health.

Internet Public Health Resources

Administration on Aging

www.aoa.dhhs.gov/

Information on referral services, job and volunteer opportunities, adult day care center programs, and transportation. Includes useful state data.

Centers for Disease Control and Prevention (CDC)

www.cdc.gov

Includes a traveler's health section as well as training and employment resources. With links to state (e.g., New Mexico and Louisiana) and some local health department Web sites.

Department of Health and Human Services

www.os.dhhs.gov/

Links to research institutes, with press releases and extensive consumer information on matters such as aging.

Department of Veterans Affairs

www.va.gov/

Index to press releases, benefits, facilities, special programs, organizational structure, and data.

Environmental Health Perspectives

ehis.niehs.nih.gov

EHPnet publications relating to scientific and social environmental health issues.

Family Health International (FHI)

www.fhi.org/fhi1.html

Family Health International works on improving maternal and child health around the world through biomedical and social science research, health service delivery, training, and information programs.

Food and Drug Administration

www.fda.gov

Wide-ranging resources to everything from foods, cosmetics, and human drugs to toxicology and biologics.

Global Child Health Society

edie.cprost.sfu.ca/gcnet/

Uses the Internet to disseminate child health information from around the world. Includes a bibliographic database.

Hazard Net

hoshi.cic.sfu.ca/hazard/

Directory to government and international agencies and services relating to hazards and disasters.

Health Policy Page

www.epn.org/ideacentral/health/

Articles on health insurance legislation, medical savings accounts, recent trends in HMOs, and Medicaid proposals.

Health Resources and Services Administration

www.hrsa.gov/

HRSA directs national health programs to improve access to health care in the area of HIV/AIDS, primary health care to medically underserved people, maternal and child health through state programs, and health professions training.

Hospital Infections Program

www.cdc.gov/ncidod/hip/DEFAULT.HTM

> This site for the Division of Healthcare Quality Promotion discusses infection control in hospitals and clinics. Includes information on nosocomial infections and management of infection outbreaks.

Indian Health Service

www.ihs.gov/

> The Indian Health Service (IHS) is an agency within the U.S. Department of Health and Human Services and is responsible for providing federal health services to American Indians and Alaska Natives.

International Federation of Red Cross

www.ifrc.org/

> Index to world situation reports, annual world disaster reports, NGO Code of Conduct, and links to national chapters.

The National Association of Community Health Centers

www.nachc.com/

> This is the national trade association representing America's community health centers. The site includes some state profiles of health care resources and programs for underserved populations.

National Center for Health Statistics

www.cdc.gov/nchs/

> NCHS is the federal government's principal vital and health statistics agency. The agency provides a wide variety of data to monitor the nation's health.

National Institute for Occupational Safety and Health (NIOSH)

www.cdc.gov/niosh/homepage.html

> Web site for the federal agency responsible for conducting research and making recommendations for the prevention of work-related disease and injury.

National Institutes of Health

www.nih.gov

> Excellent source of FAQs on almost any illness, from one of the world's foremost biomedical research centers.

National Safety Council

www.nsc.org/

> Explains what the council does and what its major campaigns are. Includes research, statistics, and library and training resources.

NIH Clinical Alerts

www.nlm.nih.gov/databases/alerts/clinical_alerts.html

> Links to alerts since 1993. Alerts are provided where the release of trial findings could significantly affect health.

NIH Consensus Development Program

text.nlm.nih.gov/nih/nih.html

> Organizes major conferences on controversies in medicine, providing statements, conference schedules, and related materials. Conferences are convened to evaluate available scientific information and resolve safety and efficacy issues related to biomedical technology.

Occupational Safety and Health Administration (OSHA)

www.osha.gov

> Site provides information on OSHA's mission of establishing and enforcing protective standards for worker health and safety.

Public Health—Martindale's
www-sci.lib.uci.edu/HSG/PHealth.html.

> Extensive site with glossaries, journals, databases, and information about courses and textbooks.

Reproductive Health Information Source
www.cdc.gov/nccdphp/drh/

> Maternal and child health data and information from CDC.

SatelLife
www.healthnet.org/

> Reports on public health, medicine, and the state of the environment in developing countries.

Social Statistics Briefing Room
www.whitehouse.gov/fsbr/ssbr.html

> Easy access to current federal social statistics including annual health care expenditures and the use of health services.

Trauma Foundation
www.traumafdn.org/

> Aims to reduce injury and death by focusing on policy development. Includes information on injury prevention, statistics, and public health. (Web site under construction.)

UN Food and Agriculture Organization
www.fao.org/

> Information that features a food suppliers index, food quality reports, events calendar, and documentation services.

United Nations Children's Emergency Fund
www.unicef.org/

> Lists information resources including statistical information on the situation of women and children, by country.

World Health Organization (WHO)
www.who.int/

> Links to major programs, an archive of WHO statements, and guidelines for international health and travel.

Statistical Sources

Adolescent and School Health State Profiles
www.cdc.gov/nccdphp/dash/ahson/profiles.htm

> Provides access to state-by-state and national data and graphics on a variety of health issues relevant to school-age children.

Bureau of Labor Statistics
stats.bls.gov/

> Includes regional and state data.

Census Bureau
www.census.gov

> The latest statistics on populations, with links to other useful sites.

Demographics and Health Surveys

www.measuredhs.com

>A wide variety of publications that provide country-specific and comparative data on population, health, and nutrition in developing countries based on the results of the demographic and health surveys.

Fedstats

www.fedstats.gov

>The Federal Interagency Council on Statistical Policy maintains this site to provide access to the statistics and information of interest to the public produced by more than 70 agencies in the U.S. federal government.

Health Resources and Services Administration (HRSA)

www.hrsa.gov/

>Lists state health workforce profiles, county demographics, and community health status indicators.

NIOSH: State Profiles

www.cdc.gov/niosh/statepro.html

>Occupational safety and health profiles are available for all fifty states.

The Prevention Guidelines Database

aepo-xdv-www.epo.cdc.gov/wonder/PrevGuid/PrevGuid.shtml

>A compendium of all the official guidelines and recommendations published by the U.S. Centers for Disease Control and Prevention (CDC) for the prevention of diseases, injuries, and disabilities, regardless of when and where they were originally published.

Rehydration Project

www.rehydrate.org/index.html

>Provides information on diarrhea, dehydration, and oral rehydration for developing countries.

State Child Care Profiles

www.nccic.org/statepro.html

>National Child Care Information Center State Child Care Profiles. State profiles include demographic information about the children, families and child care in each state, and contact information for different state agencies.

State Health Departments

www.rho.arizona.edu/ph/depts.htm

>Links to fifty state health departments and Guam. Last updated September 3, 1999. There is no link for the District of Columbia. Some states such as Montana, West Virginia, and Virginia need updating, but links often provide access to state data.

Trends in Indian Health

www.ihs.gov/PublicInfo/Publications/trends97/trends97.asp

>Tables and charts describing the health status of American Indians and Alaska Natives, including information about IHS structure, American Indian and Alaska Native demography, patient care, and community health.

CHAPTER 3

Oral Presentations in Public Health Settings

Presenting information orally requires careful thought. As you advance in your career, you will increasingly be called on to speak to others. For example, you may need to persuade higher management to adopt a new policy, to present a grant proposal to the board of a philanthropic organization, or to discuss a service area status report with your employees. Whether you are presenting information to a group of your peers, your supervisor, a group of community leaders, or members of the health care profession, effective oral communication involves three major steps: planning, organizing, and delivering the subject matter.

Plan Your Presentation

Several factors must be considered before you can plan a presentation effectively. You must determine the type of presentation you will make, analyze your audience, gather information, and consider the logistics of the speaking site.

Determine the Type of Presentation You Will Make

The first step in planning is to examine what you hope to accomplish with the presentation. Your goals will determine the type of presentation you will make.

This chapter was written by Gary F. Kohut and Carol M. Baxter, the University of North Carolina at Charlotte.

Generally, oral presentations are divided into two broad categories: informative and persuasive. *Informative presentations* convey information or ideas, whereas *persuasive presentations* sell an idea or a service to an audience. Informative presentations include progress reports, instructions, and explanations. For example, you may give a progress report to your supervisor detailing your efforts on an assigned project, or you may give similar information to a small group if it is a team-related task. On the other hand, you may be directing a group of volunteers in a fund-raising effort, and as coordinator you may inform them about their responsibilities.

Many presentations in the health care field are instructional. For example, you might instruct individuals on how to obtain services for a special group of clients, how to administer a new drug, or how to complete a new form required by a governmental agency. Another variation of the informative presentation is the explanatory presentation, very common in the health care industry. For example, you may be asked to explain to the media the features of a plan to cut the teen birthrate among Hispanic women. Other examples of explanatory presentations include informing family members of a patient's condition and orienting new employees to the policies of the agency.

The second category, persuasive presentations, includes proposals and requests. For example, you may have to make a persuasive presentation to obtain authorization to purchase an expensive piece of equipment, or you may present a proposal to your supervisor to conduct research about ways to reach a resistant group of clients. Similarly, in the classroom, when you analyze a case, you are attempting to persuade your audience to understand the logic of your arguments and accept your recommendations. Once you have decided on the type of presentation needed to accomplish your goals, you are ready to consider the audience who will hear your presentation.

Analyze Your Audience

Audience analysis is a conscious method of examining the knowledge, interests, and attitudes of the people who will hear your presentation. Your analysis will help you determine how best to appeal to their concerns, needs, and values; how to organize your material; how to select supporting information; how to choose the appropriate wording; and how to select or produce appropriate visual aids.

Audience analysis is critical to ensuring that your information is accepted. Many presentations might be well delivered, but they fail because speakers do not anticipate audience reaction. You need to consider such characteristics as the size of the group, the audience members' level of knowledge about your subject, their interest in the material, their attitude and predispositions toward the subject, and their organizational relationship to you. For example, if your audience consists of five people, select a site that is small and personal when you present the information. If your audience is large, make sure all members can both hear and see the information you are presenting.

Although individuals within the health care industry tend to be well educated, their technical expertise usually is very specific. Therefore, when planning a presentation, you must ask, "What does this audience already know about this subject?"

Never assume that your audience is as knowledgeable about the topic as you are. When analyzing the prospective audience, you may want to ask yourself the following questions: "What information will I use to impress my audience? Will I employ technical data, demonstrations, or statistical comparisons?"

Whatever information you use, you should take care to reach your intended audience. This is particularly true when presenting ideas to laypeople, who generally know much less about the material than health care professionals. Choose your vocabulary and your examples to meet the audience's needs. Within the industry, people tend to have high interest in their respective areas but may have less interest in subjects that affect them less directly. Similarly, laypeople are often especially interested in their own health but may be easily confused concerning the technical details about it.

Every audience is unique because all audience members have different perceptions based upon personal experiences, which influence their attitudes about any subject. Understanding these predispositions will prevent you from making bold assumptions that may offend the audience. For example, if your audience consists of people sixty to seventy-five years of age, avoid any current slang lest you appear flippant and uncaring. Similarly, if your audience consists of young adults, avoid examples that they cannot understand because they have not experienced them. Because experience is such an important factor in understanding perceptions, you would not use the same explanations and examples with an audience of parents as you would with a childless audience. Good questions to ask when analyzing an audience include "What does this group want/need/expect from me?" and "How can I give that to them?"

Once you have answered some of the questions about who your audience is, next ask yourself what type or types of appeal will reach them. These include ethical, emotional, and logical appeals, or any combination of them.

The *ethical appeal* addresses the speaker's or the organization's credibility. It is impossible to separate the speaker's effect on an audience from the content of a message. If listeners regard the speaker highly, they will adopt a more favorable attitude toward the service or idea than if they have a negative impression of the person. Consequently, a speaker must bring to the platform a strong, positive, personal style. Credibility hinges on believability. You may have a high ethical appeal to members of an audience if they perceive that you have acted with integrity in the past. If, in previous dealings with this audience, you have acted rudely, unethically, or unprofessionally toward them, your ethical appeal will be very low. Many characteristics, such as honesty, dependability, and expertise, help to develop credibility. Although it takes some time to establish credibility, it takes only an instant to lose it by saying or doing something unexpected or inappropriate.

With the *emotional appeal*, the speaker uses the audience's motivations to change their thinking or behavior. Because emotion provokes action, speakers often seek to arouse the feelings of their listeners. The emotional appeal is characterized by the use of fear, sympathy, love, jealousy, sex, the desire for attention, the desire for security, or a host of other emotions to persuade the audience. To use the emotional appeal, first analyze the specific emotions to which the audience will respond. Then determine which words, pictures, or actions you can use to best evoke the desired emotion. Once members of the audience are drawn into the persuasion by the emotional "hook," it is easy to ask them to take action to meet the need or to satisfy the emotion that was touched. For example, most people are touched by the vulnerability of children, so when you show them a cute or sad photograph of a child, you may be able to capitalize on their emotions to persuade them to do whatever you suggest, such as financially supporting research on childhood diseases. Speakers should be aware, however, that excessive attempts to arouse emotions can lead to a rejection of their arguments by an audience. Thus, the emotional appeal should be used with restraint.

The *logical appeal* draws on an audience's ability to think and reason. This appeal uses sound reasons to show members of an audience why they should change their opinions or actions. The reasoning process and the supporting materials used to give credence to an argument are the elements of the logical appeal. For example, if you needed to persuade an audience to reengineer their department, you might stress making work more meaningful, more client-friendly, and more cost-effective. Often, the use of facts and figures is the most effective way to reach audiences that are accustomed to the logical approach in their own work environments.

Gather Information

Your effectiveness as a speaker depends on what you say about the topic you have selected. For case analyses in a classroom setting, a thorough understanding of the case is crucial. Knowing where to look is a starting point for finding the best possible information on your topic, whether it is a classroom case or a work setting. Sometimes the information will come from your personal knowledge, experience, or research. At other times, you may use information collected by others, such as census data, admissions/discharge records, inventory records, or pricing information. Information from electronic databases or from the Internet can provide current data that may enhance the quality of your presentation.

Your credibility as a speaker—your ethical appeal—will be determined largely by the quality of the information you present. For example, if you are talking about recent trends, data from the 1990 census would damage your credibility unless you want to compare it to 2000 census data. Conversely, up-to-date health care reform legislation passed by various states would be beneficial to an audience that needs to plan strategy in an unstable legislative environment. Always ask yourself what kind of material will best promote the desired audience response.

Consider the Logistics of Your Speaking Site

Before you can finalize the organization of your presentation, you must consider some logistical concerns. First, how much time will you need to give the presentation? Sometimes you have no control over how long you will speak: You are told the specific amount of time available to you. In such cases, it is imperative that you stay within your time limit. When the time is exceeded, the audience becomes less receptive to your ideas. When given some choice over the length of a presentation, most speakers take too much time. Remember that it is difficult to hold people's attention beyond twenty to thirty minutes. To improve effectiveness, speakers also need to watch the audience for verbal and nonverbal feedback to evaluate whether their message is being comprehended and accepted.

Second, you need to know where you will make the presentation. Will it be made in a conference room, a traditional classroom, a large auditorium, an office, or a dining hall? The location of your presentation will determine the kind of delivery and the types of visual aids that you will use as well as how you set up the room. Some guidelines for setting up the speaking site are to

- Arrange seating so that every member of the audience can see and hear you; the horseshoe arrangement is preferred if the room and the size of the audience will allow for it.
- Check the lighting, temperature, and noise level of the site to ensure that your audience will be comfortable.
- Avoid high-traffic areas, such as a room next to a kitchen or one off a busy hallway, that will present distractions to your audience.
- Check any equipment you intend to use to be sure that it can be easily viewed or heard by your audience.
- Remember that if anything can go wrong, it generally will.

Try to anticipate any problems before they occur. For example, when using any kind of projected visual aids, you should carry an extra bulb or have alternate visual aids in case the equipment breaks down. If you are speaking at a site that you have not visited previously, you may even want to bring an extension cord and an adapter plug, tape, push pins, or other supplies that may not be available at the site.

Organize Your Presentation

Once you have determined the type of presentation, analyzed your audience, gathered information, and considered the logistics of the speaking site, you are ready to organize your information logically. Effective organization and appropriate repetition are two of the most powerful keys to audience comprehension and retention. Most experts recommend the following pattern:

- Tell your audience what you are going to say
- Say it
- Tell your audience what you have just said

In other words, repeat the main points in the introduction, body, and conclusion of your presentation. Although it may sound simple, this strategy works surprisingly well. Construct the three parts of your presentation and add appropriate material to ensure that your listeners understand and remember your material.

Introduction

Because people tend to remember the beginning and end of a presentation, prepare a strong introduction. The opening of your presentation should accomplish three specific goals: (1) capture your listeners' attention, (2) establish your credibility and goodwill with the audience, and (3) preview your main points.

Your first obligation as a speaker is to get the audience interested in your subject. If you are able to attract the audience's attention from the start, you are more likely to hold their attention until the finish. Attention grabbers may include the following:

1. A promise. Begin with a promise that keeps the audience expectant. For example, "By the end of this presentation, I will show you how you can improve pulmonary diagnoses by 50 percent."
2. A reference to the event or the occasion. "On Friday, December 12, Sonoma Valley clinics treated more than 11,000 patients. Although this may be indicative of the recent flu outbreak, the stress on our clinics continues to grow. We need to build a strategic plan for the next decade. That is what I'd like to talk about today."
3. A brief story that relates to the topic. "On June 5, Paula Torres survived complications from an automobile accident the night before. Medical personnel at the Robinson County health center diagnosed her condition and the potential for complications with a CRX-14 medical scanner. This presentation will review the life-saving qualities of this miracle of modern science and its potential for the coming year."
4. A quotation by a recognized authority on the subject. "The Surgeon General of the United States has recommended that we reduce our fat intake by 40 percent. Three out of four Americans have too much fat in their diets. This serious problem is one of many reasons why we need to begin our health awareness program."
5. A thought-provoking question that requires the audience members to participate by answering the question or to get involved by raising their hands. "How many of you have been hospitalized in the past year? (Pause for an audience response.) If you have, you know the importance of having state-of-the-art health facilities in Mentuk Valley. Today, I'm going to talk about what patients value in our facilities."
6. A startling statement; it may or may not be a statistic. "If our costs continue to increase over the next three years at the rate they have been over the past decade, we will have to increase our treatment fees by 200 percent. Today, I will present five strategies for reducing costs in . . ."
7. A personal story or reference about the topic. "Seven years ago I suffered from a serious disease. Metaburen was prescribed to treat my illness. I'm happy to say that I am fully recovered and owe much of my recovery to this miracle

drug. Metaburen was just one of the drugs we developed in the past decade. We continue to add new products. This presentation will preview two of them: Zacatril and Premaris."

8. A joke. This can be particularly tricky in public health settings because most people feel that poor health is not a joking matter. The key is to know your audience and, when in doubt, avoid humor.

Audiences respond to things that are familiar to them. Events in their hometown, individuals they know, and problems faced by their employers attract their attention. From your audience analysis, you may be able to make a specific reference to an event or person familiar to this particular audience. Audiences react to the new, the unusual, or the exotic. A promise of new information or treatment, or the description of something beyond their experience, will hold their attention. In other words, show them how they will learn something new as a result of your presentation.

Stating the thesis is the second function of an effective introduction. Once you have successfully chosen an attention-getting statement, tell the audience the purpose of your presentation by stating the thesis. The thesis is a statement that tells what you want to accomplish in the presentation. The relationship of your purpose to your audience members and their interests is an important consideration. They will listen more attentively if the topic is vital to them and if it is near in time and in place. Although the introduction is designed to get the audience members to think about the topic, you must be sure that they understand what you intend to do with the topic. The thesis statement helps focus the entire presentation. Below are examples of thesis statements from two team members making a case analysis presentation to the class.

Speaker One: Our team believes that the Almira Clinic should pursue aggressive preventive strategies to improve our community health statistics and become a major player in the treatment of STDs.

Speaker Two: Our team proposes an alternative strategy of improving community health statistics. We believe that to compete in the regional health care environment, the Almira Clinic should provide the total continuum of care for STDs.

Previewing the main points of your presentation keeps your audience attuned to what you are saying. Audiences will listen more attentively if they know where you are going, the appearance of organization will increase your credibility, and the repetition of main ideas will increase the likelihood that they will be remembered. Recognize that the attention span of an audience varies from one occasion to the next. Following are two examples of previews that come after the thesis statement in a case analysis by team members.

Speaker One: We need to take immediate action to maintain our visibility in the area. Because health care options are increasing, we have a number of empty beds, and HCA—The Healthcare Company just purchased the Sisters' Hospital.

Speaker Two: Our caseload has been decreasing. Providing the complete continuum of care means that we must become more than merely a local clinic. We need to establish a "face" in the community. Also, because recruiting is becoming more difficult, our patients need an individual who can offer the quality care they need.

Later, during the body of the presentation, you will develop in more detail each point mentioned in the preview.

Body

The biggest problem with most oral presentations is a failure to focus on a few principal ideas. The body of your presentation should include a limited number of main points. Next, you should develop each main point with adequate, but not excessive, explanation and details. Too many details can obscure the main message, so keep your presentation simple and logical. Remember, listeners may have no pages to review should they become confused.

Various methods are available to develop the body of the presentation. Below are some common ones.

1. Use statistics or other facts.
2. Cite quotations or expert testimony.
3. Employ examples, real or hypothetical.
4. Refer to personal experiences.
5. Use comparisons, contrasts, or analogies to the audience's experiences.

Whatever method you choose to employ, smooth transitions are a key aspect of organization. A link must be established between one idea or issue and another so the audience sees the relationship. This link may take the form of a short summary that simply states that a new point will now be discussed. It might contrast what has just been presented with that which is to follow. Another technique is the repetition of key words or phrases for emphasis. Some examples include the following:

- "The first way Zacatril differs from our earlier products is . . ."
- "Now for the second difference . . ."
- "Also . . ."
- "To begin . . ."
- "Finally . . ."

Conclusion

You should prepare your conclusion carefully because this is your last chance to drive home your main points. Good speakers leave a favorable impression in the minds of the audience. An effective conclusion must accomplish this objective. For example, don't end limply with comments like "I guess that's about all I have to say." Too often, speakers just trail off with a "That's all. Thank you very much" ending. Whatever the specific nature of your conclusion, it should clearly communicate that the speaker is ending.

Skilled speakers use the conclusion to review the main points of the presentation and focus on a goal. They concentrate on what they want the audience to do, think, or remember. Although they were mentioned earlier, important points must be repeated. Do not introduce any new information in your conclusion lest you appear unfinished. If some action is expected from the audience, the speaker's expectations should be made clear and easy to follow.

A presentation can have an excellent introduction and body but still not be effective. Conclusions can be developed in a number of ways:

- Summarize your main points.
- Ask the audience to take some action, such as visiting your health care facility or contributing to a particular cause.
- Recall the story, joke, or anecdote in the introduction and elaborate on it or draw a "lesson" from it.

Now that you have structured your presentation, you must find ways to enhance it further. Visual aids are the tools to accentuate the information you want to share.

Prepare Your Visual Aids

Because your goals as a speaker are to make listeners understand, remember, and act on your ideas, include visual aids to get them interested and involved. Some experts suggest that we acquire 85 percent of all of our knowledge visually. Research also indicates that audiences remember only 10 to 20 percent of what they hear but 80 percent of what they see. Therefore, an oral presentation that incorporates visual aids is far more likely to be understood and retained than one lacking visual enhancement.

Because we live in a visually oriented society, we expect to see as well as hear information. Effective speakers show as well as tell their points. Remember that your audience must understand the material that is being presented to remember it. Visual aids help maintain audience attention and involvement. Two broad categories of visual aids are available to enhance presentations. One category, direct viewing visuals, includes such things as real objects, models, flip charts, handouts, and chalkboards or whiteboards. The second category, projected visuals, includes slides, videotapes, overhead transparencies, and computer presentations.

Direct Viewing Visuals

Real objects are often the best visuals when the audience is small and when seeing "the real thing" will be more convincing than viewing a drawing, diagram, or photograph. For example, if you are touting the quality of a product, it might be good to show how a particular component is manufactured—what it looks like, feels like, sounds like, and so forth. This can best be done by using real items.

Models are very effective for showing how a dialysis unit, operating room, or visitor waiting room will look. This type of visual can be very persuasive if the audience is small enough that everyone can see the model as it is being discussed.

Flip charts are excellent for use with audiences that are small enough to see the information on the chart. Most speakers "write as they talk" when using flip charts. This flexibility gives an informal, conversational tone to a presentation. However, some information, such as key words, may be put on the chart ahead of time and elaborated on during the speech. If this method is used, the words should be covered by leaving the top page blank and lifting it when ready to show the key words.

Handouts allow you to fit more information on a printed page than with other visuals, but avoid doing so. Keep handouts simple. Summarize major points, but do not provide the audience with your entire presentation. If possible, distribute the handout when it is needed rather than at the beginning of the presentation. Otherwise, the audience may read the handout while you are explaining background information needed to understand the ideas presented in the handout.

Chalkboards or whiteboards are useful for presenting informal visuals to small groups. Some major problems presented by chalkboards and whiteboards are the time necessary to write the information, lack of cleanliness of some boards, poor penmanship of the user, and failure of the user to erase items once they have been considered. If you plan to use a board, practice and make certain you have all the necessary equipment (appropriate markers, eraser, and so on). If your visual is complex, you may find it helpful to place it on the board before your presentation. Many portable chalkboards or whiteboards have two sides, thus permitting you to keep your material from view until you need it.

Projected Visuals

Slides can be effective when showing how something looks at particular phases, such as the stages in the progress of a disease. Of course, slides should be organized before they are loaded into the projector. The speaker should practice using them so none are in upside-down, backward, or out of sequence. Remember to allow enough time to develop the slides if you are producing them yourself.

Videotapes are effective if you need to show a process. Few other types of visuals can capture the drama of a videotape. For example, if you were demonstrating a surgical procedure, a videotape could be excellent. It could show exactly how to perform the surgery and could even be done in slow motion or freeze-frame to allow surgeons to see particularly delicate processes. Or it could be used to demonstrate the ease of a minor surgical procedure to a patient to dispel anxiety.

Overhead transparencies work best when a large amount of material must be presented and there is little time or money for a more sophisticated type of presentation. Overheads give you a great deal of flexibility. For example, you can circle an important point or change a number or label. In addition, you can place one transparency over another to create a multilayered look. Prepared overheads, such as charts or diagrams, can offer a neat appearance and a more polished presentation.

The use of overheads also allows you to vary the size of the image through adjusting the distance from the projector to the screen. Finally, even if a transparency is created "on the spot," it still has the advantage of giving you the opportunity to face the audience. You can maintain eye contact and observe audience feedback while you talk about your material.

Computer presentations are being prepared by increasing numbers of speakers. When using presentation software such as Microsoft, PowerPoint®, Lotus, Freelance®, and Corel "Presentation"®, speakers should consider the following points:

1. Input your ideas into a built-in outliner that will help you organize your thoughts. On-screen assistance generally is available to those needing help with various organizational plans.
2. Select features for displaying your text (font, type size, color, texture, border, and so on).
3. Edit each visual, indicating the exact sequence and special effects (graphics, transitions, sounds, and motion).
4. Generate printed handouts, slides, transparencies, or a slide show for an on-screen presentation.

Many programs provide templates (prepared designs) that suggest features and colors that work well together. You simply select the template, and your information (text or graphics) is formatted automatically. After viewing the results, you can revise the format if you wish. These templates help the novice presenter resist the temptation to create overwhelmingly complex visuals simply because the technology is available.

Running an on-screen presentation takes some practice. Depending on the length of your presentation, it may be difficult to remember what information is on each slide. Experience will teach you to rehearse the material to help develop a verbal introduction, develop effective transitions from one slide to another, and conclude effectively.

Although they are very effective for large audiences, on-screen presentations may overwhelm a smaller audience. Rather than focusing on the material, the audience may be distracted by the special effects used to move from one idea to another. In addition, on-screen presentations limit audience interaction, which may be an important part of your presentation.

Guidelines for Selecting Visual Aids

Visual aids attract and hold attention, clarify the meaning of your points, emphasize ideas, or prove a point. Several factors must be considered in selecting the appropriate visual aid:

1. The constraints of the topic. Some topics will limit your choice of visual aids. For example, if you were explaining to a group of laypeople how microsurgery is performed on a hand, you would not use a flip chart because it would

be ineffective. You would probably not show a videotape of the surgery being performed because the sight of blood may upset some individuals. Instead, you might use a model of the hand. However, a videotape might be very effective in teaching surgeons how to perform the procedure.

2. The availability of the equipment. If the speaking site does not have an overhead projector, you could not use transparencies. Similarly, if the site does not have an electrical outlet near the podium, you would not be able to use a projected visual. Always check to see what equipment is available or bring your own. Also, verify that your computer presentation will run on the version of software installed on the available equipment.

3. The cost of the visual. If your budget is very small, a transparency, flip chart, or handout may be preferable to the more elaborate types of visual aids such as slides or videotapes.

4. The difficulty of producing the visual. If you have only two days to prepare for your presentation, it may be impossible to assemble a scale model of a labor/ delivery room interior or process slides of a sequence of cancer growth.

5. The appropriateness of the visual to the audience. The type of audience and the nature of the presentation affect the choice of visual aids. Some charts, graphs, and diagrams may be too technical for anyone but specialists to grasp. Detailed and complicated tables and charts that require considerable time to digest should be avoided. When in doubt, keep your visuals short and simple.

6. The appropriateness of the visual to the speaker. Visual aids require skill to be presented effectively. A speaker must be able to write in large, legible letters and draw well-proportioned diagrams to use a flip chart. Projected visuals require skill in handling slides, videotape, or film. Unless you feel comfortable with a particular visual medium, avoid using it.

7. The appropriateness of the visual to the time limit. The speaker should carefully check the time required to display and explain a visual aid to make sure the main ideas of the presentation will not be neglected. Any visual aid that needs too much explanation should be avoided. An appropriate visual aid should be simple, clear, and brief.

Once you have planned and organized the content of your presentation and prepared your visual aids, you are ready to deliver your presentation.

Beginning Your Presentation

During the first few minutes of a presentation, the audience "sizes up" the speaker and draws conclusions about his or her credibility. Because credibility is essential to achieving their goals, speakers should understand how to gain it.

Establish Credibility

The factors that determine credibility include the speaker's enthusiasm, expertise, and trustworthiness. *Enthusiasm* is conveyed through tone of voice, eye contact, and energy. Clearly, the major ways speakers can display these characteristics are by believing in the subject and acting as if they enjoy conveying the information. For example, at the beginning of the presentation, look directly at the audience, give a sincere smile, and say the first few words with energy and excitement. Your credibility will be off to a great start.

Expertise is conveyed through the accuracy of your information, the amount of experience you have had with the subject, and the confidence with which you speak. To guarantee this aspect of your credibility, check your facts, refer to your personal experience with the topic, and talk about your personal experiences with confidence.

Trustworthiness refers to the audience's perception that the speaker is unbiased. Consistency in dealing with people over a period of time is important to establish trust. If the audience members have had positive dealings with or have heard good things about the speaker, they are likely to perceive him or her as trustworthy.

Reduce Speech Anxiety

One factor that detracts from credibility is speech anxiety. Several techniques can relieve this problem with a small investment of time. The first technique is borrowed from athletes. Before major events, they mentally see themselves doing all the correct things to ensure a win; then they picture themselves winning the event. Speakers should do the same thing. For several nights before the presentation, just before falling asleep, you should close your eyes and picture yourself making a great speech. This positive mental preparation actually works!

Another characteristic of speech anxiety is a lack of control of one's breathing. Again, this can be corrected by practicing an exercise several days before the speech. Select a quiet place where you can sit. Place both feet on the floor and put one hand on your stomach. Take a deep breath, then exhale deeply (you have done this correctly if you can feel your hand rise and fall on your stomach). Clear your mind of other thoughts and start to focus on the breathing. Continue the deep breathing. Think about how it feels to have the air pass through your nostrils. Think about the pressure on your eyes, the sound of your breathing, and so on. If other thoughts intervene, banish them and return to focus on your breathing. Perform this exercise a minimum of five minutes before you quit. Do this as many times a day as you can to gain control of your breathing. On the day of the presentation, you can do the same exercise for a few seconds just before you speak. You have just done an exercise that relaxes not only your breathing but your whole body as well. A relaxed speaker is a more credible speaker.

If you suffer greatly from speech anxiety and these exercises do not help you, perhaps some work with a therapist will help you uncover the root of your severe anxiety.

Use Your Visual Aids

The use of effective visual aids can enhance your presentation and improve your credibility. Conversely, poor use of visual aids can detract from your presentation. Some guidelines for using visual aids follow.

1. Avoid turning your back on the audience while you look at or point to a visual aid. Talk to the audience, not to your visuals.
2. Show the visual aid only when you are talking about it; otherwise, the audience may be distracted from what you are saying. For example, if you are using transparencies, cover everything except what you are talking about at the moment.
3. Refrain from removing the visual before the audience members have had an opportunity to look at the information for themselves. To guarantee that you do not speed past the visuals, make it a point to go over orally everything that is on your visuals.
4. Organize the visuals in the order in which you will use them so you will appear prepared and confident.

Manage Your Nonverbal Communication

Several dimensions of nonverbal communication related to speaking include (1) kinesics, the way people use their bodies to communicate; (2) proxemics, the way people use space to communicate; and (3) paralanguage, the way people use their voices to enhance the verbal message.

Two of the most important types of kinetic behavior in a presentation are gestures and eye contact. Speakers are rarely credible when they stand rigidly behind a podium, grasp it as if it were a crutch, and seldom glance up from their notes to look at the audience. Similarly, poor posture, hands in pockets, and playing with objects, such as chalk or pointers, lessen a speaker's credibility.

Speakers who recognize that "space communicates" will use it wisely. For example, if the audience is small, it may be better to sit at the head of the group than to "stand over them" to deliver the information. Also, if you must deliver unfavorable information, stand close to the audience to appear more sincere and understanding.

Aspects of the voice that affect credibility include volume, rate, pitch, tone, and voice quality. The "sound" of the voice (voice quality), such as raspiness or a nasal sound, evokes images in the minds of the listeners; however, it is very difficult to change the voice quality you have. On the other hand, tone, pitch, rate, and volume are easily changed. For example, the person who has a monotone can make his or her voice seem less monotonous by saying some words softly and others loudly. Even though the tone hasn't changed, the audience perceives that the tone is varied. A low pitch is viewed as more credible in our culture, and a high pitch is often associated with nervousness. Speakers should start talking at the lowest pitch they can achieve. Then, if it rises a little during the speech, it will seem less offensive than if the speaker begins with a high pitch.

Delivering Your Presentation

The situation, the audience, and the speaker determine the type of delivery. The formality or informality of the situation greatly affects delivery. The more formal it is and the larger the audience, the fewer gestures and movements speakers make. They limit themselves more to their position behind the lectern and use a more emphatic speaking voice to compensate for fewer gestures. In very informal situations, speakers are free to move away from the podium and interact with the audience, even strolling between tables or down aisles.

The available equipment will also determine delivery. For instance, if the size of the audience necessitates a microphone, speakers should not move away from it. They may also need to adapt themselves to various tables or other unusual speaking platforms that will hold their notes, visuals, or other forms of support.

The larger the audience, the louder speakers must talk unless there is a microphone. Likewise, eye contact is more challenging with large groups. Delivery to small groups therefore can be more informal and conversational than to large groups; however, speakers should always look at the audience even if it is impossible to make direct eye contact with members.

Determine the Type of Delivery You Will Use

Several methods for delivering material can be employed, and each has its unique advantages. The four methods of delivery are impromptu, manuscript, memorized, and extemporaneous.

Impromptu delivery requires speaking spontaneously on a topic. This type of delivery generally is inappropriate for technical or complex material because you may forget crucial information if the presentation has not been carefully planned. Impromptu delivery is often used at social occasions such as introductions at an after-dinner speaking engagement or at a professional meeting where you are asked to "sit in" for someone who was going to introduce a speaker but was called out because of an emergency.

Manuscript delivery requires that the speaker read from a prepared text. This type of delivery is ineffective in most presentations because audiences generally prefer more eye contact (they also dislike having material read to them). Manuscript delivery is necessary in one particular situation: when a crisis has occurred. For example, if a client receives the wrong medication and dies as a result, the media are quick to "look for the story." The spokesperson for the organization should never deliver the information in an impromptu manner. Rather, the response should be carefully prepared and read to the media because any misstatement in such a situation could result in litigation against the organization or, at the least, a change in the public's perception of the agency or organization.

Memorized delivery is self-explanatory. In most cases, it is discouraged because memorized presentations usually sound "canned" rather than natural. Worse yet, the speaker may forget part of what was memorized and may lose confidence in himself or herself to remember the rest of the presentation. This type of delivery might be appropriate in situations where the presentation will be only a few minutes long, such as introducing a speaker or "saying a few words" about someone at a retirement party.

Extemporaneous delivery is the preferred approach for most presentations because it helps build the speaker's credibility in the eyes of an audience. This type of delivery allows the use of notes or an outline to deliver the information. The speaker should talk in a conversational tone but refer periodically to notes to be sure that all the information is covered. Some people prefer following a precise outline, whereas others prefer using note cards to deliver a presentation. With the use of presentation software such as PowerPoint®, speakers can even show the audience their "notes" by making them part of certain slides. Each person must find what works best for him or her. Although notes can be a valuable resource for a speaker, they can easily become a psychological crutch. To make sure that they do not become a crutch, remember to use notes only when absolutely necessary.

Rehearse Your Delivery

Preparation influences a speaker's delivery. A speaker who is well prepared and has something valuable to communicate will be more comfortable physically and vocally. If speakers are unsure of themselves and the material, they may be tempted to read word for word from their outlines. Being too self-conscious or nervous can create physical and vocal qualities and mannerisms that detract from the message. Too much concern with oneself or the ideas and too little concern for the audience will also hinder a speaker's delivery.

Always practice aloud what you want to say. You don't need an audience; you can talk aloud to yourself, to your dog or cat, or to the trees. Rehearsing not only will give you confidence but also will help you to hear any awkward phrasing or words that are hard to pronounce. If possible, practice with your visuals so you will know when to use them and how much time it takes to discuss them.

Delivery is not something added to a speech but an integral part of it. Consider the following when rehearsing your presentation:

1. Practice how you will stand to open the presentation. Will you use a podium or hold your notes?
2. Practice what to do with your hands, but keep them at or above the waist. Gestures give credibility unless they are erratic or overly large and dramatic. Notice if you do anything distracting such as repeatedly scratching your nose or fiddling with your hair.
3. Rehearse projecting your voice. If you will be using a microphone, practice positioning it correctly and holding it to avoid feedback. Practice articulating your words and pronouncing them correctly. A speaker who puts the full "ing" endings on words will seem more educated than one who leaves off the "g."

4. Practice sounding positive and enthusiastic. In a sense, a speaker is a momentary actor and sometimes has to "act" more enthusiastic than his or her normal speech patterns would reflect.

5. Rehearse ways to differentiate the main points in some way. Perhaps you will hold up your fingers as you say point 1, point 2, and so on. Or perhaps you will say the points louder or softer or more slowly than the rest of the speech. Or maybe you will pause in some places for emphasis or effect.

6. Involve the audience by practicing eye contact with imaginary audience members in all parts of the room.

After you have rehearsed your speech, you will be prepared to make a dynamic presentation. Before we leave the subject of delivery, we will discuss how to prepare for questions that may arise from your presentation.

Manage Questions From the Audience

Many presentations are followed by a question-and-answer period, which gives a speaker some indication of whether or not the audience received the message. This period is a continuation of the presentation, albeit in a more informal, give-and-take manner. Answering questions provides the presenter with the opportunity to clarify points and to reinforce parts of the presentation that may have seemed less convincing to listeners. Any question-and-answer period should be well organized and brief. To make the most of the available time, follow these guidelines:

1. Repeat the question. Except in small groups or settings, it is a good idea to repeat the question as you heard it. Repeating the question ensures that you understand the question that is being asked. In addition, not everyone may have heard the question. Repeating it makes sure that everyone understands the question you are answering, and repeating it gives you an opportunity to organize an answer.

2. Ask for questions in a positive way. For instance, you could say, "Who has the first question?" If no one asks a question, you may say, "You may be wondering . . ." or "I am often asked. . . ." After supplying an answer to the question you have asked, you may ask, "Are there any other questions?"

3. In general, you should try to frame your answer so that it is of general interest to the whole group. This technique can also prevent the setting up of a continuing dialogue between you and the questioner, leaving the rest of the audience out of the conversation. You are addressing everyone, not just the person asking the question.

4. Keep your answers concise and to the point; do not give another speech. You risk losing the audience's attention as well as discouraging further questions.

5. Cut off a rambling questioner politely. If the person starts to make a speech without getting to the question, wait until he or she takes a breath and then interrupt with, "Thanks for your comment. Next question." Then look to the other side of the room.

6. Postpone questions that are of individual or very special concern. Some questions interest only one person, the questioner, or may require an answer that should be presented only to that particular person: "Why was I charged $119 for pain medication last month?" Suggest that the individual see you immediately after the formal question-and-answer period for a personal response.

7. Say "I don't know" when that is the case. It usually is not a good idea to try to bluff your way through answers when you are not sure. When you have to say that you do not have an answer, give a good reason why you don't and indicate how the questioner can obtain a satisfactory answer to that question. For example, you may point out that in your part of the operations you don't deal with the relevant subject area: "Well, Mr. Jones, I am in the counseling area, so I don't really get involved in prescribing pain medications. I know who can answer your question, however, and I'll see that she gets in touch with you."

8. Remain in control of the situation. Establish a time limit for questions and answers and announce it to the audience before the questions begin. Anticipate the types of questions your audience may ask and think how you will answer. Never lose your temper as you respond to someone who is trying to make you look bad. You may respond with something like, "I respect your opinion even though I don't agree with it." Then restate your response to the issue.

9. Watch your nonverbal communication when answering questions. For example, pointing a finger at the audience, putting your hands on your hips, or raising your voice above the pitch of the presentation may give the appearance of authoritarianism and rudeness.

Because your presentation does not end when you finish your speech, your credibility can be enhanced or lost in the question-and-answer period. Prepare intelligently and establish strategies for handling difficult situations.

Developing the skills needed to present your point of view in a convincing manner is essential to reaching your personal and career goals, and presenting information orally is a challenging task. However, if you follow the guidelines suggested, your presentation will be rewarding to both you and your audience.

Evaluate Your Presentation

Some organizations that provide speakers also distribute questionnaires to the whole audience after a presentation. Such formal procedures usually are effective for providing specific kinds of observable information, such as whether the speaker was on time or whether he or she spoke on the subject expected. Such instruments can provide information on how much the group felt they learned, or how much they changed position on the topic. Although such tools work well for external, more formal presentations, they are less likely to be useful for internal, or in-house, presentations; informal feedback may be more typical for in-house presentations.

Conclusion

Effective speaking means that you should be yourself. You express yourself best when you are natural and conversational, and you can be most naturally conversational when you are highly familiar with the content and delivery of your presentation. The only way to test an oral presentation is to rehearse it several times. At this rehearsal, you should use your notes and visual aids to check your use of pauses, eye contact, transitions, and so on. This will give you more confidence and help you estimate the total amount of time necessary to deliver the final presentation. Rehearsal can go a long way toward making your presentation a success by giving you an opportunity to evaluate, revise, and consider all aspects of your presentation.

CHAPTER 4

Financial Analysis for Health Care Organizations

The purpose of this chapter is to explain some basic concepts of finance. Financial analysis as it is conducted in for-profit and not-for-profit health care organizations is not often used in public health agencies. Financial analysis in public health does not require different methods, but it does require thinking in a different context. Unlike most other sectors of the economy, public health is composed primarily of government organizations or voluntary not-for-profit organizations. In addition, it is heavily regulated by government. These special characteristics of the industry should not preclude innovative and sound financial planning and analysis.

In addition, it is important to recognize that public health leaders do compete for financial resources with other sectors of the economy. Such competition takes many forms, including lobbying at the federal, state, and local levels for financial appropriations; seeking grants and contracts from government and foundations; competing for labor to staff public health programs; negotiating with government financial officials and vendors; and, for some public health agencies, competing with the private sector to deliver primary care services. Understanding how these competitors will analyze their financial situation is fundamental for making critical leadership and management judgments in public health. The financial analysis methods used in various types of health care settings are presented in this chapter to encourage creative thinking about these methods as they relate to, and can be used by, public health managers and leaders.

To analyze the financial health of any organization, you need to understand how to read the financial statements. The income statement and balance sheet are the two

This chapter was written by Mahmud Hassan, Rutgers University.

Exhibit 4.1. Memorial Hospital Consolidated Statement of Income (in thousands of dollars except per share amounts)

	1998	1999	2000
Revenues	$2,973,643	$3,435,397	$4,087,994
Operating expenses	2,340,178	2,786,230	3,401,884
Depreciation and amortization	180,197	195,651	209,469
Interest expense	154,156	145,938	138,477
Interest income	(30,923)	(46,064)	(60,570)
	2,643,608	3,081,755	3,689,260
Income before income taxes	330,035	353,642	398,734
Provision for income taxes	147,196	126,602	142,747
Income before extraordinary items and cumulative effect of a change in accounting principle	182,839	277,040	255,987
Extraordinary loss on early extinguishment of debt, net of income tax of $9,597	—	(16,133)	—
Cumulative effect on prior years of a change in accounting principle for retirement plan actuarial gains, net of income tax of $9,645	—	16,214	—
Net income	$ 182,839	$ 277,121	$ 255,987
Earnings per common share:			
Income before extraordinary item and cumulative effect of a change in accounting principle	$1.86	$2.30	$2.56
Extraordinary loss on early extinguishment of debt	—	(.16)	—
Cumulative effect on prior years of a change in accounting principle for retirement plan actuarial gains	—	.16	—
Net income per share	$ 1.86	$ 2.30	$ 2.56

most important financial reports of an organization. Not-for-profit and government organizations do not produce income statements, but they may prepare balance sheets for internal use. In this chapter, we will compute financial ratios, net income, and other financial performance figures for Memorial Hospital, a for-profit hospital company, for the years 1999 and 2000. The detailed financial statements are available in the Annual Report of Memorial Hospital. Copies of these statements are shown in Exhibits 4.1 and 4.2.

As previously mentioned, not-for-profit organizations are not required to prepare balance sheets or income statements. However, some not-for-profit health care organizations do prepare balance sheets to satisfy requirements of the Securities and Exchange Commission (SEC) and the rating agencies (Moody's or Standard and Poor's) when they borrow money by selling bonds. For example, University Hospital

Exhibit 4.2. Memorial Hospital Consolidated Balance Sheet (in thousands of dollars)

	1999	2000
Assets		
Current assets		
Cash and cash equivalents	$140,201	$105,340
Marketable securities	106,490	79,104
Accounts receivable less allowance for loss of $157,505–2000 and $110,909–1999	507,141	616,210
Inventories	69,786	80,632
Other current assets	104,788	133,615
Total current assets	928,407	1,014,901
Property and equipment, at cost		
Land	168,761	177,275
Buildings	1,678,685	1,759,959
Equipment	1,086,374	1,211,401
Construction in progress (estimated cost to complete and equipment after August 31, 2000–$114,000)	41,729	57,719
Gross fixed assets	2,975,549	3,206,354
Less accumulated depreciation	987,790	1,154,868
Net fixed assets	1,987,759	2,051,486
Investments in insurance/health plan subsidiaries	315,875	462,541
Other assets	189,921	167,646
Total assets	$3,421,962	$3,696,574
Liabilities and common stockholders' equity		
Current liabilities		
Trade accounts payable	$107,666	$115,338
Salaries, wages, and other compensation	82,184	95,760
Other accrued expenses	173,956	229,201
Medical claims reserves	141,773	194,925
Income taxes	95,475	106,241
Long-term debt due within one year	32,680	35,045
Total current liabilities	633,734	776,510
Long-term debt	1,210,618	1,140,366
Deferred credits and other liabilities	422,993	452,722
Common stockholders' equity		
Common stock, 16 2/3¢ par; authorized 200 million shares; issued and outstanding 98,438,852 shares–2000 and 97,886,147 shares–1999	16,314	16,406
Capital in excess of par value	233,898	243,398
Other adjustments	(11,047)	(11,029)
Retained earnings	915,452	1,078,201
Stockholders' equity	1,154,617	1,326,976
Total liabilities and stockholders' equity	$3,421,962	$3,696,574

(a not-for-profit organization) borrowed money in 2001 from the capital market by selling bonds. It had to prepare a balance sheet for three years, 1998 through 2000, to have its bonds rated. The balance sheet for University Hospital is shown in Exhibit 4.3. Publicly traded for-profit hospitals are required by their charters to produce balance sheets and income statements each year. As mentioned earlier, we will analyze the financial statements of Memorial Hospital in this chapter.

The contents of balance sheets vary by company depending on the nature of the business and the type of ownership. Memorial Hospital's balance sheet contains some information regarding investments in subsidiaries, whereas the not-for-profit University Hospital reported a trustee fund in its balance sheet. Not-for-profit organizations show their equity or ownership share as a fund balance. For University Hospital, the amount of equity investment in 2000 was more than $185 million, as shown in Exhibit 4.3 under "fund balance." All other items in Exhibit 4.3 are comparable with those in Exhibit 4.2.

Financial ratios for University Hospital can be computed using the same formulas as shown for Memorial Hospital, but some financial ratios will require information from income statements. Because not-for-profit hospitals do not prepare income statements, the ratios for days in accounts receivable, average payment period, days' cash on hand, times interest earned, debt service coverage, operating margin, markup, return on assets, and so on cannot be computed for University Hospital.

In addition to the analysis of the income statement and balance sheet, an analysis of the cost of capital is provided. This is an important topic for the health care industry because of its dependence on technology and because of reimbursement issues involving third-party payors. The cost of capital for an organization is important because of its use as the discount rate in the analysis of investment projects.

The Income Statement

Income statements are prepared by proprietary hospitals for the computation of net profit and incurred tax. (A not-for-profit hospital is not required to prepare an income statement, but it may choose to do so to keep its various constituencies informed. The IRS does require "informational reports" to be filed for not-for-profit organizations generating more than $25,000 in revenue.) Public health agencies, because they are generally part of the state government, are not subject to federal IRS regulations. However, public health may want to consider "informational reports" as a means of improving financial thinking within the organization.

The income statement shows all revenue receipts and expenditures during a year. Receipts usually are shown as gross revenue and net revenue. Net revenue is equal to gross revenue minus any uncollectibles such as contractual allowances, bad debt, charity care, and business discounts. In the case of Memorial Hospital, the net revenue for 2000 was (all figures for Memorial are in thousands of dollars):

Net revenue: $4,087,994

Exhibit 4.3. University Hospital Balance Sheet

	Fiscal Year Ended September 30		
	1998	*1999*	*2000*
Assets			
Current assets			
Cash and short-term investments	$5,768,785	$7,184,131	$2,084,610
Accounts receivable	51,415,071	40,085,497	53,338,410
Inventory	1,518,012	2,097,327	2,677,247
Prepaid expenses and other current assets	6,971	0	0
Total current assets	58,708,839	49,366,955	58,100,267
Property, plant, and equipment	171,270,793	197,572,904	212,140,823
Less accumulated depreciation	61,175,801	72,626,040	85,433,535
Net property, plant, and equipment	110,094,992	124,946,864	126,707,288
Capital fund	23,233,852	26,730,346	20,657,000
Trustee funds	6,992,981	6,731,182	7,034,719
Total assets	$199,030,664	$207,775,347	$212,499,274
Liabilities and fund balance			
Current liabilities			
Accounts payable	$2,684,893	$3,911,504	$2,638,836
Accrued salaries	462,326	663,161	1,084,692
Advances from third-party payors	1,051,000	0	0
Deferred revenue	61,561	85,554	85,554
Current portion of long-term debt	2,022,140	2,068,744	1,659,565
Other current liabilities	69,623	17,038	561,853
Accrued interest expense	983,277	805,688	768,511
Total current liabilities	7,334,820	7,551,689	6,799,011
Long-term debt	21,792,410	21,525,786	19,866,221
Fund balance	169,903,434	178,697,872	185,834,042
Total liabilities and fund balance	$199,030,664	$207,775,347	$212,499,274

Memorial does not report gross revenue or uncollectibles.

Operating expenses represent selling, general, and administrative expenses.

Operating expense: $3,401,884

Depreciation and amortization are non-cash expenses due to wear and tear or decline in the useful life of an asset. (There is no cash payment for these items, but a for-profit company uses them as expense items to compute taxable income. Public health agencies do not pay income taxes; however, public health may want to consider maintaining such financial records because they can assist in planning for the replacement of high-cost assets as they wear out.) Depreciation can be on a straight-line basis or an accelerated basis. For straight-line depreciation, the assumption is that there will be equal wear and tear on the asset each year of its useful life. Accelerated depreciation assumes the wear and tear is high during initial years and declines over time.

Depreciation and amortization: $209,469

Interest expense is the amount paid to creditors on the total amount of debt the organization holds.

Interest expense: $138,477

Interest income is computed by subtracting dividends and capital gains from the investment income. In the case of Memorial Hospital, this amount is a positive quantity for 2000 and hence entered as a negative quantity in the expense category (see Exhibit 4.1).

Interest income: $60,570

Income before income taxes can be computed by subtracting operating expenses, depreciation, amortization, interest expense, and interest income from net revenue.

Income before income taxes: $398,734

Provision for state and federal taxes is computed at the statutory rate (35.8 percent for Memorial) on the income before income taxes.

Provision for income taxes: $142,747

Net income is computed by subtracting provision for income taxes and other adjustments from the income before taxes.

Net income: $255,987

The Balance Sheet

A balance sheet is a statement of the financial status of an organization at a particular point in time (date). It is divided into two sides: assets are shown on the left side and liabilities and owners' equity are shown on the right side. Assets are divided into current assets and fixed assets. Current assets include cash, marketable securities, accounts receivable (less uncollectibles), inventories, and other current assets. Marketable securities are short-term government securities. Other current assets include prepaid expenses such as insurance premiums, advertising charges for the next year, and so on.

In the case of Memorial Hospital in 2000:

Cash and cash equivalents:	$ 105,340
Marketable securities:	79,104
Accounts receivable less uncollectibles:	616,210
Inventories:	80,632
Other current assets:	133,615
Total current assets:	$1,014,901

In this case, cash equivalents include investments in securities with a maturity of three months or less. Fixed assets are land, buildings, equipment, and construction in progress.

Land:	$ 177,275
Buildings:	1,759,959
Equipment:	1,211,401
Construction in progress:	57,719
Gross fixed assets:	$3,206,354

Accumulated depreciation is the sum of all the depreciation expenses (as found in the income statement) since the inception of the organization.

Accumulated depreciation:	$1,154,868

Net fixed assets are computed by subtracting the accumulated depreciation from the gross fixed assets.

Net fixed assets:	$2,051,486

Memorial Hospital shows investments in its subsidiaries in a separate category:

Investments in insurance/health plan subsidiaries:	$ 462,541
Other assets:	167,646
Total assets:	$3,696,574

On the other side of the balance sheet, liabilities include current liabilities, long-term liabilities, and other liabilities. Current liabilities are accounts payable, salaries, wages and other compensation payable, other accrued expenses, medical claims reserves, income taxes payable, and that portion of long-term debt due within one year. Other accrued expenses include any other unpaid amounts. Medical claims reserves include outstanding claims from Memorial Hospital's insurance business.

Total current liabilities: $776,510

All debts not due within one year are listed under long-term debt.

Long-term debt: $1,140,366

Owners' equity includes the value of common stock outstanding (at face value or "par value"), the value of the stocks in excess of par value, other adjustments in the value of stocks, and retained earnings. For not-for-profit hospitals, the owners' equity is represented by a fund balance. Retained earnings are the accumulated net income minus the amount of any dividends paid to shareholders.

Stockholders' equity: $1,326,976

Financial Ratios

Thus far, different items on Memorial Hospital's income statement and balance sheet have been explained. Now we can proceed with the computation of different financial ratios that are used to evaluate the financial health of an organization. The four types of financial ratios usually computed are liquidity ratios, capital structure ratios, activity ratios, and profitability ratios.

Liquidity ratios consist of different measures of liquidity (how rapidly a non-cash asset can be converted into cash without losing its value) and the cash position of an organization. Capital structure ratios include measures of leverage (the amount borrowed compared to the amount invested by owners) and equity (investment or ownership). Different types of efficiency measures are included in the activity ratios, and a variety of profitability measures (the extent to which income exceeds expenses) are included in the profitability ratios. Each of these four types of ratios is computed and described below. The first example is for 2000, and the second example is for 1999.

Liquidity Ratios

Current Ratio

$$\frac{\text{current assets}}{\text{current liabilities}} = \text{current ratio}$$

$$\frac{1,014,901}{776,510} = 1.31 \ (2000)$$

$$\frac{928,407}{633,734} = 1.46 \ (1999)$$

Current ratio is one of the most widely used financial ratios. It represents the firm's ability to pay current financial obligations out of current assets. A higher value of current ratio is better than a lower value. A value of 1.31 in 2000 means that for every dollar of current liability, Memorial Hospital had $1.31 in current assets. The value declined from 1.46 in 1999. This means that Memorial Hospital's liquidity (ability to pay financial claims) deteriorated in 2000. It is possible for a firm with a high current ratio to experience payment problems if its current assets are not available in liquid form (cash or short-term investments) in time to meet the current obligations. A large current ratio may also imply idle cash, too much investment in inventory, or bad collection policies resulting in large accounts receivable. To verify the possibility that a high current ratio may indicate overinvestment in current assets or a high number of days in accounts receivable, the current-asset turnover and inventory ratios should be analyzed. Organizations with low current ratios can reduce the probability of short-term liquidity problems by carrying larger balances of liquid assets.

Quick Ratio

$$\frac{\text{current assets} - \text{inventory}}{\text{current liabilities}} = \text{quick ratio}$$

$$\frac{1,014,901 - 80,632}{776,510} = 1.20 \ (2000)$$

$$\frac{928,407 - 69,786}{633,734} = 1.35 \ (1999)$$

The quick ratio is a more stringent test of liquidity than the current ratio. A higher quick ratio implies a better liquidity position for the organization. However, because it includes accounts receivable, a high value could indicate a bad collection policy, and a low quick ratio is not necessarily indicative of a future liquidity problem. For example, a large accounts payable (due to construction, for example) might result in a lower quick ratio, but the construction accounts payable does not require payment from the current assets. It is paid out of construction-in-progress assets. In the case of Memorial Hospital, the quick ratio declined from 1.35 in 1999 to 1.20 in 2000. This says that Memorial Hospital can pay off its current liabilities from its current assets without liquidating inventory, even though the quick ratio declined between 1999 and 2000.

Acid Test Ratio

$$\frac{\text{cash plus marketable securities}}{\text{current liabilities}} = \text{acid test ratio}$$

$$\frac{105,340 + 79,104}{776,510} = 0.24 \ (2000)$$

$$\frac{140,202 + 106,490}{633,734} = 0.39 \ (1999)$$

The acid test ratio is the most stringent test of liquidity. It measures the firm's ability to pay its current liabilities out of cash and marketable securities only. A high value is a good indication of a favorable liquidity position, although a very high value may imply too much idle cash and inefficient investment-portfolio management. The primary source of funds for paying current liabilities is usually collections from accounts receivable. Firms with large variances in collection of accounts receivable should maintain higher levels of cash and short-term investments, which would result in a higher acid test ratio. Memorial Hospital's acid test ratio declined from 0.39 in 1999 to 0.24 in 2000. This means that in 2000 Memorial Hospital could pay off $0.24 of every dollar of its current liabilities from its cash and marketable securities. An increase in the quick ratio and a decrease in the acid test ratio indicate an increase in the days in accounts receivable ratio.

Days in Accounts Receivable (A/R) Ratio

$$\frac{\text{net accounts receivable}}{\text{net revenue}} \times 365 = \text{days in A/R ratio}$$

$$\frac{616,210}{4,087,994} \times 365 = 55.02 \ (2000)$$

$$\frac{507,141}{3,435,397} \times 365 = 53.88 \ (1999)$$

This ratio represents the average collection period. The value for this ratio provides a measure of the average time that receivables are outstanding. A value of 55 in 2000 implies that a patient discharged from Memorial Hospital pays the bill on the fifty-fifth day from the date of his or her discharge. High values imply a longer collection period and thus a greater sum in accounts receivable. An increase in the number of days in the collection period may result in a shortage of cash. The short-term solution would be to borrow or to liquidate a part of the investment portfolio. A continuing increase in the collection period would require an increase in operating margin or equity financing. To reduce the A/R collection period, the health care organization might improve management of the business office and improve third-party payor relationships.

Average Payment Period Ratio

$$\frac{\text{current liabilities}}{\text{operating expenses} - \text{depreciation}} \times 365 = \text{average payment period ratio}$$

$$\frac{776,510}{3,401,884 - 209,469} \times 365 = 88.78 \ (2000)$$

$$\frac{633,734}{2,786,230 - 195,651} \times 365 = 89.29 \ (1999)$$

The average payment period ratio is the counterpart to the days in accounts receivable ratio. The average payment period provides a measure of the average time that elapses before current liabilities are paid. A high value for this ratio indicates a liquidity problem. Low values for this ratio may not always imply a good liquidity position; they might simply be due to a change in policy. For example, changing payroll from biweekly payments to weekly payments will decrease the value for this ratio. A very low value for this ratio might also indicate poor cash management, including poor investment-portfolio management. In both 1999 and 2000, Memorial Hospital took about eighty-nine days to pay off its current liabilities.

Days' Cash-on-Hand Ratio

$$\frac{\text{cash} + \text{marketable securities}}{\text{operating expenses} - \text{depreciation}} \times 365 = \text{days' cash on-hand ratio}$$

$$\frac{105,340 + 79,104}{3,401,884 - 209,469} \times 365 = 21.09 \ (2000)$$

$$\frac{140,202 + 106,490}{2,786,230 - 195,651} \times 365 = 34.76 \ (1999)$$

The days' cash-on-hand ratio measures the number of days of average cash expenses that a firm maintains in cash and marketable securities. A high value for this ratio implies a greater ability to meet short-term financial obligations. High values for the days' cash-on-hand ratio, however, are not always in the best interest of the organization. They may imply over investment in liquid assets that have a very low rate of return.

An increase in the days in accounts receivable ratio may be associated with a reduction in the days' cash-on-hand ratio. If the increase in the days in accounts receivable ratio is permanent, some alternative financing may be necessary. In 2000, Memorial Hospital had twenty-one days of operating expenses in cash and marketable securities.

Capital Structure Ratios

Equity Ratio

$$\frac{\text{fund balance or stockholders' equity}}{\text{total assets}} = \text{equity ratio}$$

$$\frac{1,326,976}{3,696,574} = 0.36 \ (2000)$$

$$\frac{1,154,617}{3,421,962} = 0.34 \ (1999)$$

The equity ratio measures the proportion of total assets that have been financed with equity. High values for this ratio imply that a greater amount of equity relative to debt has been used to finance the total assets. Creditors usually consider this a sign of good financial health because it means less debt and therefore less likelihood of insolvency. A high equity ratio does not always imply solvency. Poor profitability may result in a cash-flow problem that weakens the liquidity position. Equity financing of 100 percent is not desirable because it increases the cost of capital. In practice, some mix of debt and equity is used to finance an organization's total assets. In 2000, Memorial Hospital invested $0.36 of its own funds in every dollar of total assets. The remaining $0.64 came from borrowed funds.

Long-Term Debt-to-Equity Ratio

$$\frac{\text{long-term debt}}{\text{fund balance or stockholders' equity}} = \text{long-term debt-to-equity ratio}$$

$$\frac{1,140,366}{1,326,976} = 0.86 \ (2000)$$

$$\frac{1,210,618}{1,154,617} = 1.05 \ (1999)$$

Long-term debt and equity are permanent capital because they are not repaid within one year. A higher ratio implies a greater amount of external capital in the form of debt relative to equity. This is viewed unfavorably by creditors, although a high long-term debt-to-equity ratio may not prohibit future debt financing (nor does a low ratio guarantee a favorable credit line). The ability to repay debt, rather than the amount of debt, is the important issue. A high long-term debt-to-equity ratio can be risky for an organization if it has high and stable values for debt service coverage (loan payments) and low times-interest-earned ratios. In 2000, Memorial Hospital had $0.86 in long-term debt for every dollar of its own funds. The value had declined somewhat in 2000 from $1.05 in 1999. This is an indication of a more favorable financial condition for Memorial Hospital in 2000.

Fixed-Asset Financing Ratio

$$\frac{\text{long-term debt}}{\text{net fixed asset}} = \text{fixed-asset financing ratio}$$

$$\frac{1{,}140{,}366}{2{,}051{,}486} = 0.56 \ (2000)$$

$$\frac{1{,}210{,}618}{1{,}987{,}759} = 0.61 \ (1999)$$

The fixed-asset financing ratio measures the extent of long-term debt invested in fixed assets. A high value is considered by creditors to be an indicator of future debt repayment problems. The numerator of the ratio represents a future demand for cash, and the denominator is the source to generate that cash in the form of depreciation charges. In 2000, 56 percent of Memorial Hospital's net fixed assets were funded by long-term debt.

High values for the fixed-asset financing ratio are associated with low equity financing and high long-term debt-to-equity ratios. The risk of insolvency resulting from a high value of the fixed-asset ratio can be partially offset by achieving high values for the times-interest-earned ratio and the high debt service coverage ratio.

Times-Interest-Earned Ratio

$$\frac{\text{excess of revenues over expenses} + \text{interest expense}}{\text{interest expense}} = \text{times-interest-earned ratio}$$

$$\frac{686{,}110 + 138{,}477}{138{,}477} = 5.95 \ (2000)$$

$$\frac{649{,}167 + 145{,}938}{145{,}938} = 5.45 \ (1999)$$

(Note: The excess of revenues over expenses is computed from the first two lines of Exhibit 4.1.)

The times-interest-earned ratio measures the ability of a firm to pay its interest expense obligation. The higher the value, the better the financial ability of the firm to pay its interest obligation. Note that this ratio does not measure the ability of the firm to repay the principal; therefore, it is important to consider both the times-interest-earned and debt service coverage ratios when evaluating a firm's ability to pay its total debt obligation (interest expense plus principal payment).

Debt Service Coverage Ratio

$$\frac{\text{excess of revenues over expenses} + \text{depreciation} + \text{interest}}{\text{principal payment} + \text{interest expense}} = \text{debt service coverage ratio}$$

$$\frac{686,110 + 209,469 + 138,477}{63,980 + 138,477} = 5.11 \ (2000)$$

$$\frac{649,167 + 195,651 + 145,938}{256,387 + 145,938} = 2.46 \ (1999)$$

(Note: Principal payments for 2000 and 1999, respectively, are $63,980 and $256,387. These are not shown in the financial statements provided here but are shown in the detailed cash-flow statements of Memorial Hospital's 2000 Annual Report.)

The debt service coverage ratio measures the firm's ability to pay its total debt obligation (both interest and principal). High values are considered favorably by creditors; however, this interpretation could be misleading in some cases, especially in the early years of a capital-expansion program when debt principal is not yet due but the depreciation expense has started. In this situation, the times-interest-earned and the fixed-asset financing ratios are better measures of the debt repayment ability of a firm.

It is important to maintain a high debt service coverage when new debt financing is being considered. The ability to attract debt capital with favorable terms may be related to past debt service coverage ratios.

Activity Ratios

Asset Turnover Ratio

$$\frac{\text{total revenue}}{\text{total assets}} = \text{asset turnover ratio}$$

$$\frac{4,087,994}{3,696,574} = 1.11 \ (2000)$$

$$\frac{3,435,397}{3,421,962} = 1.00 \ (1999)$$

The asset turnover ratio measures the dollar amount of revenue generated per dollar of investment. This is a measure of efficiency. Higher values for this ratio imply better usage of the available resources. In 2000, Memorial Hospital generated $1.11 in revenue for every dollar invested in assets. This ratio should not be the only criterion of efficiency because the age of the plant affects this ratio rather significantly. As the plant gets older, the book value of the asset, net of depreciation, gets smaller, resulting in a higher asset turnover ratio. The point is that the age of the plant needs to be considered when analyzing asset turnover ratios.

Fixed-Asset Turnover Ratio

$$\frac{\text{total revenue}}{\text{net fixed assets}} = \text{fixed-asset turnover ratio}$$

$$\frac{4{,}087{,}994}{2{,}051{,}486} = 1.99 \ (2000)$$

$$\frac{3{,}435{,}397}{1{,}987{,}759} = 1.73 \ (1999)$$

This ratio computes dollars of revenue generated for each dollar of investment in fixed assets. The items included in fixed assets are land, buildings, equipment, and furniture. The ratio represents those assets not intended for sale that are used over and over again to provide the services of the health care organization. High values for the fixed-asset turnover ratio are usually regarded as a positive indication of operating efficiency.

The fixed-asset turnover ratio is also likely to be affected by the age of the plant, as in the case of the asset-turnover ratio. The fixed-asset turnover ratio decreases immediately after an expansion or replacement program.

Current-Asset Turnover Ratio

$$\frac{\text{total revenue}}{\text{current assets}} = \text{current-asset turnover ratio}$$

$$\frac{4{,}087{,}994}{1{,}014{,}901} = 4.03 \ (2000)$$

$$\frac{3{,}435{,}397}{928{,}407} = 3.70 \ (1999)$$

The current-asset turnover ratio measures the dollars of revenue generated per dollar of investment in current assets. The lower the investment in current assets and the higher the current-asset turnover ratio, the more efficient the organization. This does not imply that the investment in current assets should be cut to a minimum; that would cause delivery of services to be impaired, which would create severe short-term operating problems.

A high value for the current-asset turnover ratio is better than a low value, but a lower value might be the result of an expansion program during which the organization holds more liquid assets. A low or high value for the current-asset turnover ratio can be further investigated and diagnosed by analyzing the days' cash-on-hand ratio, the days in accounts receivable ratio, and the inventory turnover ratio.

Inventory Turnover Ratio

$$\frac{\text{total revenue}}{\text{inventory}} = \text{inventory turnover ratio}$$

$$\frac{4,087,994}{80,632} = 50.70 \ (2000)$$

$$\frac{3,435,397}{69,786} = 49.23 \ (1999)$$

An inventory turnover ratio measures the dollars of revenue generated per dollar of investment in inventory. A higher value for this ratio indicates operating efficiency because the organization is not tying up a lot of money in inventory. However, possible impacts on customer service, such as being out of stock, are not considered.

An organization using just-in-time (JIT) inventory management would have a high inventory turnover ratio. Other reasons for low investments in inventory (resulting in a high inventory turnover ratio) include geographic location, access to suppliers, unavailability of quantity discounts, and so on.

Profitability Ratios

Deductible Ratio

$$\frac{\text{gross revenue} - \text{net revenue}}{\text{gross revenue}} = \text{deductible ratio}$$

(Note: Memorial Hospital does not report gross revenue.)

The deductible ratio measures the proportion of gross revenue that is not expected to be realized because of contractual allowances, bad debts, charity care, volume discounts, and so on. In the hospital industry, this ratio is very important because of the widespread presence of contractual allowances for insurors, health maintenance organizations, preferred provider organizations, and charity care to indigent patients. From a profitability point of view, increasing values of the deductible ratio result in lower profitability. A high deductible ratio may not imply poor profitability if the organization has a high markup or a large amount of non-operating revenue (for example, philanthropic donations). The deductible ratio should be monitored closely against changes in the collection process, reimbursement management, or the organization's charity care policy.

Markup Ratio

$$\frac{\text{gross revenue}}{\text{operating expenses}} = \text{markup ratio}$$

(Note: Memorial Hospital does not report gross revenue.)

The markup ratio measures the multiples by which prices are set above expenses. Higher numbers for this ratio imply a higher price per dollar of expenses and the likelihood of achieving greater profitability. If a high markup ratio is associated with a high deductible ratio, then the organization may not be any better off. Organizations with relatively old plants and a high debt-to-principal payment schedule may need to maintain relatively high markup ratios. However, if markups are too high, the organization may lose clients and eventually become insolvent. If it is too low, then the organization may become insolvent. The markup ratio is directly related to the operating margin ratio, the return on total asset ratio, the return on equity ratio, the debt service coverage ratio, and the times-interest-earned ratio. An increase in prices may improve profitability, but depending on the third-party payor mix, it may also increase the deductible ratio, driving profitability downward.

Operating Margin Ratio

$$\frac{\text{net income}}{\text{total revenue}} = \text{operating margin ratio}$$

$$\frac{255,987}{4,087,994} = 0.06 \ (2000)$$

$$\frac{227,121}{3,435,397} = 0.07 \ (1999)$$

This ratio is a measure of profitability. Net income is before any extraordinary items. Alternative measures of profitability include return on total assets or return on equity. A low operating margin is not necessarily an indication of poor profitability if the organization has significant non-operating revenue from investment income, philanthropic donations, or any other sources. Improvement in the operating margin usually results in higher working capital, which in turn improves liquidity ratios.

Operating Margin Price-Level Adjusted Ratio

$$\frac{\text{net income} + \text{depreciation} - \text{price-level depreciation}}{\text{total revenue}} = \text{operating margin price-level adjusted ratio}$$

$$\frac{255,987 + 209,469 - 242,984}{4,087,994} = 0.05 \ (2000)$$

$$\frac{227,121 + 195,651 - 219,129}{3,435,397} = 0.06 \ (1999)$$

(Note: The age of the plant in 2000, as computed earlier, is six years. This indicates that investments in plant assets were made in 1994. Price-level depreciation is defined as the amount of annual depreciation expressed in the year of the investment. In this case, because the investments were made in 1994, the annual depreciation for 1999 and 2000 should be expressed in 1994 dollars. Assume the purchasing power of the dollar declined to 0.88 and 0.84 in 1999 and 2000, respectively, using 1994 as the reference year. Thus, a dollar in 1994 is worth only $0.88 in 1999 and $0.84 in 2000 because of inflation. The Consumer Price Index [CPI] for 1999 and 2000 was 1.12 and 1.16, respectively, using 1994 as the reference [base] year. The price-level depreciation for 1999 and 2000 is computed as the product of annual depreciation expenses and the CPI of each year.)

This ratio is the same as the operating margin ratio except the depreciation expenses are adjusted for inflation. When equipment is purchased, a depreciation schedule is developed that identifies the future deductions from the operating revenue for the depreciation expense. The dollar values posted are based on the year the equipment was acquired. Because of inflation, those posted dollar values may be worth less than the original estimate. Therefore, the operating margin should be computed to reflect the inflation-adjusted depreciation, not the originally estimated depreciation.

Higher inflation translates into higher inflation-adjusted depreciation, and hence the lower the operating margin in the price-level adjusted ratio. In 2000, Memorial Hospital's operating margin ratio was 6 percent, but after the depreciation expense was adjusted for inflation, the operating margin dropped to 5 percent.

Return on Total Assets (ROA)

$$\frac{\text{net income}}{\text{total assets}} = \text{return on total assets}$$

$$\frac{255,987}{3,696,574} = 0.07 \ (2000)$$

$$\frac{227,121}{3,421,962} = 0.07 \ (1999)$$

The return on total assets measures the amount of net income earned per dollar of investment in total assets. It is a measure of profitability. This ratio is affected by the age of the plant. An organization with a relatively old and largely depreciated plant may show a higher return on assets ratio. If the organization is planning a major replacement, this high profit rate may be misleading for creditors.

Return on Equity (ROE)

$$\frac{\text{net income}}{\text{fund balance or shareholders' equity}} = \text{return on equity}$$

$$\frac{255{,}987}{1{,}326{,}976} = 0.19 \ (2000)$$

$$\frac{227{,}121}{1{,}154{,}617} = 0.20 \ (1999)$$

This ratio, similar to the return on assets ratio, measures the extent of profitability but uses return on equity investment instead of total assets. Many analysts consider the return on equity as the primary test of profitability. Unless a satisfactory return on equity is generated, the organization may find it very difficult to raise future equity capital by selling new shares.

A high return on equity may not imply sound financial health because the organization might have huge debt and earned the profit on monthly debt-financed (leased) assets. Further analysis of the return on equity ratio compared to the return on assets ratio would indicate the effect of debt-financed assets. If replacement needs are expected to be financed from operating income, the return on total assets ratio may be a better indicator of profitability than the return on equity ratio.

Other Financial Information

Age of the Facility

$$\frac{\text{accumulated depreciation}}{\text{depreciation expense}} = \text{age of the facility}$$

$$\frac{1{,}154{,}868}{209{,}469} = 5.51 \ (2000)$$

$$\frac{987{,}790}{195{,}651} = 5.05 \ (1999)$$

This is a very crude formula to estimate the age of the plant in years. This measure is more reliable if straight-line rather than accelerated depreciation is used. With the accelerated depreciation method, this formula tends to underestimate the age of newer plants and overestimate the age of older plants. When inflation is occurring, the formula underestimates the age of the plant because the annual depreciation expense increases with inflation.

Working Capital

$$\begin{aligned}
\text{current assets} + \text{current liabilities} &= \text{working capital} \\
\$1,014,901 + 776,510 &= \$1,791,411 \ (2000) \\
\$ \ \ 928,407 + 633,734 &= \$1,562,141 \ (1999)
\end{aligned}$$

The amount of working capital, defined as current assets plus current liabilities, is very important for an organization in its day-to-day operations. An organization's liquidity depends on the amount of working capital.

Net Working Capital

$$\begin{aligned}
\text{current assets} - \text{current liabilities} &= \text{net working capital} \\
\$1,014,901 - 776,510 &= \$238,391 \ (2000) \\
\$ \ \ 928,407 - 633,734 &= \$294,673 \ (1999)
\end{aligned}$$

Many analysts want to find out the net liquidity position (net working capital) of an organization. Net liquidity is computed by subtracting current liabilities from current assets. If the organization were to pay its current obligations (current liabilities), how much working capital would be left? The answer is the net working capital.

Limitations of Ratio Analysis

The financial ratios we have discussed provide valuable information concerning the financial health of an organization. We computed different ratios for Memorial Hospital for two consecutive years, and these indicate changes in financial performance by the organization. In addition, every ratio can be compared with national or regional averages that are available annually from the Financial Analysis Service (FAS) of the Healthcare Financial Management Association (HFMA). These national or regional averages are called the standards of the industry. Public health does not have a widely accepted set of standard financial ratios; hence, no national or regional comparative standards for the financial performance of a public health agency exist.

An individual hospital's ratios are compared with these standards, and financial performance is evaluated. If a hospital is older or newer than the rest of the hospitals in the region, then comparing its financial ratios with the regional averages is not quite as meaningful. Financial ratios reflect the activities of the organization in the past year or years; however, financial ratios do not reflect strategic planning by the organization. It is possible that a hospital is going through a structural change to achieve future benefits, which would affect many of the ratios. Thus, the long-term planning of the hospital must be considered as well as the financial ratios. Using financial ratios alone may give the wrong signal to analysts.

The presence of severe inflation in the early or later years of a trend analysis makes the analysis less reliable. In addition, values for the financial ratios depend on the accounting practices and policies of the organization. For example, the value of investment in inventory depends on the valuation policies of the organization (first in, first out or last in, first out) and the depreciation policies (straight-line or accelerated), which in turn determine the value of net assets, and so on. To the extent that these policies vary, financial ratios will vary as well.

Cost of Capital

When organizations borrow money, they have to pay interest on the debt. If an organization chooses to use its own funds for the acquisition or replacement of an asset, an opportunity cost is associated with that decision, called the *cost of equity*. In many cases, some combination of debt and equity is used to finance a capital investment. The weighted average cost of capital (WACC) is derived as an average cost of debt (k_d) and cost of equity (k_e). (A numerical example follows later in the section.)

$$\text{WACC} = Dk_d + (1 - D)k_e$$
where D is the ratio of debt to assets

Some insurors reimburse hospitals on a cost basis so that a portion of the cost of debt (k_d) is considered a pass-through. Assuming M is the proportion of cost-based reimbursement, the cost of debt is $(1 - M)k_d$. Some insurors pay on a cost-plus basis to for-profit hospitals, where the payment above the cost represents some agreed to (or at least known) return on equity. For-profit hospitals pay taxes on income at the current tax rate (t_c). Interest payments by for-profit hospitals work as a tax shield because tax liability decreases with an increase in interest payments. However, for-profit organizations have to pay taxes on any return they earn on their equity investment. Assuming k_e^m as the return on equity and m' as the proportion from the payor that uses the cost-plus basis, then the WACC for not-for-profit (np) and for-profit (fp) institutions can be written as

$$\text{WACC}_{np} = D(1 - M)k_d + (1 - D)k_e$$
$$\text{WACC}_{fp} = D(1 - M)(1 - t_c)k_d + (1 - D)(k_e - m'[1 - t_c]k_e^m).$$

Cost of Debt

To compute the cost of debt (k_d), data must be collected on the types and amount of debt and the corresponding interest rates for different hospitals over several years. For each year, a weighted average cost of debt can be computed using the individual debt information. Assume that the cost of debt (k_d) for not-for-profit and for-profit hospitals in 2000 is 5.4 percent and 7.5 percent, respectively. Further assume that the proportion of payors who pay cost-based reimbursement (M) are 10 percent and 8 percent for not-for-profit and for-profit hospitals, respectively. The effective corporate tax rate (t_c) for the for-profit hospitals in 2000 is assumed to be 22 percent.

The cost of debt for the not-for-profit and for-profit hospitals can then be computed as

$$
\begin{aligned}
\text{Not-for-profit cost of debt} &= (1 - M)k_d \\
&= (1 - 0.10)5.4 \\
&= 4.86 \text{ percent} \\
\text{For-profit cost of debt} &= (1 - M)(1 - t_c)k_d \\
&= (1 - 0.08)(1 - 0.22)7.5 \\
&= 5.38 \text{ percent}
\end{aligned}
$$

The cost of debt is usually available from the for-profit hospital's annual reports. The cost of debt for not-for-profit hospitals is usually lower than that of for-profit hospitals. The reason is that the not-for-profit hospitals use tax-exempt revenue bonds to borrow money from the capital market.

Medicare Reimbursement Under the Prospective Payment System

On October 1, 1983, Medicare started reimbursing hospitals for inpatient non-physician services under a DRG-based prospective payment system (PPS). Several types of hospitals were exempt from DRGs (diagnosis related groups), including psychiatric, rehabilitation, children's, and long-term-care hospitals. About 500 DRGs have been identified from the International Classification of Diseases, 9th Revision, Clinical Modification (ICD-9-CM). Total payments made to a hospital under Medicare include two components: prospective payment and reasonable cost payment. Prospective payment is further divided into operating payment and capital payment. (Effective October 1, 1992, Medicare began using prospective payments for capital payments. Prior to this date, capital payments were paid on a reasonable cost basis.) Reasonable cost payment includes direct medical education costs, kidney acquisition costs, and some outpatient services.

Each of the DRGs has been assigned a weight to indicate the relative resource requirement to provide the service. For example, DRG 103 (heart transplant) has a weight of 14.0323 and DRG 320 (kidney and urinary tract infection) has a weight of 1.0002. This means that DRG 103 is about fourteen times as expensive as DRG 320. When the Health Care Financing Administration (HCFA) announced a nationwide payment for the labor and nonlabor component of the operating payment, every hospital in the country was preassigned a wage index for the labor component. Reimbursement for a particular DRG is computed as follows:

Reimbursement = DRG weight × [(labor amount × wage index) + (nonlabor amount)]

The reimbursement may be further increased by an additional payment to cover the costs of indirect medical education, disproportionate share, and outlier payments. Teaching hospitals incur additional costs because of extra laboratory and other teaching demonstrations. The allowance for indirect medical education covers these additional costs. Hospitals that treat a large percentage of Medicaid patients receive an additional payment under PPS. This additional payment is referred to as a disproportionate share payment. The outlier payments are additional payments for patients who use an unusually large amount of resources, indicated by high cost of care.

The capital component of the prospective payment that began on October 1, 1992, had a ten-year phase-in period, blending federal and hospital components of payments. The hospital component of the capital costs includes interest, depreciation, and lease costs. In addition, taxes and insurance are considered capital costs if they are related to capital assets. There is a federal payment for capital costs that is similar to the national rates for labor and nonlabor costs discussed earlier.

Physician Reimbursement Under the Resource-Based Relative Value Scale

Beginning in January, 1992, Medicare started paying physicians using a resource-based relative value scale (RBRVS). Physician services are categorized into approximately 7,000 different codes using the current procedural terminology (CPT). Resource-based relative value (RBRV) has three components: (1) a work unit that represents physician time, level of stress, and skill; (2) a unit of practice expense representing the costs of support personnel and office expense; and (3) a unit of cost that represents the cost of malpractice insurance.

The level of RBRV for a particular CPT code is obtained by adding the products of each of the three components and multiplying the RBRV by a conversion factor, determined by the Health Care Financing Administration each year. The products of the three factors are generated by multiplying the work unit, practice cost expense, and malpractice insurance cost by the regional cost index for each. The regional cost index is based on the difference in costs geographically as well as the inflation rate.

In Exhibit 4.4, Medicare's RBRV reimbursement for an office visit is computed. The physician's level of work depends on the predetermined CPT codes. The example is for a CPT designated "midlevel" office visit (other options would include minimum-level and extensive office visits) for a San Francisco physician in 2000. The $103.11 reimbursement is significantly less than what the physician charged self-pay or insured patients. For this reason, many physicians limit the number of Medicare

Exhibit 4.4. Physician Reimbursement for an Office Visit

1. Relative Value

Physician's work (based on CPT code)	1.71	
× Cost index	× 1.068	
Adjusted value		1.826
Practice expense (based on CPT code)	0.78	
× Cost index	× 1.330	
Adjusted value		1.037
Malpractice insurance (based on CPT code)	0.08	
× Cost index	× 0.596	
Adjusted value		0.048
Total value		2.911

2. Conversion factor (determined by HCFA each year) — × 35.42

3. Medicare's office visit reimbursement — $103.11

patients they accept; too many patients paying below practice costs means they close the practice.

Capitation

The health care industry has experienced a tremendous increase in managed care insurance plans in recent years. These types of plans are expected to have even higher *rates of penetration* (defined as the percentage of population covered by managed care plans) in the future. Managed care plans consisting of health maintenance organizations (HMOs) and preferred provider organizations (PPOs) negotiate with health care providers to arrive at a predetermined price schedule. Many of the negotiations conclude with contracts between the plans and health care providers for a fixed monthly payment per insured individual. Because the providers receive only a fixed amount of revenue from the managed care plans for a given number of insured individuals (known as enrolled members), financial risk of a shortfall in revenues over expenses is shifted from the insuror to the provider. The providers receive their revenue in the form of capitation—a set sum of money received based on membership rather than services delivered, usually expressed in amounts per member per month (PMPM). Under capitation, profit accrues by controlling costs as well as utilization of services. Because revenue is fixed, profit is maximized by either cutting unit cost or controlling utilization of services, or some combination of both. This section discusses several methods of determining the capitation amount in the form of a monthly payment for each enrollee (PMPM). In negotiating the capitation rate, providers typically use the fee-for-service (FFS) rate as the basis of calculation. Specifically:

$$PMPM = \frac{\text{forecasted annual utilization rate} \times \text{FFS rate}}{12 \text{ months}}$$

Suppose an HMO is negotiating the capitation rate with a hospital for the inpatient care of its members. Past utilization of hospital inpatient services by the enrollees of the HMO show that for every 1,000 enrollees, 350 inpatient days were used in a year and the average charge was $1,050. Thus, the corresponding PMPM rate is

$$PMPM = \frac{(350 \text{ inpatient days/1,000 members}) \times \$1,050}{12 \text{ months}} = \$30.63$$

Similarly, the capitation rate can be determined for any specific service (i.e., outpatient, dental, surgical, drug, and others). As an example, assume an HMO randomly selected 1,000 of its members to monitor their utilization of inpatient hospital care for medical and surgical services separately, and it found forty admissions for medical services and twenty admissions for surgical services during a one-year period. Assume the length of stay for medical service equals 3.5 days at an average daily cost of $1,050, and the length of stay for surgical service equals 4.8 days at an average daily cost of $1,800. Now, the capitation rates for medical and surgical services can be computed as follows:

$$\text{Medical: } \frac{(40 \times 3.5/1,000) \times \$1,050}{12} = \$12.25 \text{ PMPM}$$

$$\text{Surgical: } \frac{(20 \times 4.8/1,000) \times \$1,800}{12} = \$14.40 \text{ PMPM}$$

Hence, the capitation rate for the total hospital inpatient care equals $12.25 + $14.40 or $26.65 PMPM.

Let us now compute the capitation rate for a primary care physician (PCP). Assume the physician's fee for an office visit is $50. A random sample of 1,000 members of an HMO show a total of 3,500 visits to physicians during a one-year period. That is, on the average, each member has 3.5 visits in a year. Thus, the capitation rate for PCP is:

$$\frac{3.5 \times \$50}{12} = \$14.58 \text{ PMPM}$$

Obviously, the utilization rates for specialists' services is a much smaller number; therefore, the PMPM for such physicians is normally lower than their PCP counterparts. If the fee of a neurosurgeon is $900 per service and the annual average use of such service is 5 per 1,000 members, then the PMPM for such a specialist is:

$$\frac{5/1,000 \times \$900}{12} = \$0.38 \text{ PMPM}$$

The PMPM rate can be computed for each service and an aggregate PMPM calculated by adding all the services for a comprehensive capitation rate, unless the parties concerned agree on some carve-outs (i.e., to leave some services outside the capitated payments).

The aggregate capitated amount is then adjusted for the cost of reinsurance, cost of administration, and margin. The final amount is risk adjusted for age, gender, and family status.

Medicare is now experimenting with capitated payment by contracting with federally approved HMOs in many states for the health care services of a defined population of Medicare enrollees in a market. Under the contract, HMOs receive a fixed amount of payment from the Health Care Financing Administration for each Medicare enrollee in each month. The HMO is responsible for all the Medicare-approved health care services for the enrolled members. The Medicare PMPM is based on the adjusted average per capita cost (AAPCC) of the Medicare patients in the county of the HMO location. The actual expenses of this population (as paid by HCFA in the previous time period on the DRG-based system) are adjusted for age, gender, welfare status, and geographic location of the enrollees to compute the AAPCC.

Medicare's Reimbursements for Outpatient Services

On June 1, 2000, Medicare began reimbursing outpatient care by hospitals using its ambulatory payment classification (APC) system. The classification of services is based on current procedures terminology (CPT) codes and the HCFA common procedure coding system (HCPCS). The payments are determined on a prospective basis by HCFA. An APC payment is supposed to cover the cost of equipment, supplies, and drugs, in addition to the cost of professional time measured in relative value units (RVU). This system of reimbursement replaced the traditional cost-based and fee-for-service system for outpatient services.

Medicare's Reimbursements for Skilled Nursing Facilities

Under the Balanced Budget Act (BBA) of 1997, Medicare began reimbursing skilled nursing facilities (SNFs) based on resource utilization groups (RUGs). SNF patients are classified into one of forty-four resource utilization groups to reflect the level of resources required to treat patients. The RUG system determines a per diem rate for each patient for reimbursement by Medicare.

Conclusion

This chapter provides an introduction to thinking financially in the context of health care organizations. Financial analysis is not widely used in the management and leadership of public health programs, often placing public health agencies at a competitive disadvantage. Used creatively and adapted to the public health context, the methods presented in this chapter not only make public health leaders more effective competitors for the limited financial resources that fund public sector programs but also improve the overall financial performance of the public health sector. Some of the cases in this book present financial issues whose analysis will benefit from use of these methods. Public health leaders need to practice making the critical leadership judgments that guide the allocation of financial resources to protect and improve the public's health.

Bibliography

Asper, Elaine, and Mahmud Hassan, "The Impact of PPS Legislation on the Systematic Risk of Hospitals," *Journal of Economics and Finance* 17, no. 3 (Fall 1993), pp. 121–135.

Cleverley, William O., and Paul C. Nutt, "The Decision Process Used for Hospital Bond Rating— And Its Implications," *Health Services Research* 19, no. 5 (December, 1984), pp. 615–637.

Cleverley, William O., and W. H. Rosegay, "Factors Affecting the Cost of Hospital Tax-Exempt Revenue Bonds," *Inquiry* 19 (Winter, 1982), pp. 317–326.

Sloan, Frank A., Joseph Valvona, Mahmud Hassan, and Michael A. Morrisey, "Cost of Capital to the Hospital Sector," *Journal of Health Economics* 7, no. 1 (March, 1988), pp. 25–45.

PART II

Public Health—Context

P art II contains two "Industry Notes" that provide the backdrop or decision context for making health care and public health decisions. The first industry note, "The U.S. Health Care System," traces health care's important historical events, describes the industry's major characteristics, and discusses the key factors for success in the industry. In addition, the note examines central health care organizations and professional participants. The second industry note, "The U.S. Public Health System," explores the colorful history of public health, its legal framework, expenditures, function, and current trends.

The U.S. Health Care System

An understanding of the health services environment is provided as a background for the public health leadership and management cases presented in this book. An Industry Note describes key historical events, major characteristics, and key factors for success in the industry as well as the most significant organizational and professional participants.

History of the Health Services Environment

Over the past fifty years, the history of the health services environment has been characterized by three basic trends:

1. Growth in the scientific knowledge that underpinned professional practice in health care,
2. Growth in the percentage of U.S. financial resources allocated to the provision of health services, and
3. Change in the relationships among health care professionals, health service organizations, payors for health services, and health care clients.

This Industry Note was prepared by Stuart A. Capper, the University of Alabama at Birmingham. It is intended as a basis for classroom discussion rather than to illustrate effective or ineffective handling of an administrative situation. Used with permission from Stuart A. Capper.

These trends did not proceed consistently over time. Rather, growth in scientific knowledge accelerated over time; growth in financial allocations was rapid between 1950 and 1990 but leveled during the 1990s; and changes in organizational relationships were a more recent trend. Each trend significantly affected the health care environment that emerged in the beginning of the twenty-first century.

Growth in Scientific Knowledge

Prior to the 1940s, medical armamentarium and medical research were limited. World War II marked the beginning of a dramatic expansion of both medical knowledge and federal medical research funding.[1] Prior to the War, federal funding of medical research was almost entirely intramural. That is, federal money was used to fund research in federal labs, and few grants were awarded to outside organizations for research projects. Most private not-for-profit research was foundation funded, and the amount was not highly significant. Beginning in the late 1940s, a consistently growing program of federally funded grants for medical research outside federal labs emerged. The national priority given to innovations in medical care generated a steadily increasing scientific base for medical practice and a rapidly diversifying technology for application in patient care. Exhibit IN 1-1 illustrates the growth in federal funding for medical research.

The impact of this extraordinary increase in scientific knowledge on the health care industry was multifaceted. First, the adult life span increased about two years per decade during each decade following the 1950s. This represented a significant change. Prior to the 1950s, life expectancy increased as a result of decreases in infant deaths. After the 1950s, in part because of expanded medical knowledge, life expectancy increased because of years added at the end and middle of life.

Second, the growth in medical specialization was likely related to the increasing amount of medical knowledge that had to be mastered initially as well as the substantial continuing education required to remain current in any given specialty. Also, increasing technological options created economically viable specialty areas where none existed previously.[2] In 1950, there were twenty-eight different specialty and subspecialty residency programs in the United States. As of 2000, the number had grown to 103.[3]

Finally, data from the Health Care Financing Administration (HCFA) suggested that the increase in medical knowledge contributed to the rapid cost escalation in medical care. The most recent HCFA analysis, for fiscal 1997–98 indicated that 39 percent of the 5.2 percent increase in medical care expenditures for that year could be attributed to increased intensity—"changes in the use of kinds of services and supplies"—of medical services.[4]

Growth in Health Care Spending

The second trend delineated was growth in the percentage of U.S. financial resources allocated to the provision of health services compared to the percentage

Exhibit IN 1-1. National Institutes of Health Grants for Medical Research (dollar amounts per year, selected years 1940–1995)

SOURCE: *NIH Almanac 1999,* www.nih.gov/about/almanac/index.html

spent by other developed countries in the world. In 1999, the United States spent about $4,000 per person annually on health care, significantly more than other industrialized nations (Exhibit IN 1-2).

Some analysts suggested that the stabilization of expenditure growth relative to GDP during the 1990s was a result of the third trend, the changing relationships among health services providers and health care organizations, payors, and patients.[5]

Changing Relationships

Prior to World War II, there was little experimentation with organizational design in the health services industry, resulting in a relatively simple and stable market. After World War II, a small number of large new health plan organizations developed, covering substantial groups of enrollees. Examples of this type of organization included Group Health Cooperative of Puget Sound and Kaiser Permanente in California. This type of "prepaid" and "capitated" health plan, rather than the traditional

Exhibit IN 1-2. Per Capita Health Spending in Industrialized Nations, 1997

Australia	$1,909
Austria	1,905
Belgium	2,175
Czech Republic	943
Denmark	2,042
Finland	1,525
France	2,047
Germany	2,364
Greece	1,196
Hungary	642
Iceland	1,981
Ireland	1,293
Italy	1,613
Japan	1,760
Korea	870
Luxembourg	2,303
Mexico	363
Netherlands	1,933
New Zealand	1,357
Norway	2,017
Poland	386
Portugal	1,148
Spain	1,762
Switzerland	2,611
Turkey	259
United Kingdom	1,391
United States	**3,912**

SOURCE: National Center for Health Statistics, *Health, United States, 2000, With Adolescent Health Chartbook* (Hyattsville, MD: National Center for Health Statistics), Table 321, p. 114.

"fee-for-service" system, was strongly opposed by organized medicine, and such plans developed in only a limited number of states.

In capitated systems, providers were prospectively paid a fixed premium per person or per family that covered specified benefits, and the payment was independent of the amount of service provided. Fee-for-service was the more traditional method of payment for health care services; a specific payment was made for a specific service rendered. In 1973, the Health Maintenance Organization (HMO) Act was passed by Congress and signed by President Nixon. This law created a set of subsidies

Exhibit IN 1-3. Health Service Spending as a Percentage of After-Tax Profit, Selected Years 1965–1987

SOURCE: Adapted from D. R. Levit, M. S. Freeland, and D. R. Waldo, "Health Spending and Ability to Pay: Business, Individuals, and Government," *Health Care Financing Review* 10, no. 3 (Spring, 1989), Table 5, p. 9.

and standards that encouraged this capitated or "managed care" form of health care delivery organization to grow. Although encouraged by the legislation, growth in enrollment in managed care plans was slow during this period.

A factor that spawned more growth in the managed care industry was the rapid health care price inflation of the 1980s and early 1990s. Many employers saw employee health care costs become their largest single uncontrolled expenditure. Exhibit IN 1-3 illustrates the concern that developed for private employers.

Between 1965 and 1987, employee health benefit spending rose from about 14 percent of after-tax profits to nearly 100 percent of after-tax profits. This situation caused employers to look for ways to stabilize and possibly reduce the costs of health care benefits. Employers began to experiment with and embrace new organizational relationships with their employees as payors and clients, and with health care organizations, providers, and insurors. A diverse array of organizational arrangements evolved, with most of them generally under the rubric of "managed care." These new organizational forms, with their emphasis on efficiency and cost containment, appeared to be succeeding, at least in the short run. During the 1990s, health care cost inflation, measured as a percentage of GDP, stabilized. Some events late in 2000 suggested that this cost-stabilizing effect of managed care might be temporary. Analysts' projections again suggested that increasing proportions of U.S. financial resources would be devoted to health care over the next decade.

Exhibit IN 1-4. Significant Health Care Events

1940s	Introduction of antibiotics, penicillin, and sulfonamides gave physicians their first effective therapies for treating infectious diseases. These drugs accelerated the shift from infectious diseases to chronic diseases as the chief source of mortality in the United States.
1946	Passage of the Hill-Burton Act for Health Facilities Construction stimulated the first major involvement by the federal government in a national program to allocate resources to health services. Over the next thirty years, the program provided billions of dollars in construction subsidies, primarily to hospitals. Between 1940 and 1987, community hospital beds per capita increased 25 percent, although some areas of the country, such as the East South Central Region, experienced as much as a threefold increase.[a]
1950s	Development of modern anesthesiology, particularly the introduction of synthetic agents for anesthesia, led to significantly reduced risks in surgery, especially for higher risk patients.
1960s	Extension of the adult life span by about two years per decade during each decade subsequent to the 1950s.
1963	Passage of the Health Professionals Education Assistance Act enabled forty-one new medical schools to be opened in the United States (a 48 percent increase).
1964	The Surgeon General's Report on Smoking and Health identified cigarette smoking as one of the primary preventable causes of morbidity and premature death.
1965	Passage of Medicare and Medicaid (The Social Security Amendments of 1965) marked the first large-scale federal initiative to provide health insurance for major segments of the population. The elderly, and to some extent the poor, became beneficiaries of congressionally mandated health insurance programs. Between 1967 and 1997, total expenditures for Medicare enrollees increased from $4.74 billion to $213.58 billion. During the same period, per capita fee-for-service payments for enrollees increased nearly twenty-five-fold, from $217 to $5,314.[b]
1972	Passage of Social Security Amendments created Professional Standards Review Organizations (PSROs), the first direct intervention by the federal government into medical practice, by mandating the creation of "standards of care."[c]
1975	The Supreme Court decision in Goldfarb vs. Virginia Bar (421 U.S. 713) effectively removed the traditional "learned professions" exemption from antitrust laws. Professional practices were no longer immune from price-fixing restrictions, and professional associations could not mandate bans on professional advertising.
1983	Passage of Social Security Amendments that created the prospective payment system (PPS) for hospital services to Medicare beneficiaries. Financial incentives for hospital care providers were significantly changed.
1992	Medicare introduced the resource-based relative value scale (RBRVS) system for determining physician payments. Rather than basing payments on reasonable, customary, and prevailing charges in the community, Medicare based its payments to physicians on RBRVS. In addition to Medicare, RBRVS became the leading methodology used by most managed care companies. The system incorporated three basic relative value units (RVUs) to determine the physician's reimbursement: (1) an RVU for physician work time, (2) an RVU for practice expense, and (3) an RVU for malpractice expense.
2000	Scientists announced they had mapped a first draft of the entire human genome. This achievement created the promise of significant advances in treatment and cure of many genetically based diseases. In addition, it introduced an array of unresolved philosophical and ethical questions for policy makers, health insurors, and health care providers.

a. National Center for Health Statistics, *Health, United States, 1992* (Hyattsville, MD: Government Printing Office, 1993), Table 110, p. 156.

b. National Center for Health Statistics, *Health, United States, 2000, With Adolescent Health Chartbook* (Hyattsville, MD: National Center for Health Statistics, 2000), Table 134, p. 350.

c. George J. Annas, S. A. Law, R. E. Rosenblatt, and K. R. Wing, *American Health Law* (Boston: Little, Brown and Company, 1990), pp. 526–527.

Significant Events Affecting Health Care Trends

During the past fifty years, many significant events contributed to the three trends that were discussed; however, a handful of them were particularly significant (see Exhibit IN 1-4).

Economic Characteristics of the Health Services Sector

The overall size of the nation's economy was gauged by the use of gross domestic product (GDP) statistics. GDP measured the value of all goods and services produced by all sectors of the economy from resources within the United States. The proportion of GDP contributed by the health services sector was rapidly increasing. This occurred during a period when the GDP itself increased sixteen-fold, from $527 billion to $8.5 trillion. Health services were constituting an increasingly significant proportion of a rapidly growing United States economy. The growth in health expenditures per capita was dramatic. Per capita health care expenditures between 1960 and 1998 increased nearly twenty-eight-fold.

The relationship of the health services component of GDP to other components could be illustrated by considering the sector breakdown in 1950 versus the figures for 1998. In 1950, the health services sector was $4.7 billion out of a total GDP of $294.3 billion. Numerous sectors of the economy were larger in dollar terms than health services. For example, agriculture, forestry, and fisheries was four times as large as the health services sector (Exhibit IN 1-5). Among the other sectors that were larger than health services were mining; primary metals manufacturing; machinery manufacturing; food products; transportation; gas, electric, and sanitary services; real estate; and the federal government.

By 1998, the situation had changed significantly. Health services made up $495.5 billion of a $7.66 trillion GDP. Of those sectors mentioned, the only one that remained larger than health services was real estate. Health services became larger, in GDP terms, than the entire federal government. In addition, a sector such as agriculture, forestry, and fisheries, which had been more than four times the size of the health services sector, became only 25 percent of the size of health services. In 1950, the food products sector was more than twice the size of the health services sector; however, by 1998, the food products category was only one-fourth the size of health services. Even real estate, which was nearly five times the size of the health services sector in 1950, was only about twice as large as the health services sector in 1998. The relationship of the health services industry to other sectors of the U.S. economy was significantly altered by the extraordinarily rapid growth in expenditures for health care products and services. Even rapid growth in other sectors of the economy was no match for the explosive growth in health services.

The growth in health expenditures was not consistent over time. Up until 1965, growth in health expenditures was moderate. Following the creation of Medicare and Medicaid in 1965, expenditures began to increase rapidly. This rapid growth continued until the 1990s, when expenditures as a percentage of GDP stabilized. Recent

Exhibit IN 1-5. Selected Sector Breakdown of GDP, 1950 vs. 1998 (in billions of current dollars)

	1950	1998
Total Gross National Product	294.3	7,660.0
Health services	4.7	495.5
Agriculture, forestry, and fisheries	20.7	125.2
Mining	9.4	105.9
Primary metals industries	7.5	54.8
Machinery manufacturing	7.0	153.3
Gas, electric, and sanitary services	5.5	216.6
Food products	10.7	122.0
Transportation	16.7	283.9
Real estate	23.0	967.9
Federal government	18.2	360.9

SOURCE: U.S. Bureau of Economic Analysis, Department of Commerce, Industry Accounts Data, Gross Product by Industry, www.bea.doc.gov/bea/dn2/gpoc.htm

projections suggested that expenditures would again begin to take a larger proportion of the GDP over the early years of the twenty-first century (see Exhibit IN 1-6).

Of the $1,113,700,000,000 spent on health services and supplies in 1998, more than 75 percent of these expenditures were attributable to five provider categories—hospitals, physicians, other professional services, nursing homes, and drugs. Exhibit IN 1-7 presents a percentage distribution breakdown for all major components of U.S. national health expenditures in 1998.

Hospitals

Between 1970 and 1990, the hospital sector accounted for approximately 40 percent of total expenditures for health services and supplies. The percentage of total expenditures attributable to the hospital sector declined during the 1990s. By 1998, the figure stood at 33.3 percent. This expenditure trend was related to a real decline in the use of the inpatient component of the hospital sector. Discharges from nonfederal short-stay hospitals per 1,000 population decreased significantly over the past 20 years. In 1985, there were 137.7 discharges per 1,000 population from nonfederal short-stay hospitals. By 1998, this number decreased to 103.0 discharges per 1,000. During the same period, the actual hospital days of care provided per 1,000 population declined from 872.1 to 508.1.[6]

Exhibit IN 1-6. National Health Expenditures, Selected Years 1970–2005 (percentage of GDP)

SOURCE: U.S. Health Care Financing Administration, www.hcfa.gov/stats/NHE-Proj/proj1998/tables/table1.htm

As inpatient utilization of hospitals declined, outpatient utilization increased. Between 1985 and 1998, the number of visits to nonfederal hospital outpatient departments more than doubled. Total outpatient visits in hospitals increased from 230 million in 1985 to more than 482 million in 1998.[7]

Physicians

In terms of national expenditures for health services, physicians made up the largest single professional service component of the health services sector. Payments to physicians accounted for 20 percent of total health services expenditures in 1998. Physicians were the only professionals in the health services sector who were broadly licensed to perform any medical procedure. Thus, they had significant influence over the allocation of most health care resources.

Physicians generally were considered to be either doctors of medicine or doctors of osteopathy; however, osteopaths represented only about 5 percent of all active physicians in the United States. The number of physicians in patient care practice in 1998 was approximately 667,000, or 22.5 doctors per 10,000 population.[8]

Expenditures for physicians' services grew at an average annual rate of 12.3 percent from 1965 through 1985; however, the decade of the 1990s experienced much

Exhibit IN 1-7. National Health Expenditures, 1998 (percentage distribution, selected categories)

SOURCE: National Center for Health Statistics, *Health, United States, 2000, With Adolescent Health Chartbook* (Hyattsville, MD: National Center for Health Statistics, 2000), Table 118, p. 326.

slower growth of expenditures for physician services. From 1990 through 1998, the average expenditure growth for physician services was 5 percent.[9] As a result of the overall slowdown in the growth of the health services sector during this period, physicians maintained approximately a 20 percent share of the total expenditures for health services and supplies.

Other Professional Services

In general, the "other professionals" category included chiropractors, optometrists, podiatrists, and licensed medical practitioners other than physicians and dentists.[10] In addition, this category included allied health services, such as kidney dialysis centers and specialty outpatient facilities for mental health and substance abuse, as well as ambulance services. Although the proportion of health care expenditures attributable to dental services declined (7.3 percent in 1960 to 4.7 percent in 1998), the proportion attributable to services from other types of health care professionals steadily increased. In 1960, the proportion of the health care dollar spent on other professional services was only 2.3 percent. By 1998, this proportion had increased to about 5.8 percent.

One reason for this trend was the rise of independent practices by nurse practitioners. Nurse practitioners in full-time independent practice in the United States numbered more than 50,000. The majority of these individuals were family nurse practitioners, adult nurse practitioners, and pediatric nurse practitioners. Forty-six states required nurse practitioners to be certified. Data from the American Nurses Credentialing Center (ANCC) suggested that the number of nurses entering private practice each year was increasing.

In 1995, more than 3,000 family nurse practitioners were certified. By 1997, this figure had risen to more than 4,500. The growth trend in independent nurse practices was likely to continue. In 1998, less than 15 percent of all nurse practitioners had decided to operate independent practices.[11]

Nursing Homes

Nursing home services accounted for 7.6 percent of national health care expenditures in 1998. This was a significant increase over 1960, when nursing home care used 3.2 percent of the health care dollar. In the decades of the 1960s and 1970s there were large increases in average annual expenditures for these services. During that twenty-year period, the average annual percentage increase in nursing home expenditures exceeded 15 percent. The rate of annual increase began decreasing during the 1980s to the 10 to 11 percent range and subsided further during the 1990s to less than 8 percent per year and as low as 5.3 percent in 1998.[12]

Between 1976 and 1998, the number of nursing homes increased from 14,133 to 17,259. In the same period, the inventory of nursing home beds grew from 1.292 million to 1.812 million; however, the availability of beds decreased, as measured by the ratio of nursing home beds to population eighty-five years of age and over. In 1976, there were 681 beds per 1,000 residents eighty-five years of age and older. By 1998, that ratio had decreased to 446.9 beds per 1,000 population eighty-five and over.[13]

Drugs

Major international corporations such as Merck, Pfizer, Johnson & Johnson, and American Home Products represented the drug and medical supply industry. Between 1960 and the mid-1980s, the portion of the domestic health care dollar devoted to products from suppliers such as these actually declined. In 1960, drugs and other medical nondurables accounted for 15.8 percent of health care expenditures. By 1985, the proportion had decreased to 8.6 percent. However, during the decade of the 1990s this trend reversed. In 1990, the proportion of the health services dollar devoted to drugs and other medical nondurables was still 8.6 percent; however, in 1998 the proportion was 10.6 percent.[14]

The elderly purchased the largest share of prescription drugs. By one estimate, people sixty-five years of age and older used three times as many prescription drugs as all other age groups. The 13 percent of the population who were sixty-five and over accounted for 42 percent of expenditures on prescription drugs.[15]

Although each of the five components of the health services sector—hospitals, physicians, other health professionals, nursing homes, and drugs—had its own organizations, advocacy groups, and legal and economic structures, by and large physicians controlled the allocation of resources on behalf of patients. Obviously, physicians controlled the 20 percent of the health care resources that paid for their services; however, they substantially influenced the allocation of resources in many other components of the health sector as well. For example, hospitals were not licensed to practice medicine; rather, hospitals approved physicians for a medical staff, and the medical staff physicians allocated the 30 to 40 percent of health care dollars that purchased hospital resources for patient care. Physicians admitted patients to the hospital, discharged patients from the hospital, and made the resource allocation judgments in between. In addition, the influence by physicians on resource allocations was substantial in the prescription drug component and to some degree in the nursing home and home health care component.

Understanding the nature and extent of physician influence over the health sector's resource allocation was important. Regulatory and competitive forces that influenced physician behavior might have resource allocation outcomes that were not immediately obvious. Physician choices, when considered in the aggregate, were strategically important for the health care system and public health practice.

Paying for Health Services

In general, health service payor organizations could be dichotomized into those in the private sector and those in the public sector. In 1965, 61.5 percent of all payments for health care goods and services were made directly by private households. By 1995, this percentage dropped to 33.8 percent. For the latest available thirty-year period, there was a significant change in the distribution of payments among payor categories in the health services sector. Payors were generally categorized as household payors, private business payors, federal government payors, state government payors, and non-patient sources.

Household Payors

Various categories of payment from individual households in the United States made up the largest single payor category. In 1995, individual households paid out over $323 billion of the $958 billion expended on health care goods and services. There were four ways households paid for health services: (1) direct out-of-pocket health spending by individuals, (2) premiums paid by employees and the self-employed into the Medicare Hospital Insurance Trust Fund, (3) premiums paid by individuals to the Medicare supplemental medical insurance trust fund, and (4) the employee-paid share of private health insurance premiums and individual health insurance policies. In 1995, the first category—out-of-pocket spending—was more than half of all dollars expended by households on health services.

Private Business

Payments made by private businesses accounted for 26 percent of all expenditures for health care goods and services in 1995. Of this $249 billion, employers spent $184 billion for private health insurance premiums. These premiums were paid both for traditional indemnity types of insurance and, to an increasing degree, for employer self-insurance programs. In addition, private employers contributed more than $43 billion into the Medicare Hospital Insurance Trust Fund and another $19 billion for workmen's compensation and various forms of disability insurance. A small portion of the private expenditures ($3.3 billion) was made for in-house health services provided by companies at the workplace.

Non-Patient Revenues

The final category of private payments for health care goods and services was non-patient revenues. Such revenues accounted for between 2 and 3 percent of health resources. The sources of these revenues included philanthropy and other enterprises for which no patient care services were delivered. Although the dollar amount of such revenue steadily increased, its role in terms of all payments for health care goods and services was becoming less significant. Non-patient revenue increased from $0.5 billion in 1965 to nearly $25 billion in 1995. However, in terms of the percentage of the total, non-patient revenue decreased from 3.2 percent in 1985 to 2.6 percent in 1995.

Public Payors

Public expenditures from all levels of government accounted for more than 37 percent of the payments for health services and supplies in 1995. The largest portion of these public payments, $203.4 billion, was from the federal government. The federal government contributed to the health insurance programs for its own employees and expended general tax revenues for various health services programs such as health services for some poor individuals, the health services system of the Veterans Administration, the Indian Health Service that provided health care services to native Americans (American Indians and Alaska Natives), and an extensive military health service operated by the various branches of the U.S. armed services.

State and local governments contributed in excess of $157 billion to total payments for health care goods and services in 1995. In addition to health services programs provided directly by these governmental entities, this figure included state and local government contributions to private health insurance programs for their

Exhibit IN 1-8. Expenditures for Health Services and Supplies, by Type of Payor: United States, Selected Calendar Years 1990–1995 (in billions of dollars)

Type of Sponsor	1990	1991	1992	1993	1994	1995
Private						
Private business						
Employer contribution to private health insurance premiums	138.4	148.2	162.4	172.3	177.1	183.8
Employer contribution to Medicare Hospital Insurance Trust Fund[a]	29.5	32.7	34.3	36.0	40.2	43.1
Workers Compensation and Temporary Disability Insurance	15.7	16.7	18.5	18.4	18.6	19.3
Industrial in-plant health services	2.2	2.4	2.6	2.8	3.1	3.3
Total private business	185.8	200.1	217.9	229.5	239.0	249.4
Households						
Employee contribution to private health insurance	51.3	56.8	62.6	66.4	66.0	68.5
Employee and self-employment contributions and voluntary premiums paid to Medicare Hospital Insurance Trust Fund[a]	35.5	39.7	41.7	43.8	50.3	55.9
Premiums paid by individuals to Medicare Supplementary Medical Insurance Trust Fund	10.1	10.3	12.1	11.9	14.4	16.3
Out-of-pocket health spending	148.4	155.0	165.8	171.6	176.0	182.6
Total households	245.3	261.8	282.2	293.7	306.7	323.3
Non-patient revenues	19.8	21.6	22.4	23.8	23.7	24.7
Total private	450.8	483.4	522.4	547.0	569.5	597.4
Public						
Federal government						
Employer contribution to private health insurance premiums	9.2	9.8	10.7	11.5	11.9	11.3
Employer contribution to Medicare Hospital Insurance Trust Fund	2.1	2.2	2.2	2.3	2.3	2.3
Adjusted Medicare	29.8	32.0	41.2	49.8	52.1	62.7
Medicaid[b]	43.4	57.8	69.2	78.2	83.2	88.7
Other programs[c]	30.6	34.0	35.8	37.8	39.6	40.7
Total federal government	115.1	135.7	159.1	179.5	189.1	203.4

Exhibit IN 1-8. Continued

Type of Sponsor	1990	1991	1992	1993	1994	1995
State and local government						
Employer contribution to private health insurance premiums	33.5	37.5	41.2	45.2	47.7	47.1
Employer contribution to Medicare Hospital Insurance Trust Fund	4.0	4.4	4.8	5.0	5.3	5.6
Medicaid[b]	33.2	37.9	39.2	43.9	49.8	55.6
Other programs[d]	36.3	37.8	40.0	42.6	45.5	48.8
Total state and local government	107.0	117.6	125.2	136.6	148.1	157.0
Total public	222.1	253.3	284.2	316.1	337.3	360.4
Total	672.9	736.8	806.7	863.1	906.7	957.8

SOURCE: Health Care Financing Administration, Office of the Actuary; data from the National Health Statistics Group: www.hcfa.gov/pubforms/actuary/bus95/p2.htm

a. Includes one-half of self-employment contribution to Medicare Hospital Insurance Trust Fund benefits.

b. Includes Medicaid buy-in premiums for Medicare.

c. Includes maternal and child health, vocational rehabilitation, Substance Abuse and Mental Health Services Administration, Indian Health Service, federal workers' compensation, and other miscellaneous general hospital and medical programs, public health activities, Department of Defense, and Department of Veterans Affairs.

d. Includes other public and general assistance, maternal and child health, vocational rehabilitation, public health activities, and hospital subsidies.

employees as well as their contributions as employers to the Medicare Insurance Trust Fund (see Exhibit IN 1-8).

Exhibit IN 1-9 shows the changing relationship over time of the major payor organizations. This figure suggests a rationale for why it was difficult to gain a political consensus for substantial changes to the health care system despite rapidly escalating costs.

Most individuals in the United States had some form of health insurance. Individual out-of-pocket expenditures for health care as a percentage of total expenditures declined consistently over time since the mid-1960s. Hence, although health care costs escalated dramatically, the impact on individual households was muted. Government and private business became responsible for increasing proportions of the cost, and therefore individual households did not feel the entire financial impact of the rapidly increasing costs. From the viewpoint of most U.S. households, the quality of health care increased, health care providers offered more in terms of palliative and curative services, and the cost increases were moderate. It was difficult to gain a political consensus for change when most Americans maintained positive perceptions about their health services.

Exhibit IN 1-9. Expenditures for Health Services and Supplies, Payor Categories (percentage distribution, selected years)

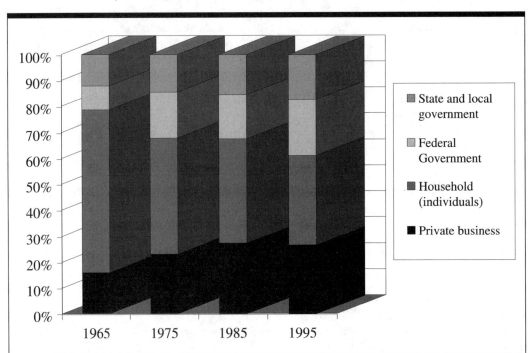

SOURCE: Health Care Financing Administration, Office of the Actuary; data from the National Health Statistics Group: www.hcfa.gov/pubforms/actuary/bus95/

Government Public Health Activities

Public health is the focus of this book and will be discussed in substantial detail in the next Industry Note. In general, government-provided public health services did not fit neatly into any individual category within the health care sector of the economy. Public health was a provider of personal health services, a regulator of service providers, a payor for services, and a major source of health-related research. Federal, state, and local governments all conducted public health activities and expended resources for public health services; however, the services were highly variable from state to state and from locality to locality within states. These services amounted to 3.2 percent of total health expenditures in 1998.[17] The largest component of this 3 percent share was used to deliver personal health services, often to the medically indigent (Exhibit IN 1-10).[18]

Exhibit IN 1-10. State Public Health Agency Expenditures by Program Area (percentage distribution, fiscal year 1991)

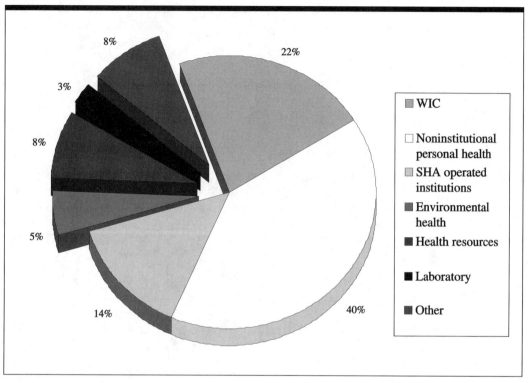

SOURCE: National Center for Health Statistics, *Health, United States, 1996–97* (Hyattsville, MD: U.S. Government Printing Office, 1997), Table 130, p. 264.

Selected Environmental Trends

Important trends in the health care environment had significant implications for the future of the health care system and public health. The external environment essentially created the rules that must be understood for leaders to make sound judgments on behalf of the public's health. Numerous environmental trends should be considered when assessing the environment. The ability to explain important environmental trends and their impact on the nation's health was a fundamental part of being accountable for the decisions made. Three important health care environmental trends serve as illustrations.

Trends in Hospital Utilization

Because the percentage of U.S. health care expenditures devoted to the use of hospital services was declining, the availability of hospital inpatient beds diminished as

Exhibit IN 1-11. Short-Term Nonfederal Hospitals, Number of Beds and Percentage Occupancy, 1985–1998

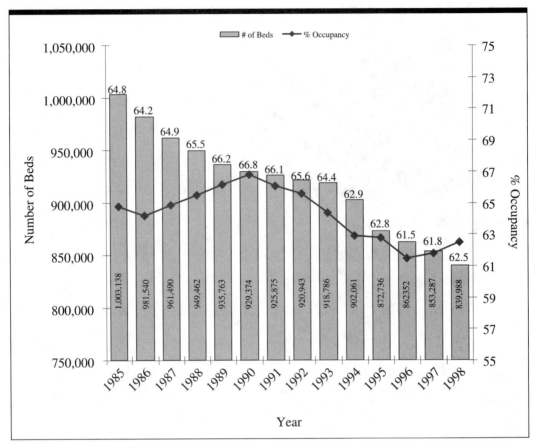

SOURCE: National Center for Health Statistics, *Health, United States, 2000, With Adolescent Health Chartbook* (Hyattsville, MD: National Center for Health Statistics, 2000), Table 109, p. 315.

well. In fact, hospitals across the country took beds out of service each year since the mid-1980s. The number of beds taken out of service since 1985 was equivalent to closing sixteen 200-bed community hospitals in every state—a substantial reduction in bed capacity.

The main reason hospitals were taking beds out of service was the declining occupancy rates for in-service beds. There were several reasons for declining use of inpatient hospital service, including changes to hospital payment methods that encouraged earlier discharge of inpatients as well as increasing outpatient alternatives to inpatient care. Exhibit IN 1-11 shows the reductions in the number of inpatient hospital beds over time and the accompanying impact of these bed reductions on the use of the remaining inpatient beds for each year. It was evident that the substantial reductions in inpatient beds had little impact on the utilization of the remaining beds. Hospital inpatient bed use was declining as fast as the hospitals took beds out of service.

Hospitals, just like hotels, must have a reasonable occupancy rate to efficiently utilize available resources. On a typical day in the United States, community hospital beds were approximately 40 percent empty. Hence, a substantial oversupply of hospital beds continued despite the extraordinary closure of hospital inpatient facilities over the past fifteen years. Additional hospital bed closures were likely until hospital inpatient beds achieved an efficient occupancy rate.

Trends in Managed Care

In general, managed care was considered to be any system of health payment or delivery arrangement where the plan attempted to control or coordinate use of health services by its enrolled members as a means of containing health expenditures, improving quality, or both. Managed care was a broad term that encompassed many different types of relationships among health care professionals, health service organizations, payors for health services, and health care clients, generally referred to as managed care organizations (MCOs). Typically, the term "managed care organization" referred to the entity that managed risk, contracted with providers, was paid by employers or patient groups, and handled claims processing.[19]

As previously discussed, the rapid rise of health care costs for private employers during the 1980s encouraged many large employers to adopt some type of managed care arrangement for employee health benefits. This led to a rapid growth of managed care organizations and numbers of enrollees during the 1990s. Between 1990 and 1999, enrollment in health maintenance organizations (HMOs), a major type of MCO, grew from 33 million to 81.3 million.[20]

Government health insurance programs such as Medicare and Medicaid were rapidly moving enrollees into managed care arrangements. Projections suggested that about 25 percent of seniors would be in Medicare HMOs by 2002 and 33 percent would be in such organizations by 2007. Projections for Medicaid, the federal/state health insurance program for the poor, were more dramatic. They suggested that 63 percent of all Medicaid enrollees would be in managed care arrangements within a few years.[21]

Enrollment in managed care organizations was clearly growing and was likely to continue to absorb a growing proportion of Americans with health insurance. The trend relative to the number of managed care organizations themselves was not as clear. The number of MCOs actually appeared to be decreasing (see Exhibit IN 1-12).

Increasing enrollment in MCOs with decreasing numbers of MCOs resulted in larger numbers of enrollees in each MCO. Such a trend suggested increasing bargaining power for MCOs when they negotiated with providers such as physicians and hospitals. This trend did not go unnoticed by provider organizations. The U.S. House of Representatives considered physician-backed legislation, the "Quality Health Care Coalition Act," that would provide self-employed physicians an exemption from federal antitrust laws. This act would confer upon physicians and other health care professionals who were engaged in negotiations with an MCO the same

Exhibit IN 1-12. HMO Enrollment and Number of Plans, 1987–1999

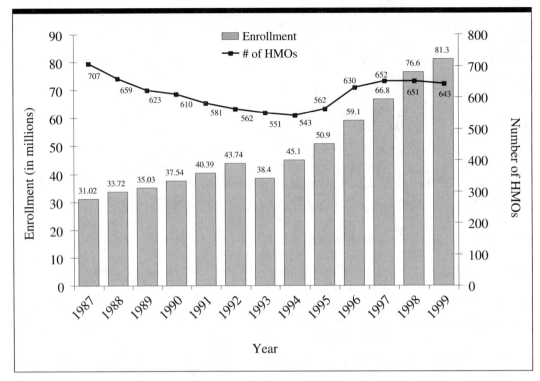

SOURCE: National Center for Health Statistics, *Health, United States, 2000, With Adolescent Health Chartbook* (Hyattsville, MD: National Center for Health Statistics, 2000), Table 131, p. 345.

treatment under antitrust laws as collective bargaining units received under the National Labor Relations Act.

Trends in the Physician Workforce

In 1980, there were 427,000 active physicians in the United States. This number for the year 2000 was projected to be 740,900. On a population basis, the availability of active physicians increased from 190 per 100,000 population in 1980 to 268 per 100,000 in 2000.[22]

To consider the strategic importance of this trend, it might be useful to view the physician to population ratio differently. Exhibit IN 1-13 presents population per active physician for selected years between 1970 and 2000. During that period, the number of people available, on average, in the United States for each physician to seek as clients decreased from 641 to 372.

This trend was primarily because of substantial increases in the number of medical schools and medical school class sizes in the United States since the passage of the Health Professions Education Assistance Act in 1963. Between 1960 and 1988, the number of first-year enrollees in U.S. medical schools more than doubled.

Exhibit IN 1-13.   Population per Active Physician in the United States (selected years; 2000 projected)

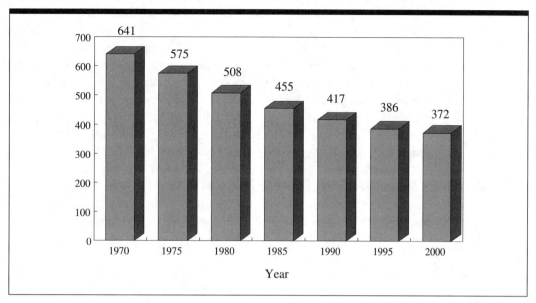

SOURCE: *Physician Characteristics and Distribution in the U.S.*, 2000 edition (American Medical Association), p. 352.

Exhibit IN 1-14.   Federal and Nonfederal Physicians by Age Group for Selected Years

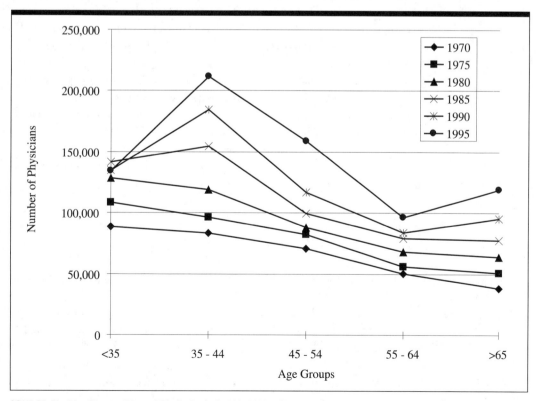

SOURCE: *Physician Characteristics and Distribution in the U.S.*, 2000 edition (American Medical Association), p. 340.

Although a future oversupply of physicians was widely projected, it was unlikely that any medical schools would close or that class sizes would decrease meaningfully; therefore an oversupply of physicians was expected to continue, at least for the foreseeable future.

New physicians were entering the workforce at about three times the rate that older physicians were leaving practice.[23] Given the approximately eight-year time lag between a student entering medical school and that student completing training and entering the workforce, this trend was expected to continue for at least a decade.

Exhibit IN 1-14 presents federal and nonfederal physicians by age group for selected years beginning in 1970. This exhibit suggests that there will be substantial increases to the supply of physicians in the near future.

Although there are some countervailing trends, such as greater requirements for physician services created by the aging of the U.S. population and increased demands of sophisticated medical technology, it was unlikely that these trends would offset the explosive growth in the supply of physicians. The strategic implications of a large oversupply of physicians for public health practice needed to be carefully considered.

Conclusion

This chapter attempted to provide an introduction to the U.S. health care system as background for the public health practice leadership and management cases in this book. It should be apparent that the health care system has undergone significant change in the past fifty years and that the near future is likely to undergo even more change. The health care environment was often described as undergoing "white water" change. Decision making in such an environment required managers to handle many judgmental challenges. Decisions made by public health professionals would directly affect the future health of our nation. Explaining decisions to various stakeholders in the community required expertise in sound decision making. That decision making must be done in the context of the general health care environment as well as the public health environment.

Notes

1. Paul Starr, *The Social Transformation of American Medicine* (New York: Basic Books, 1982), pp. 338–339.
2. N. L. Keating, A. M. Zaslavsky, and J. Z. Ayanian, "Physicians' Reports of Focused Expertise in Clinical Practice," *Journal of General Internal Medicine* 15 (2000), pp. 417–420.
3. F. G. Donini-Lenhoff and H. L. Hedrick, "Growth in Specialization in Graduate Medical Education," *Journal of the American Medical Association* 284, no. 10 (September 13, 2000), pp. 1284–1289.

4. National Center for Health Statistics, *Health United States 2000* (Hyattsville, MD: Government Printing Office, 2000), Table 119, p. 324.

5. Scientific American, "By the Numbers: Health Care Costs" (April, 1999), p. 36.

6. *Health United States 2000,* Table 90, p. 285.

7. *Ibid.,* Table 95, p. 297.

8. *Ibid.,* Table 101, p. 304.

9. *Ibid.,* Table 118, p. 325.

10. "Other professional services" covers services provided in establishments falling into SIC 804—Offices and clinics of other health practitioners (such as chiropractors, optometrists, podiatrists, and other licensed medical practitioners, not elsewhere classified) and SIC 809—Miscellaneous health and allied services (such as kidney dialysis centers and specialty outpatient facilities for mental health and substance abuse). Ambulance services paid under Medicare are also included here. Health Care Financing Administration Web site: www.hcfa.gov/stats/nhe-oact/articles/quickref.htm

11. Lynda Flanagan, "Nurse Practitioners: Growing Competition for Family Physicians?" *Family Practice Management* 5, no. 9 (October, 1998). www.aafp.org/fmp/98100fm/nurse.html

12. *Health United States 2000,* Table 118, pp. 325–326.

13. *Ibid.,* Table 113, pp. 319–320.

14. *Ibid.,* Table 118, pp. 325–326.

15. Families USA, "Growth in Drug Spending for the Elderly, 1992-2010" (July, 2000), p. 2.

16. Data on payors is excerpted from C. A. Cowan and B. R. Braden, "Business, Households, and Government: Health Care Spending, 1995," Office of the Actuary, Health Care Financing Administration. Available: www.hcfa.gov/pubforms/actuary/bus95/bus95.pdf

17. *Health United States 2000,* Table 118, p. 325.

18. Public Health Agencies, *Inventory of Programs and Block Grant Expenditures* (Washington, D.C.: Public Health Foundation, 1991).

19. Excepted from "Glossary of Terms in Managed Health Care," www.pohly. com/terms_m.shtml

20. *Health United States 2000,* Table 131, p. 345.

21. Institute for the Future, *Health and Health Care 2010* (San Francisco: Jossey Bass, 2000), pp. 43–44.

22. National Center for Health Statistics, *Health United States 1996–1997,* (Hyattsville, MD: Government Printing Office, 1997), Table 101, p. 232.

23. Institute for the Future, p. 5.

The U.S. Public Health System

In 1988, the Institute of Medicine, as part of a landmark study *The Future of Public Health*, defined the mission of public health as "fulfilling society's interest in assuring conditions in which people can be healthy."[1] This Industry Note is provided for a historical perspective of public health in the United States. Because many of public health's roles were defined by government through law, an understanding of the legal framework that defined the scope of activity and authority for public health agencies was required.

Governments made policy in several ways. One of the most important was by designating the way government funds were to be spent. Once areas of need were established and money was allocated, people were designated to carry out the work of public health. The people working in public health often had certain elements in common and performed a variety of activities to achieve the goal of healthier populations. Polls suggested that few members of the general public had the same understanding of public health as professionals working in the field. These and other general trends provided the environment of the public health system in the United States.

Brief Historical Perspective of Public Health

The origins of public health activity coincided with the evolution of human communities. George Rosen, in his well-known *History of Public Health*, originally published in 1958, stated, "Throughout human history, the major problems of health that men faced have been concerned with community life. . . . Evidence of activity connected with community health has been found in the very earliest civilizations."[2] Historical writings provided evidence that communities used isolation to prevent the spread of contamination. It was clear that these early writings, no matter their

This Industry Note was prepared by Ray M. Nicola, Centers for Disease Control and Prevention, Atlanta, Georgia. It is intended as a basis for classroom discussion rather than to illustrate effective or ineffective handling of an administrative situation. Used with permission from Ray M. Nicola.

original purpose, became the basis for some very early forms of community health promotion and health education.

For example, in an attempt to combat leprosy (Hansen's Disease) in 583, the Roman Catholic Church adopted the precepts delineated in the Old Testament book of Leviticus and restricted association with lepers. These methods of isolation or "quarantine" were refined and expanded. Lepers were considered a public menace and were expelled from the community to protect healthy citizens. For a community to decide that someone was suffering from leprosy was not a simple matter, as other skin conditions were similar in appearance and no scientific basis for causation was known. A community council of clerics and other citizens often was used to make the significant decision to declare a person a leper and remove him or her from the community. Essentially, a community decision was made to take a public health measure. Examples of protection of the public's health through community organization and education thus date back more than 1,000 years.

As active colonizers, the Greeks were aware that environment and lifestyle influenced the potential for disease in a community. The famous Hippocratic book *Air, Water, and Places* was, in part, written to assist new colonies in selecting sites that would be healthful. During the time of Emperor Augustus in Rome, certain public health services began to develop a formalized governmental administration. The "civil servants" of this era could forbid the sale of spoiled food and supervise homeowners in cleaning the streets in front of their dwellings.[3]

The Industrial Revolution was one of the more significant factors in the growth of communities in size and public health complexity. The eighteenth and nineteenth centuries saw profound economic changes that radically altered the nature, structure, and size of cities and increased the need for organized community effort to protect health. For example, in a brief span of forty years, from 1801 to 1841, the population of London increased from 958,000 to nearly 2 million. Congestion and lack of organized sanitation, as well as poor nutrition, created highly effective vectors for communicable disease. The incidence of cholera, typhoid, tuberculosis, and other diseases increased rapidly in the filthy and crowded conditions of English cities in the early 1800s. Not only were lives shortened and living conditions deteriorating, but the ability of the workforce to endure long hours in the factories was decreasing.

One of the most famous and influential governmental reports of this era was written by Edwin Chadwick. His *Report on an Inquiry Into Sanitary Conditions of the Labouring Population of Great Britain* was considered to be one of the defining documents of modern public health. It articulated not only the basis for the environmental causation of disease but also the relationship between disease prevention, governmental action, and financial well-being. One notable outcome from Chadwick's report was the establishment in 1848 of a General Board of Health for England. Chadwick was among those appointed to the board.

In his book, Rosen quoted the following passage from the 1840 British report of the Select Committee on the Health of Towns discussing the impact of disease on workers:

> The property which the country has in their useful labours will be so fare lessened, and the unproductive outlay necessary to maintain and restrain them so

far augmented . . . some such measures are urgently called for, as claims of
humanity and justice to great multitudes of our fellow men, and as necessary
not less for the welfare of the poor than the safety of property and the security
of the rich.[4]

Although many other countries had important public health activity before Great
Britain, the British experience had a major impact on the development of the public
health system in the United States. The same industrial development, lack of sanitation, and disease contagion that evoked organized community responses in Britain
provoked similar responses in the colonies of the new world. English common law
was the basis for much of American law.

As early as the mid-seventeenth century, there were instances of colonies (and
later states) establishing governmental acts with the purpose of preventing disease.[5]
The causes of disease were not well understood, and prevention activities during this
period focused on quarantine and hygiene.[6] Exhibit IN 2-1 describes some of the
more significant events in the United States that established the foundations for
public health practice.

The Current U.S. Public Health System

Activities designed to improve the health of the population in the United States were
carried out by government agencies, by the health care sector, by voluntary health
agencies, and increasingly by various other segments of society such as school systems, faith communities, law enforcement agencies, and businesses. As the major
causes of disease and death changed over the years, the role of government changed
as well. Although some analysts pointed to a trend in the privatization of governmental public health activities, it was clear that there were certain functions that only
government could perform, labeled by the Institute of Medicine in *The Future of
Public Health* as assessment, policy development, and assurance.[7]

Federal Level

Principal responsibility for assessment, policy development, and assurance
within the federal government fell to the Public Health Service, a part of the U.S.
Department of Health and Human Services. Exhibit IN 2-2 describes key public
health agencies at the federal level.[8]

More than a dozen agencies at the federal level had some environmental health
roles. These included the Departments of Transportation, Labor, Health and Human Services, Commerce, Energy, Defense, the Interior, Agriculture, and Housing
and Urban Development; the Environmental Protection Agency; the Consumer
Product Safety Commission; and the Nuclear Regulatory Commission.[9]

Exhibit IN 2-1. Significant Public Health Events in U.S. History

1794	The Act of June 9, 1794, authorized the appointment of a health officer for the Port of Baltimore, Maryland. Because of the maritime nature of commerce and national defense, port cities were magnets for industrial growth and epidemic contagion.
1796	The Act Relative to Quarantine directed revenue officers to execute health and quarantine regulations at U.S. ports of entry.
1798	The Act for the Relief of Sick and Disabled Seaman imposed a twenty cent tax per month against seamen's wages to provide for their health care. This act led to the creation of the Marine Hospital Service, considered by many to be the genesis of the U.S. Public Health Service. An act of Congress in 1902 changed the name of the Marine Hospital Service to the Public Health and Marine Hospital Service and created the Hygienic Laboratory that became the National Institutes of Health in 1930.
1845	Publication of *Census of Boston* by Lemuel Shattuck laid the foundation for the accurate reporting of vital statistics in the United States. The census revealed high general mortality, especially among infants and new mothers. Communicable diseases such as scarlet fever, typhus, diphtheria, and tuberculosis were widespread. The highly unsanitary and crowded living conditions of lower socioeconomic groups were documented. Five years later, Shattuck authored one of the most famous documents in U.S. public health history, the *Massachusetts Sanitary Commission Report* known simply as "the Shattuck Report." It recommended most of the public health policies that were later implemented; it had little impact at the time it was published.[a]
1860–1865	The U.S. Civil War fostered a new consciousness of infectious disease. Between two-thirds and three-fourths of all casualties during this war were due to disease and not to battle-related injury.
1869	Functioning state boards of health began. By 1875, boards of health existed in Massachusetts, California, the District of Columbia, Virginia, Minnesota, Maryland, and Alabama.
1879	The Act to Establish a National Board of Health was passed. A serious yellow fever epidemic in 1879 encouraged Congress to create a federal board to cooperate with state and local boards of health on "all matters affecting the public health." This body attempted to formulate quarantine regulations that involved commerce and travel between the states. The board was soon involved in bitter states' rights battles and was disbanded in 1883.
1880s	The "new bacteriology" identified the organisms responsible for tuberculosis, cholera, typhoid, and diphtheria. By the mid-1890s, laboratory tests had been developed to detect these and other diseases.[b] These developments led to a dominance of the disease-oriented approach to public health. Strong advocates also existed for the importance of nutrition, environment, and education in public health practice.
1890s	Early efforts were made to improve infant mortality and child health. They dealt primarily with infant nutrition but expanded into maternal education.
1908	New York City established the first unit within a health department to deal specifically with infant health. The Division of Child Hygiene in the New York City Health Department demonstrated the importance of prevention in reducing the number of infant deaths.
1921	The Sheppard-Towner Act, the first federal measure to appropriate funds for a health and social welfare purpose, provided matching funds to states for prenatal and child health clinics. After seven years, well-organized opponents of this type of government action succeeded in persuading Congress to discontinue the program.[c]

Exhibit IN 2-1. Continued

1935	The Social Security Act again added grant-in-aid functions to the Children's Bureau for maternal and child health activities and created federal assistance for rehabilitation of crippled children, general public health activities, and aid to dependent children under the age of sixteen.
1940s	Antibiotics, penicillin, and sulfonamides were introduced. These drugs enabled physicians for the first time to treat infectious diseases effectively and accelerated the shift from infectious diseases to chronic diseases as the chief source of mortality in the United States.
1948	The Water Pollution Control Act authorized the U.S. Public Health Service to help states develop water pollution control programs and to aid in the planning of sewage treatment plants.
1955	The Air Pollution Control Act provided aid to states, regions, and localities for research and control programs to protect air quality.
1960s	Researchers recognized extension of the adult life span. The twentieth century increase in life expectancy in the United States was more than thirty years, twenty-five of which were because of public health interventions and improvements.[d]
1965	Passage of Medicare and Medicaid as part of the Social Security Amendments marked the first large-scale federal initiative to provide health insurance for major segments of the population.
1970	The Public Health Cigarette Smoking Act banned cigarette advertising from broadcast media—radio and television.
1970	The Occupational Safety and Health Act provided federal programs of standard settings and enforcement to ensure safe and healthful conditions in the workplace.
1972	The National School Lunch and Child Nutrition Amendments added federal funds to support nutritious diets for pregnant and lactating women and for infants and children (the women, infants, and children's or WIC program).
1977	The world's final case of smallpox was identified in Merka, Somalia. This marked the ultimate success of the world's first disease eradication program, begun by the World Health Organization in 1967.
1981	The Public Health Service Hospital System was closed. The health care entitlement program for merchant seamen ended.
1981	The first acquired immunodeficiency syndrome (AIDS) case was reported.
1985	Reported cases of tuberculosis rose sharply. Drug-resistant tuberculosis was reported in the eastern United States.
1990s	Severe infectious diseases emerged, including *Hantavirus* in the Southwest United States, *Escherichia coli* 0157:H7 in hamburgers, and *Cryptosporidium* in drinking water.
1999	Tobacco companies were required to pay $2.4 billion annually, as a result of a lawsuit, for at least twenty-five years to forty-six eligible states for tobacco-related illnesses and injuries.[e]

a. George Rosen, *A History of Public Health* (New York: MD Publications, 1958), pp. 217–218.

b. Paul Starr, *The Social Transformation of American Medicine* (New York: Basic Books, 1982), pp. 137–138.

c. *Ibid.*, p. 261.

d. From *USA Today*. Retrieved from the World Wide Web on September 13, 2000: http://www.usatoday.com/news/smoke/smoke278.htm

e. J. P. Bunker, H. S. Frazier, and F. Mosteller, "Improving Health: Measuring Effects of Medical Care," *Milbank Quarterly* 72 (1994), pp. 225–258.

Exhibit IN 2-2. Key Federal Public Health Agencies

Centers for Disease Control and Prevention (CDC). CDC conducted epidemiologic surveillance and researched communicable and chronic diseases, injuries, and occupational illnesses throughout the world. CDC worked with public health agencies and others at the state level to operate prevention programs for communicable and chronic diseases, injuries, and occupational illness. The Epidemic Intelligence Service trained epidemiologists to assist in these many activities. In addition, CDC worked to strengthen the infrastructure of public health at the state and local levels. CDC headquarters was in Atlanta, Georgia, but field staff worked with state and large local public health agencies throughout the United States.

Health Resources and Services Administration (HRSA). HRSA provided health services for special populations, such as maternal and child health, rural health care, care for the underserved through the National Health Services Corps and Community Health Center support, and care for persons with HIV/AIDS. In addition, HRSA monitored the training, supply, and distribution of health professionals in the United States, including the public health workforce.

Food and Drug Administration (FDA). FDA regulated more than one-fourth of all goods and services bought and sold in the United States. FDA researchers and regulators evaluated new products in development before they were brought to market, including experimental drugs, cosmetics, food additives, radiation-emitting devices, and new medical devices.

Substance Abuse and Mental Health Services Administration (SAMHSA). SAMHSA organized and supported a wide range of services for the prevention and treatment of substance abuse and mental impairments. Programs were focused on both prevention and treatment of conditions.

Agency for Toxic Substances and Disease Registry (ATSDR). Administered by the CDC Director, ATSDR investigated the effects of toxic materials on humans. The agency trained local and state public health agency personnel in investigating toxic chemical exposures.

Indian Health Service (IHS). IHS operated health care facilities for Native American populations that were administered by the IHS or by the tribes.

National Institutes of Health (NIH). NIH funded basic biomedical research done through major medical teaching centers. NIH had a large in-house research program.

Agency for Health Services Research (AHSR). AHSR improved the quality and effectiveness of health care services including research into health services delivery, medical effectiveness, and health outcomes.

Health Care Financing Administration (HCFA). HCFA administered 84 percent of the Department of Health and Human Services's budget through the Medicare and Medicaid programs, funding health care for elderly and indigent persons.

Key federal environmental statutes included the Clean Air Act (CAA); Clean Water Act (CWA); Comprehensive Environmental Response, Competition and Liability Act (CERCLA) and Superfund Amendments and Reauthorization Act (SARA); Federal Insecticide, Fungicide, and Rodenticide Act (FIFRA); Resource Conservation and Recovery Act (RCRA); Safe Drinking Water Act (SDWA); Toxic Substance Control Act (TCSA); Food, Drug, and Cosmetic Act (FDCA); Federal Mine Safety and Health Act (MSHA); and Occupational Safety and Health Act (OSHA).[10]

State Level

By 1900, forty states had health departments that made advances in sanitation and microbial sciences available to the public. Later, states provided other public health interventions such as personal health services (e.g., services for disabled children, maternal and child health care, and sexually transmitted disease treatment), environmental health (e.g., waste management and radiation control), and health resources (e.g., health planning, regulation of health care, emergency services, and health statistics). Nearly all states had public health laboratories that provided direct services and oversight functions.[11]

Each state had a lead agency for health—the state health agency (SHA)—but additional state agencies had responsibilities for health at the state level. SHAs were free-standing agencies in about two-thirds of the states and were part of a larger health and social services organization in the remainder.[12]

In the environmental arena, SHAs mirrored the diverse federal system of agency responsibility, but there was no consistency in assigning the implementation of federal environmental laws to state agencies. Only a few states assigned the state's lead for environmental laws to the SHA. Since the establishment of the Environmental Protection Agency on December 2, 1970,[13] the monitoring of environmental concerns shifted to state environmental protection agencies, with a focus on regulatory activities. State health agencies, for the most part, were still called on to link human health issues with environmental concerns even when they did not have the regulatory responsibility in their state.

At the state level, a major issue was the fragmentation of public health concerns among a large number of "non-health" state agencies. Fragmentation complicated and exacerbated the coordination role within state public health systems.

Fundamental changes in the way public health services were organized, administered, financed, and delivered by the state health agency have occurred.[14] A survey of all fifty states by the National Governors' Association in 1996 reported that thirteen states (26 percent) were in the planning stage or the implementing stage of interagency restructuring; an additional fifteen (30 percent) were undertaking only intra-agency restructuring, and the remainder had no formal plans for restructuring. The report suggested that the restructuring involved not only changes in administrative structures but also a change in basic ways of doing business. Common themes in the restructuring initiatives included

- Integrating service delivery by moving from a categorical approach to a functional orientation
- Encouraging agency creativity and innovation by accepting risk taking
- Integrating social support services with public health and medical services
- Providing flexibility so that lessons learned during the early implementation stages were incorporated into the restructuring effort

States that were restructuring their SHAs chose one of four basic strategies: They were continuing the same broad organizational structure but combining or separating certain organizational units, combining the Medicaid program with public health functions into one entity, consolidating multiple government agencies into one umbrella agency, or transferring public health functions outside the umbrella organizational structure.

Local Level

During 1910–11, the success of a county sanitation campaign to control a severe typhoid epidemic in Yakima County, Washington, created public support for a permanent health service, and a local health department was organized on July 1, 1911.[15] Concurrently, the Rockefeller Sanitary Commission began supporting county hookworm eradication efforts. By 1920, 131 county health departments had been established.[16] By 1931, 599 county health departments were providing services to one-fifth of the U.S. population. In 1950, 86 percent of the U.S. population was served by a local health department and 34,895 persons were employed full-time in public health agencies.[17]

Local public health agencies (LPHAs) were the focal point for public health. LPHAs carried out the mandates of state and local health ordinances and delivered personal and population-based public health services to their local communities. Local agencies had to be considered in the context of the state public health system because state laws established the existence and types of agencies that were allowed. The disposition of public health functions between the state and local units varied widely across the nation based on history, legal frameworks, and political forces.

If LPHAs were defined as "an administrative and service unit of local government, concerned with health, employing at least one full-time person, and carrying responsibility for health of a jurisdiction smaller than the state," there were 2,888 local health agencies operating in 3,042 U.S. counties in 1993.[18] The organization and governance of state and local public health systems could be categorized as

- Centralized: The LPHAs were directly operated by the state.
- Decentralized: LPHAs were formed and managed by local government.
- Shared: The state had some control over the LPHA, for example, appointing the health officer or reviewing the annual budget.
- Mixed: Both centralization and decentralization occurred when a local jurisdiction chose not to form an LPHA and the state provided services.[19]

LPHAs were established by governmental units—including counties, cities, towns, townships, and special districts—by one of two general methods: through enactment of a resolution or through a referendum. Both patterns were common. Resolution health agencies were often funded from the general funds of the jurisdiction, whereas referendum health agencies often had a specific tax levy available to them. A resolution health agency was simpler to establish and developed closer working relationships with the local legislative body that created it. Referendum agencies reflected the support of the local electorate and might have access to specific tax levies that avoided the need to compete with other local government funding sources.[20]

About three-quarters of LPHAs were organized at the county level, serving a single county, a county-city, or several counties. More than half (56 percent) were single-county LPHAs. Counties were legally responsible for indigent health care in more than thirty states and paid a portion of the nonfederal portion of Medicaid in about twenty states.[21]

Cities had the ability through home rule powers to take on functions not prohibited by the state. Cities could choose to have a health department or could rely on their county or the state for public health functions. City LPHAs often had a wider array of public health programs and services because of this autonomy.[22] Many big city LPHAs took on the issue of health care for indigent residents because of home rule and because of increased demands and expectations from populations in need.

Seven percent of LPHAs operated at the city level, with 11 percent at the town or township level or other levels (primarily state).[23] Two-thirds of LPHAs served populations of 50,000 or fewer. Eighteen percent of LPHAs served a population of 100,000 or more, and only 4 percent served populations of one million or more.

A full-time top agency executive was employed by 79 percent of LPHAs.[24] LPHAs serving larger populations were more likely to have a full-time agency executive than those serving smaller populations. In the 1960s, 80 percent of LPHAs had full-time or part-time physicians as top agency executives; however, in the 1970s that percentage dropped to approximately 65 percent, and in the 1990s the percentage dropped further, to 32 percent.[25] Of the physician executives, 30 percent had advanced public health degrees in addition to MD degrees.

In 1940, the American Public Health Association published a report recommending a minimum population size for LPHA jurisdictions that would lead to improved ability to provide population health services such as disease investigation and health education. Other reports recommended consolidation of the smallest LPHAs, but little overall change occurred in numbers because of issues of local political autonomy.

Another component of many local public health systems was the local board of health. In a recent survey sponsored by the National Association of Local Boards of Health and CDC, 3,186 local boards of health were identified in the United States. Eighty-five percent of survey respondents indicated affiliation with an LPHA. Most boards (88 percent) served populations of fewer than 100,000, and 57 percent served populations of fewer than 25,000. Most local boards of health performed multiple functions, including advisory (80 percent), policy making (76 percent), and governing (71 percent). More than 70 percent of local boards reported that they had responsibilities for recommending public health policy; proposing, adopting, and enforcing public health regulations; and recommending health department budgets and priorities. Although 80 percent of boards reported having authority for environmental health programs, only 16 percent reported having authority for mental health programs.[26]

In 1993, 72 percent of all local public health departments (2,079 of 2,888 LPHAs) responded to a survey on program activities.[27] Nearly all LPHAs provided vaccination services (96 percent) and tuberculosis treatment (86 percent), but few provided substance abuse services (21 percent) or mental health services (12 percent). LPHAs serving jurisdictions greater than 100,000 in population were more likely to provide sexually transmitted disease control services (94 percent), HIV/AIDS testing and counseling (94 percent), and laboratory services (84 percent) than were smaller jurisdictions (66 percent, 63 percent, and 55 percent, respectively). In addition, environmental health services were somewhat more likely to be provided by larger jurisdictions. For example, 69 percent of larger LPHAs provided vector control services, whereas 55 percent of smaller jurisdictions provided such services.

At the beginning of the twentieth century, many public health initiatives were started and supported by nongovernment organizations such as the Rockefeller Sanitary Committee's Hookworm Eradication Project, conducted during 1910–1920. Other early efforts to promote community health included the National Tuberculosis Association's work for TB treatment and prevention, the National Consumers League's support of maternal and infant health in the 1920s, the American Red Cross's sponsorship of nutrition programs in the 1930s, and the March of Dimes's support for research in the 1940s and 1950s that led to a successful polio vaccine. In addition, professional organizations and labor unions worked to promote public health. Examples included the American Medical Association advocating for better vital statistics and safer foods and drugs, the American Dental Association endorsing water fluoridation, and labor organizations advocating for safer workplaces in industry.[28]

As the federal, state, and local public health infrastructure expanded in mid-century, government's role increased and government encompassed more responsibility for public health research and programs. Although both government and nongovernment organizations were involved in public health activities, there was an effort to get nongovernment, nonhealth organizations and individuals involved in defining health priorities for communities and in advocating for better health.

Legal Framework

When the U.S. Constitution was written, powers not specifically granted to the federal government by the states were retained by the individual states. These powers were known collectively as the "police powers" of the state. Included in state police powers were the functions involved with protecting the public's health.

Legal Sources of Public Health Powers

Federal powers in public health were based on the "commerce" clause of the Constitution—the power of Congress to "regulate commerce with foreign nations, and among the several States, and with the Indian tribes"—and on the "taxing" power of the federal government. Many federal interests in public health did not involve direct regulation; rather, the taxing and spending power of government was used to establish national programs that were operated in partnership with state and local governments. For example, Congress appropriated money for the tuberculosis program to the Centers for Disease Control and Prevention. CDC operated grant programs to states for the prevention and control of tuberculosis, and states distributed funding to local governments to carry out these programs.

The Clinical Laboratory Improvement Act of 1988 was another example of the ability of the federal government to regulate. Laboratories would not be eligible for reimbursement for Medicare or Medicaid funds if they did not meet specified standards. Congress required that CDC establish standards for clinical laboratories in the United States and that the Health Care Financing Administration inspect laboratories to ensure that they met national standards.

At the state level, the power to protect the public's health was based on the "police power," an inherent power of government.[29] State constitutions, often patterned after the U.S. Constitution, specified the delegation of this power to lower levels of government including divisions of the state, counties, cities, municipalities, and villages.

Laws came from three sources: statutory, administrative, and judicial. Statutory-based laws were passed by legislative bodies at the federal, state, or local level.[30] They included a wide range of policy initiatives such as a proclamation of public health week by a city government, an annual budget for the local public health agency specifying funding for general operations, funding for a specific public health program, and a statement providing regulation of activities for the purpose of protecting the public's health (for example, laws pertaining to restaurant inspection).

Administrative law was developed by the executive branch of government based on authority delegated under constitutional or statutory law. Typically in public health practice, a state health agency, a local public health agency, and a state or local board of health were involved in drafting administrative law. Judicial law was based on decisions made in individual cases in federal and state courtrooms. When there was no defining statutory law to identify rights and responsibilities, the courts relied on judicial law.

A Basic Legal Issue in Public Health: Individual Rights Versus the Health of the Population

Public health attempted to balance the rights of an individual to enjoy the freedoms guaranteed by the U.S. Constitution with the rights and needs of society as a whole to be protected from the harm of disease and injury. The control of communicable diseases was the major example of the conflict between an individual's rights and protection of the public.

The control of infectious disease depended on identification of people who were carriers of disease. Laws imposed a requirement to report to the health officer the suspicion or diagnosis of such reportable diseases.[31] This duty applied to physicians, heads of institutions, schools, parents, the infected person, and—in some states—clinical laboratories. Length of time to report the suspicion of a disease on the list depended on the urgency of the disease epidemiology.

Laws could provide for many kinds of compulsory medical examinations and clinical tests. For example, when a public health officer had grounds for believing that a particular person had a certain communicable disease (for example, syphilis or diphtheria), the health officer could compel the suspected person to be tested or treated or even confined to a physical location or to a hospital until the individual was no longer infectious. The health officer was required to use his or her best judgment of the risks. Courts could review the legality of a person's confinement through a habeas corpus proceeding at which a judge required the health officer to review the circumstances and reasoning used to initiate a confinement. A writ of habeas corpus was a judicial mandate to a law enforcement official ordering that an inmate be brought to the court so the court could determine whether the person was imprisoned lawfully and whether he or she should be released from custody.[32]

Basic Areas of Public Health Law

As new threats to health were discovered, new public health laws emerged. Examples of common areas that were the subject of public health law included the following:[33]

- Environmental health: Food and milk inspection, drinking water treatment, and sewage and wastewater treatment were major parts of public health law. Environmental health regulations raised the issues of compensation for regulation of individual property and the circumstances surrounding the inspection of premises by health officers.
- Disease and injury reporting: Information on diseases and injuries was critical to the tracking of illness trends and epidemics in communities. The requirement to report transcended the individual's right to privacy and the confidentiality of the physician-patient relationship.
- Vital statistics: Birth and death statistics were required in all states to monitor the health status of the population.
- Disease control: Prevention of diseases by health officials frequently inconvenienced numerous individuals but was required to protect the health of the community.
- Involuntary testing: Identification of individuals with a communicable disease such as tuberculosis required involuntary testing of populations at risk. The sole purpose of this testing was to protect the health of others and not to punish the individual being tested.
- Contact tracing: Contact tracing has been used since the early part of the twentieth century to control epidemic infectious diseases by requiring individuals to name persons with whom physical contact had recently occurred. The definition of physical contact depended on the disease entity being tracked.
- Immunizations and mandated treatment: The most common example of involuntary treatment was the state-mandated immunizations required of children before they entered school.

Exhibit IN 2-3. U.S. Local Health Department Funds by Source, 1992–1993

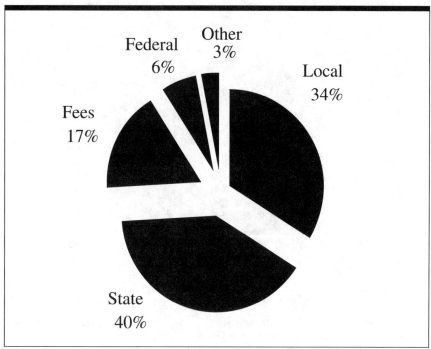

SOURCE: National Association of County and City Health Officials, *National Profile of Local Health Departments 1992–1993* (Atlanta, GA: Centers for Disease Control and Prevention, 1995), p. 37.

- Personal restrictions: Quarantine was seldom used in modern times but was occasionally necessary to prevent the spread of a very infectious disease in the case of a noncompliant patient. Directly observed therapy for tuberculosis was another example of personal restriction. Control programs in the United States required that patients with active tuberculosis ingest their medications in a setting where clinic personnel could observe them.

Public Health Expenditures

Although federal, state, and local health agencies increased in number throughout the twentieth century, public health resources represented a small proportion of overall health care costs. In 1993, federal, state, and local health agencies spent an estimated $14.4 billion on core public health functions, 1.59 percent of the $903 billion in total health care expenditures.[34] There was no existing system that captured and examined public health expenditure data comprehensively or longitudinally.

In 1993, LPHAs had approximately $8 billion in expenditures from multiple funding sources (see Exhibit IN 2-3). Most LPHAs had budgets that were less than

Exhibit IN 2-4. U.S. Local Public Health Agencies by Total Annual Expenditures, 1992–1993

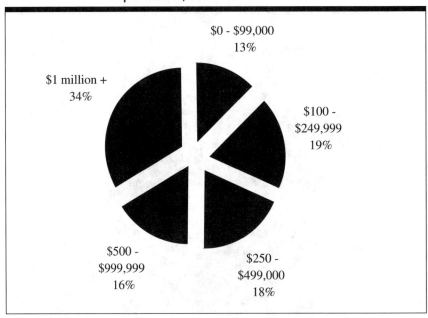

$0 - $99,000
13%

$1 million +
34%

$100 -
$249,999
19%

$500 -
$999,999
16%

$250 -
$499,000
18%

SOURCE: National Association of County and City Health Officials, *National Profile of Local Health Departments 1992–1993* (Atlanta, GA: Centers for Disease Control and Prevention, 1995), p. 34.

$1 million (see Exhibit IN 2-4). LPHA budget expenditures increased with the size of population served. In 1997, the average LPHA spent $41 per resident per year.[35]

Both city and county LPHAs relied heavily on property and sales taxes to finance health and other services, and they were struggling with the limitations of these funding sources.[36] The major limitation was political concern over increasing property and sales taxes.

Defining the Work of Public Health

The work of public health developed over time in response to community need. In 1988, after an intense study of public health in six states, the Institute of Medicine defined the basic functions of public health as assessment, policy development, and assurance.[37] CDC proposed ten organizational practices to implement the three core functions.[38] In 1994, a national working group composed of representatives of the Public Health Services agencies and the major public health organizations developed a consensus list of the "essential services of public health."[39] The consensus statement set forth a definition intended to (1) explain what public health was, (2) clarify the essential role of public health in the overall health system, and (3) provide accountability by linking public health performance to health outcomes. The new statement on essential services provided a vision for public health in America— "Healthy People in Healthy Communities"—and stated the mission of public health: "Promote physical and mental health and prevent disease, injury, and disability." The statement included two brief lists that described what public health sought to accomplish in providing essential services to the public and how it carried out these basic public responsibilities.

The Essential Services

The fundamental obligations or purposes of public health agencies responsible for population-based health were to

- Prevent epidemics and the spread of disease
- Protect against environmental hazards
- Prevent injuries
- Promote and encourage healthy behaviors and mental health
- Respond to disasters and assist communities in recovery
- Ensure the quality and accessibility of health services

Thus, part of the function of public health was to ensure the availability of quality health services. Both distinct from and encompassing clinical services, public health's role was to ensure the conditions necessary for people to live healthy lives, through community-wide prevention and protection programs.

Public health served communities (and individuals within them) by providing an array of essential services. Many of these services were invisible to the public. Typically, the public became aware of the need for public health services only when a problem developed (e.g., an epidemic occurred). The practice of public health was articulated through the list of "essential services."[40]

Assessment services included

- Monitoring health status to identify community health problems
- Diagnosing and investigating health problems and hazards in the community
- Researching for new insights and innovative solutions to health problems

Policy development services included

- Informing, educating, and empowering people about health issues
- Mobilizing community partnerships and actions to identify and solve health problems
- Developing policies and plans that supported individual and community health efforts

Assurance services included

- Enforcing laws and regulations that protected health and ensured safety
- Linking people to needed personal health services and ensuring the provision of health care when otherwise unavailable

- Ensuring a competent public and personal health care workforce
- Evaluating effectiveness, accessibility, and quality of personal and population-based health services

Providers and Organization of Essential Public Health Services

The number of full-time employees of LPHAs increased with the size of the population served. Only 9 percent of LPHAs employed 100 people or more, 24 percent had 25 to 99 employees, 25 percent had 10 to 24 employees, 20 percent had 5 to 9 employees, and 22 percent had 4 or fewer employees. The number of different disciplines was related to the size of the population served. Most common staff included nurses, environmental health specialists, physicians, nutritionists, and clerical staff.[41]

Public Health Training

Professional training in public health started early in the century and expanded slowly. The Johns Hopkins School of Hygiene and Public Health was founded in 1916.[42] Columbia, Harvard, and Yale universities established schools of public health by 1922. By 1969, the number of schools of public health had increased to twelve, and by 1999 twenty-nine universities had accredited schools of public health enrolling approximately 15,000 students.[43] Early in the twentieth century, most students in schools of public health had already obtained medical degrees. By 1978, however, 69 percent of public health students enrolled with only baccalaureate degrees. Thus, public health training evolved from a second degree for medical professionals to a primary health discipline. Schools of public health initially emphasized the study of hygiene and sanitation. Subsequently, the study of public health expanded into five core disciplines: biostatistics, epidemiology, health services administration, health education/behavioral science, and environmental science.[44]

Additional training programs in public health were available. Physicians who specialized in preventive medicine were certified by the American Board of Preventive Medicine, a member of the American Board of Medical Specialties established in 1948. Preventive medicine residency programs trained physicians in public health competency areas, and the Board of Preventive Medicine accredited providers of continuing medical education.[45] The American Nurses Credentialing Center (ANCC), a subsidiary of the American Nurses Association (ANA), certified registered nurses in community health nursing, one of twenty-nine specialty areas, through its commission on certification and boards on certification. The National Environmental Health Association (NEHA) was incorporated in 1937 to help develop standards for registered sanitarians.[46] The 5,000 member organization offered credentials in eight environmental health areas. Many other professional groups were working in public health—such as social workers, nutritionists, and lawyers—but without specific certification or training programs in public or community health.

Governmental agencies established additional public health training programs. For example, in 1951 the CDC developed the Epidemic Intelligence Service (EIS) to guard against domestic acts of biologic warfare during the Korean conflict and to address common public health threats. In 1999, 149 EIS officers were on duty responding to requests for epidemiologic assistance within the United States and throughout the world. Approximately 25 percent of them were assigned directly to state or local health departments across the nation, with an Atlanta-based supervisor to complement local supervision. The remaining were assigned to CDC headquarters.[47]

Continuing Trends in the Public Health Environment

Although many trends affected the determinants of health in the United States, such as the aging of the population, several trends directly affected the ability of public health practitioners to accomplish their work.

Intergovernmental Relationships

State primacy in public health funding in the early part of the twentieth century was superseded by the federal government. Public health programs such as immunizations and communicable disease investigation went from being funded mostly through state general funds to being funded mostly through federal funds. Federal programs were administered early in the century as block grants, then funding streams were organized as categorical grants in the middle part of the century, and in the final part of the century there was a trend back to administering program funds again as block grants.

Opinion polls illustrated that the public's view was that government—particularly at federal and state levels—was not to be trusted to do the right thing. A 1999 Harris Poll reported continuing low public confidence in the federal government.[48] Key political figures at national and state levels reflected public sentiment when they espoused minimizing government. The phrase "getting government off our backs," widely used in the 1980s and 1990s, reflected this position. Many citizen-born initiatives at the state level, with ripple effects at the local level, attempted to limit or reduce taxes and to minimize government.

Budget and personnel actions by state and local government attempted to be responsive to public feelings. Results from a 1996 telephone survey of state and selected large-city health departments indicated that the privatization of public health services increased throughout the 1990s.[49]

Privatization trends were related to personnel and funding decreases because of downsizing of government organizations. Concerns were raised that block grant funding encouraged additional contracting of public health activities and that cost savings would disappear as privatization activities matured, and that service quality would decrease.

The Changing Health System Environment

Major changes in the medical care system, driven by market forces, initiated changes in the public health system. Many state Medicaid systems across the nation moved to managed care for covered populations, and local public health systems re-evaluated their role in the provision of medical care services. Many local public health agencies shifted their role as providers of primary care to providers of more limited public health support services. Others redefined their role as a deliverer of essential public health services.[50]

Emerging Infectious Diseases

In her book *Betrayal of Trust: Collapse of Global Public Health*,[51] Laurie Garrett investigated the consequences of inadequate funding for surveillance and control of communicable diseases in the United States and around the globe. She made the point that with globalization, no person or corner of the planet was safe from epidemics, antibiotic-resistant "super-bugs," or bio-warfare. Illnesses such as plague (*Yersinia pestis*), the Ebola virus, multiple drug–resistant tuberculosis, and other equally morbid infectious disease agents were on the rise around the world. A lack of investment in public health infrastructure left a path for potential catastrophe. In the United States, new infections such as hantavirus appeared, and older infections, such as tuberculosis, made a comeback in the form of a multiple drug–resistant tuberculosis bacteria. Medical researchers previously believed that the era of antibiotics had made infectious diseases illnesses of the past. With air travel and antibiotic resistance, the resurgence of communicable diseases challenged that assumption.

Genetics

The Human Genome Project, funded by the National Institutes of Health and the Department of Energy, set a goal of mapping the twenty-three pairs of human chromosomes and sequencing the 3 billion nucleotide bases that make up the human genome. The aim of the project, according to Dr. Francis Collins, Director, was to "arm biomedical scientists with powerful gene-finding and DNA analysis tools to unravel and understand the myriad human diseases that have their roots, at least in part, in DNA."[52]

Using these tools, a researcher could track down the specific heritable causes of a genetically caused illness and had a much better chance of describing the genetic contribution to complex diseases. The tools were expected to lead to pharmacologic interventions for genetic disease and more precise screening tests for genetic disease.

Much of the challenge of genetics has been in dealing with the ethical, legal, and social implications.

Information Technology and the Internet

Electronic transmission of information provided potential for major improvements in disease surveillance and the ability to provide health alerts on disease outbreaks and health hazards. For example, in 1992 CDC—with funding from the Robert W. Woodruff Foundation—began developing the Information Network for Public Health Officials (INPHO) to create a new, integrated public health information system through advanced, electronic information tools including wide-area, connected networks; telecommunications; new software; and training.[53] In 1995, CDC's National Immunization Program funded tracking systems that supported state public health information systems. In 1999, CDC's Bioterrorism Preparedness and Response Program provided funding and technical assistance to thirty-seven state health agencies, three metropolitan health departments, and three Centers for Public Health Preparedness as part of Health Alert Network. The Health Alert Network was a nationwide, integrated information and communications system serving as a platform for distribution of health alerts, dissemination of prevention guidelines and other information, distance learning, national disease surveillance, and electronic laboratory reporting, bioterrorism alerts, and other initiatives to strengthen state and local preparedness.

Public health activities were funded largely through a variety of categorical grant programs, many of which had different data collection requirements, making integration of data difficult to achieve. CDC implemented the National Electronic Disease Surveillance System (NEDSS) to electronically integrate and link a wide variety of surveillance activities and facilitate more accurate and timely reporting of disease information.

The development of the Internet revolutionized the availability of technical medical information to the public. The National Library of Medicine (NLM) in Bethesda, Maryland, pioneered research on the uses of computer, communication, and audiovisual technologies to improve the organization, dissemination, and utilization of biomedical information. The library's major on-line database, MEDLINE, contained more than 10 million journal article references and abstracts going back to 1966. Other databases provided information on monographs, books, and audiovisual materials, and on such specialized subjects such as toxicology, environmental health, and molecular biology. Through the World Wide Web site www.nlm.nih.gov, by the end of the twentieth century some 250 million searches of MEDLINE were performed each year by health professionals, scientists, librarians, and the public. The NLM created a special Web site, MEDLINEplus, to link the general public to many sources of consumer health information.[54] The tremendous increase in activities related to information systems in public health resulted in the emergence of a new specialty area known as *public health informatics,* the systematic application of information and computer science and technology to public health practice, research, and learning.[55]

Conclusion

At the end of the twentieth century, public health was a complex partnership among federal agencies, state and local governments, nongovernment organizations, academia, and community members. In the twenty-first century, the success of the U.S. public health system will depend on its ability to change to meet new threats to the public's health.

Notes

1. Committee for the Study of the Future of Public Health, *The Future of Public Health* (Washington, DC: Institute of Medicine, 1988), p. 7.
2. George Rosen, *A History of Public Health* (New York: MD Publications, 1958), p. 1.
3. *Ibid.*, p. 25.
4. *Ibid.*, p. 188.
5. John J. Hanlon and George Pickett, *Public Health Administration and Practice*, 8th ed. (New York: Times Mirror/Mosby College Publishing, 1984), p. 30.
6. Fitzhugh Mullan, *Plagues and Politics: A History of the United States Public Health Service* (New York: Basic Books, 1989), p. 14.
7. Committee for the Study of the Future of Public Health, p. 31.
8. B. J. Turnock, *Public Health: What It Is and How It Works* (Gaithersburg, MD: Aspen, 1997), p. 140.
9. *Ibid.*, p. 155.
10. W. M. Tabb and L. Malone, *Environmental Law: Selected Statutes and Regulations*, 1997 ed. (Dayton, OH: Lexis Law Publishing, 1997); Turnock, p. 155.
11. R. Ahn, D. S. Gaylin, A. Keiller, et al., *Public Health Laboratories and Health System Change*, report prepared by The Lewin Group under the direction of the Office of the Assistant Secretary for Planning and Evaluation (ASPE), Department of Health and Human Services, Washington, D.C., October 6, 1997.
12. *Public Health Macroview* 7, no. 1 (Washington, DC: Public Health Foundation, 1997).
13. U.S. Environmental Protection Agency. Retrieved from the World Wide Web September 18, 2000: www.epa.gov/epahome/faq.htm#create
14. M. Maralit, T. Orloff, and R. Desonia, *Transforming State Health Agencies to Meet Current and Future Challenges*, paper presented to the National Governors' Association, Health Policy Studies Division, April 15, 1997, pp. 1–86.
15. Mullan, p. 55.
16. M. Terris, "Evolution of Public Health and Preventive Medicine in the United States," *American Journal of Public Health* 65 (1975), pp. 161–169.
17. J. W. Mountin and E. Flook, *Guide to Health Organizations in the United States, 1951*, PHS publication no. 196 (Washington, DC: Public Health Service, Federal Security Agency, Bureau of State Services, 1951).

18. National Association of County and City Health Officials (NACCHO), *Profile of Local Health Departments 1992–1993* (Atlanta: Centers for Disease Control and Prevention, 1995), p. 13.

19. Turnock, p. 160.

20. *Ibid.*, p. 157.

21. NACCHO, *Fact Sheet* (Washington, DC: NACCHO), 1991.

22. Turnock, p. 157.

23. NACCHO, *Profile*, p. 21.

24. *Ibid.*, p. 39.

25. R. B. Gerzoff and T. Richards, "The Education of Local Health Department Top Executives," *Journal of Public Health Management Practice 3*, no. 4, pp. 50–56.

26. National Association of Local Boards of Health (NALBOH), U.S. Department of Health and Human Services, *National Profile of Local Boards of Health* (Atlanta, GA: NALBOH, September, 1997), esp. pp. 6 and 7.

27. C. Brown, N. Rawding, and D. Custer, "Selected Characteristics of Local Health Departments—United States, 1992–1993," *Morbidity and Mortality Weekly Report 43*, no. 45 (November 18, 1994), pp. 838–843.

28. Centers for Disease Control and Prevention (CDC), "Achievements in Public Health, 1900–1999: Changes in the Public Health System," *Morbidity and Mortality Weekly Report 48*, no. 50 (December 24, 1999), pp. 1141–1147.

29. Turnock, p. 131.

30. *Ibid.*, p. 130.

31. Hanlon and Pickett, p. 274.

32. Retrieved from the World Wide Web, October 16, 2000: www.lectlaw.com/ def/ h001.htm.

33. F. Douglas Scutchfield and C. William Keck, *Principles of Public Health Practice* (New York: Delmar, 1997), pp. 46–53.

34. CDC, *Estimated Expenditures for Core Public Health Functions—Selected States, October 1992–September 1993* (Atlanta, GA: CDC, 1993).

35. G. P. Mays, *Organization of the Public Health Delivery System in Public Health Administration: Principles for Population-Based Management*, edited by L. F. Novick and G. P. Mays (Gaithersburg, MD: Aspen, 2000), p. 87.

36. Turnock, p. 158.

37. Committee for the Study of the Future of Public Health, p. 31.

38. W. W. Dyal, "Ten Organizational Practices of Public Health: A Historical Perspective," *American Journal of Preventive Medicine* 11 (Suppl. 2), pp. 6–8.

39. E. L. Baker et al., "Health Reform and the Health of the Public: Forging Community Health Partnerships," *JAMA 272*, no. 16, pp. 1276–1282.

40. *Ibid.*, p. 1280.

41. NACCHO, p. 53.

42. CDC, "Achievements in Public Health, 1900–1999."

43. W. Winkelstein and F. E. French, "The Training of Epidemiologists in Schools of Public Health in the United States: A Historical Note," *International Journal of Epidemiology* 2, pp. 415–416; Association of Schools of Public Health, *Annual Data Report* (Washington, DC: Association of Schools of Public Health, 1999).

44. CDC, "Achievements in Public Health, 1900–1999."

45. American Board of Preventive Medicine. Retrieved from the World Wide Web, September 13, 2000: www.abprevmed.org/.

46. National Environmental Health Association. Retrieved from the World Wide Web, September 13, 2000: www.neha.org/neha.html.

47. CDC, "Achievements in Public Health, 1900–1999."

48. Retrieved from the World Wide Web, October 17, 2000: www.harrisinteractive.com/harris_poll/index.asp?PID=32.

49. Division of Public Health Systems, *Environmental Scan of Privatization Activities in State and Selected Urban Health Departments*, unpublished report, Centers for Disease Control and Prevention, Atlanta, Georgia, April, 1996.

50. Baker et al.; J. A. Harell and E. L. Baker, "Essential Services of Public Health," *Leadership in Public Health* 3, no. 3 (1994), pp. 27–31.

51. L. Garrett, *Betrayal of Trust: The Collapse of Global Public Health* (New York: Hyperion, 2000).

52. F. Collins, "Statement on Genetic Testing in the New Millennium: Advances, Standards, Implications," before the House Committee on Science, Subcommittee on Technology, April 21, 1999. Retrieved from the World Wide Web, November 8, 2000: http://waisgate.hhs.gov/cgi-bin/waisgate?WAISdocID=310 6917274+38+0+0&WAISaction=retrieve.

53. K. Miner, M. Alperin, and C. Escoffery, *Lessons Learned From Georgia INPHO* (Atlanta, GA: Rollins School of Public Health, Emory University, May, 1996).

54. Retrieved from the World Wide Web, November 9, 2000: www.nlm.nih.gov/pubs/factsheets/nlm.html.

55. W. A. Yasnoff, P. W. O'Carroll, D. Koo, R. W. Linkins, and E. M. Kilbourne, "Public Health Informatics: Improving and Transforming Public Health in the Information Age," *Journal of Public Health Management Practice* 6, no. 6, pp. 67–75.

PART III

Public Health—Cases

Part III contains fifteen case studies that deal with a variety of public health management and leadership issues. The cases incorporate both the administrative disciplines (finance, marketing, human resources, information systems, and so on) and the core public health disciplines (epidemiology, biostatistics, health behavior, environmental health sciences, and health policy). Students will be required to draw on the theory and practice of all these disciplines to address the core issues and make the required decisions. Each of these cases presents students with an opportunity to make public health management and leadership decisions and develop a course of action for implementing their recommendations.

CDC and the Mantookan Blood Supply

A Tough Management Decision

Dan Hatcher had yet to make a decision concerning Jonathon Myongo. The meeting at which he would have to make the decision was due to begin in five minutes, and he still was not quite sure what he should do. He was good at working under pressure in difficult situations, and he had the reputation of being an effective, somewhat distant, but scrupulously fair manager. This decision, too, had to be completely fair, he knew. The difficulty lay in picking out the relevant information so that the right decision could be made. Dan had received input from all concerned parties via e-mail or phone. He had reviewed the policies and procedures. He had spoken with everyone except Jonathon, and in just a few minutes Jonathon would present his side of the story in person for the first time. What

would Jonathon say, Dan wondered, and would his words help to clarify the situation?

The Problem

The situation with Jonathon was first brought to Dan's attention on the afternoon of Wednesday, May 10, when he received a very unsettling e-mail:

From:	Foresyth, Dale
To:	Hatcher, Dan; Baker, Sten
Subject:	Blood transfusion related HIV in Mantooka
Date:	Wednesday, May 10, 1995 3:00 PM

Dan,

This in follow-up to your phone conversation with Sten Baker and me regarding the newspaper article that ap-

This case was prepared by Terrie C. Reeves, Texas Woman's University; Stuart A. Capper, University of Alabama at Birmingham; Arthur P. Liang, Centers for Disease Control and Prevention; and Gail W. McGee, University of Alabama at Birmingham. It is intended as a basis for classroom discussion rather than to illustrate effective or ineffective handling of an administrative situation. All rights reserved by the authors and the North American Case Research Association (NACRA). Copyright © 1999 by the *Case Research Journal* and Terrie Reeves, Stuart Capper, Arthur Liang, and Gail McGee. Used with permission from Stuart A. Capper and the *Case Research Journal*.

All the incidents in this case are real; however, all the names of individuals have been changed, and the name of the country involved in the case and its newspapers have been disguised. Throughout the case, all e-mail communication has been reproduced *verbatim*, including the spelling, grammar, and punctuation errors found in the originals, unless otherwise noted, but "CC" recipients' names are included in the e-mails only to the extent they are necessary to analyze the case. The reader may wish to have the organizational relationship charts in Exhibits 1-4 through 1-6 available to assist in identifying names in the case.

Exhibit 1-1. Dan Hatcher, MD

Dan Hatcher, MD, was the Director of the Epidemiology Program Office (EPO), one of the many offices and centers into which the Centers for Disease Control and Prevention (CDC) was divided (see the organizational chart in Exhibit 1-4). As the EPO Director, Dan reported directly to the Director of CDC, Dr. David Satcher, in the Office of the Director. Dan had been Director, EPO, since 1989, except for the two years he had spent at the National Center for Environmental Health.

Dan's EPO Office was responsible for some of the CDC services best known by the general public. For example, the EPO supervised the Epidemiologic Services (involved in prevention and control of epidemics in the United States), the coordination of CDC Surveillance Efforts (coordinated and analyzed public and private sector health data), the Epidemic Intelligence Service (EIS—trained applied epidemiology officers and sponsored the annual EIS conference), and the National Electronic Telecommunication System for Surveillance (provided transmission of data to all states and territories on infectious diseases). The EPO published the well-known *Morbidity and Mortality Weekly Report*. The EPO's Preventive Medicine Resident (PMR) program was less well known in the United States than some of the other programs in Dan's office, but it was important. Each year, the PMR program prepared thirty-two physicians and veterinarians from the United States and around the world for careers in general preventive medicine and public health in a two-year fully accredited residency program.

---

peared in the Mantookan papers "The Union" and "African Times." I have FAXed the article to you. As we explained, the article was written by Jonathon Myongo, who is Mantookan, and a CDC PMR stationed at the Georgia Dept. of Health. The basis of the article was Arturo Lorenzo's (our EIS officer) EIS conference presentation about our Mantookan blood transfusion study. The study documented HIV transmission from "screened" and unscreened blood. The results at the conference were preliminary and have not yet been published. They were due to be presented to the Minister of Health this week by our Mantookan collaborators. Afterwards, Jonathon Myongo asked Arturo on several occasions for more information, including confidential information such as the names of the hospitals where we did the study. Jonathon said that he just wanted to show some of the results to "friends in Mantooka." Arturo informed Jonathon that the information had not been presented to the Minister of Health and was preliminary. Fortunately, Arturo did not disclose further information. At no time did Jonathon say that the information was for a newspaper article.

The first we heard about the article was when it was FAXed to us by a CDC employee stationed in Mantooka who saw it in the newspaper. The article has been published in at least two Mantookan newspapers and referenced in another. We are extremely concerned about this because:

1. This jeopardizes our future collaboration with the Mantookan government. We have spent several years building trust with the Mantookans in order to do transfusion-related HIV work there. The Mantookans were trying to arrange funding to up-

grade their transfusion system through a USAID-Japanese collaboration and we had planned on evaluating the outcome. These plans may be hindered by this unauthorized release of information by a CDC employee. We also have a CDC field station in Mantooka which relies on the support of the Mantookan government.

2. CDC is mentioned numerous times throughout the article. At no time does it mention that we did the study in collaboration with WHO and the Mantookan government.

3. The article was extremely critical of the Mantookan government. This is extremely inappropriate for a CDC employee to be writing articles like this.

4. Jonathon tried to get additional confidential information from our EIS officer under false pretenses.

5. The article was not cleared through any channels.

Dan read the e-mail through twice. At the time, he thought "We have a problem. This could compromise the whole field program in Mantooka, and it could be real serious for Jonathon." Still, the e-mail seemed a bit "testy" to him, and he thought that he probably did not have the whole story. If decisions had to be made, he knew he would be the final arbiter, but he had good people working for him upon whose abilities he relied. He knew it was time to get them involved. He wanted input from the people who had the day-to-day responsi-

Exhibit 1-2. Sten Baker, MD

Sten Baker, MD, formerly Assistant Director of EPO, was thinking about the reorganization at CDC. He was now acting director of the groups coming together from other offices to form the new National Center for HIV, STD, and TB Prevention. People were nervous about the changes being made, and Sten was fully occupied with work concerning the reorganization. When Dale came to him with "the problem," his first thought was to calm an angry Dale and then to make sure that the appropriate people were informed. In his mind, four main issues were involved.

First was the ongoing viability of the Global Blood Safety (GBS) Project. Sten felt that the CDC had to preserve its role of technical assistance to Mantooka, and to contribute to the safety of the world's blood supply. Many African governments refused to admit that any of their citizens were HIV positive, yet Sten knew there was a high prevalence of HIV infection in several African countries. The objectives of the GBS Project could be summed up in three questions: First, were appropriate screens being used? Second, were appropriate transfusion methods being used, and were only the appropriate patients receiving transfusions? Third, was HIV being transmitted in the transfusion process? The GBS Project was important because blood safety was a major worldwide public health problem, because U.S. citizens abroad could be endangered, because it allowed CDC to track developments in the world's blood supply, and because it was a way for health professionals from CDC and from the host countries to develop expertise.

The second issue was the EIS conference and scientific protocol. CDC members viewed the conference as a training seminar where current and former EIS officers could present data of interest to the CDC community. The atmosphere at the conference tended to be "club-like" because all abstract presenters and most attendees were EIS members. Many participants thought of it as an "in-house" conference, but actually it was run like other scientific meetings, open to the public and the press. All involved were supposed to be fully informed before any data were presented or published in the conference proceedings. Most presenters hoped to have the results of their studies published in peer-reviewed scientific journals. Sten wanted to make sure that the Mantookan collaborators knew in advance what Arturo had included in the abstract and had agreed the material could be presented.

The third and fourth issues in Sten's mind concerned CDC and its operations. He felt that the way in which Jonathon represented himself at the EIS conference "broke the rules." PMRs were considered part of the EIS/CDC scientific community, but newspaper reporters were not members. Scientific papers were supposed to be cleared for publication through CDC. Even though he realized newspaper articles were in a "gray area," Sten thought Jonathon's articles should have been cleared because they were about HIV, and he considered articles about HIV to be scientific.

---

bility for running the PMR program, and from Jonathon himself. He composed a return e-mail to Dale that said:

From: Hatcher, Dan
To: Foresyth, Dale
Date: Wednesday, May 10, 1995

We will get on this right away. As I told Sten [Baker] [on the phone], the PMRs are in [Washington] DC this week, but I have spoken with Paula Davis and she will get to Stuart [Koeshi]. Thanks for bringing this to our attention.

Dan

Later that day, after several more phone calls, Dan composed another e-mail to Dale and Sten that said:

From: Hatcher, Dan
To: Foresyth, Dale; Baker, Sten
Date: Wednesday, May 10, 1995

Jonathon is in DC at the PMR meeting. I have spoken with Stuart and Joan as well as Darlene. I plan to meet with Jonathon on Monday unless a crisis arises before then. Could you fax the articles to me again, please? Thanks for letting me know about this serious issue. I am trying to keep this relatively quiet until I hear directly from Jonathon. I will keep you posted.

Dan

Dan certainly hoped no crisis would arise until he could speak with everyone involved.

Background

CDC

Walking into the Atlanta campus of the Centers for Disease Control and Prevention was a little like walking into another world. The language was filled with acronyms (see the glossary at the end of the case), and the prevailing attitudes appeared to be different from those in many other government agencies. The strong commitment to public health was apparent, but there was also a strong emphasis on scientific research and integrity. In addition, the organizational structure was quite complicated, and "dotted line" reporting relationships appeared frequently. (See Exhibit 1-3 for information on CDC, Exhibits 1-4 to 1-6 for CDC organization charts, and Exhibit 1-7 for information about the CDC preventive medicine residency.)

Mantooka*

Mantooka became an independent nation on December 12, 1963, and Monroe Fengattie, a member of the predominant Mikoku tribe and head of the Mantooka African National Union (MANU) became Mantooka's first president. The minority party dissolved itself voluntarily in 1964 and joined forces with MANU. However, by 1966, a small but significant leftist opposition party, the Mantooka People's Union (MPU), had emerged. After the assassination in 1969 of a government official and the resulting political unrest, the MPU was banned and its leaders detained. No new op-

position parties were formed, and at his death in 1978, Fengattie's party was the sole and ruling political party. Patrick Boyie became MANU leader, sole presidential nominee, and the new president. In June, 1982, the National Assembly amended the constitution, officially making Mantooka a one-party state. It was not until December 1991 that the constitution was again changed to allow more than one party, and by early 1992, several parties had been formed. During the December 1992 elections, President Boyie was reelected for another five-year term with about 45 percent of the parliamentary seats.

Since independence, Mantooka had remained remarkably stable politically. Despite an agenda of development, Boyie's government had pursued Africanization, but with significant participation of Asians and Europeans. Economic growth had declined since 1973 due to bad weather, inconsistent pricing and credit policies, inadequate marketing systems, periodic high inflation, a rapidly growing population (at 3.4 percent, one of the world's highest), and high unemployment (running about 30-40 percent). Pressure on social services had been intense, especially in the cities. However, the United States and Mantooka had enjoyed cordial relations, and Mantooka had been the recipient of about $350 million in U.S. direct investment, even though many companies found it difficult to transfer out dividends.

Chronological Sequence

Dan considered how he could best prepare for the meeting. He decided to arrange all the information he had in chronological order.

1989: U.S. Department of Health and Human Services issued Standards of Conduct, Personnel Pamphlet Series No. 6, March 30, 1989. Subpart F, Sections 73.735-601 through 603 dealt with Political Activities, and Subpart G, Sections 73.735-701 through 710 described Outside Activities. The CDC EIS guides referred employees to the appropriate Section in the Standards of Conduct.

---

*Although the names "Mantooka," "Monroe Fengattie," and "Patrick Boyie" are pseudonyms, all other information about the country is factual.

Exhibit 1-3. The Centers for Disease Control and Prevention (CDC)

The CDC was one of eight operating agencies in the U.S. Public Health Service (PHS). It was the focal point for national health and public safety. Headquartered in Atlanta, Georgia, the CDC developed from a World War II unit, the Malaria Control in War Areas Unit, which had the mission of protecting southeastern military bases and the southeastern part of the country from malaria epidemics. During those early years, the Communicable Disease Center, as it was first called, assisted state health departments with the control of communicable diseases when asked, but the responsibility for public health rested with the states. In 1951, during the period when concern about biological warfare was high, the Epidemic Intelligence Service (EIS) was created at the CDC. The EIS quickly became a resource to be assigned to the states or abroad in the event of an epidemic or disease outbreak. Throughout the 1950s and early 1960s, the CDC acquired broader responsibilities, including the administration of grants to the states for disease control. Gradually, in addition to the EIS collaborations, a pattern of collaboration developed whereby advisors recruited by the CDC were assigned to the states for work on a day-to-day basis.

The CDC had been instrumental in efforts to prevent malaria, poliomyelitis, smallpox, toxic shock syndrome, Legionnaires' disease, Lyme disease, and, recently, human immunodeficiency virus infection/acquired immunodeficiency syndrome (HIV/AIDS). It also worked to protect workers from environmental hazards and to prevent various chronic diseases and injuries. The CDC was charged with monitoring national disease trends and health statistics, conducting disease investigations and research, and supporting extramural research in disease and injury prevention. In addition, it provided various public health services at the local level.

The number of employees at the CDC grew from 369 in 1946 to approximately 5,600 in the mid-1990s. The budget had grown from $1,040,000 in 1946 to about $2.086 billion during the same time. HIV/AIDS prevention and immunizations were the two largest programs, together accounting for about 50 percent of the budget.

Exhibit 1-4. Centers for Disease Control Organization Chart

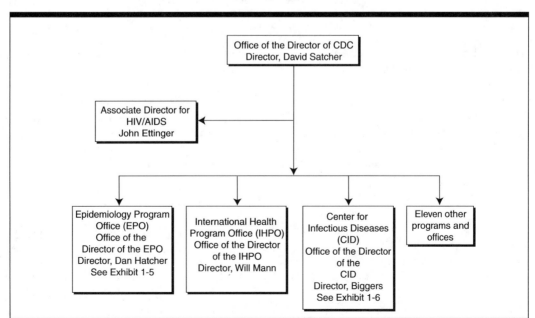

Exhibit 1-5. Epidemiology Program Office Organization Chart

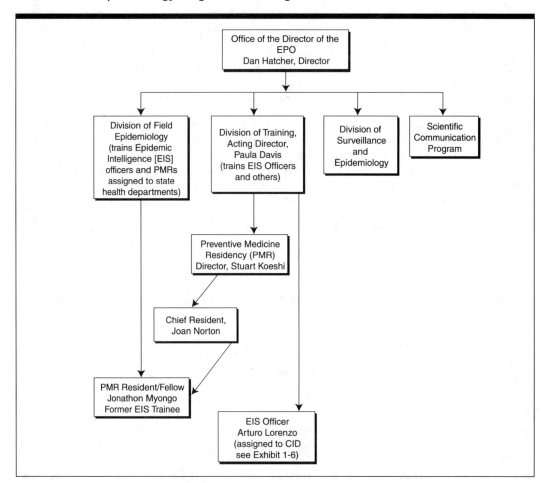

1995: CDC Human Resources policies, on writing and editing done as outside activities, required that "Appearance of governmental sanction or official support must not be expressed or implied in the material itself or advertising or promotional material . . . relating to the employee and the employee's contribution to the publication. . . . The employee may use his/her official title or position with the Department provided that the title is accompanied by a reasonably prominent disclaimer . . . [that the employee's writing was in his] private capacity." (CDC/ATSDR, September, 1995, *Human Resources Management Manual* [draft], CDC Guide to Outside Employment or Activity, p. 13; see Exhibit 1-8.)

March 27-31, 1995: EIS Conference in Atlanta, Georgia.

March 29, 1995: Arturo Lorenzo presented "Evaluation of HIV testing of the blood supply in 'Mantooka.'" Jonathon Myongo attended conference.

April 5, 1995: Arturo and Jonathon corresponded via e-mail.

Exhibit 1-6. Center for Infectious Diseases Organization Chart

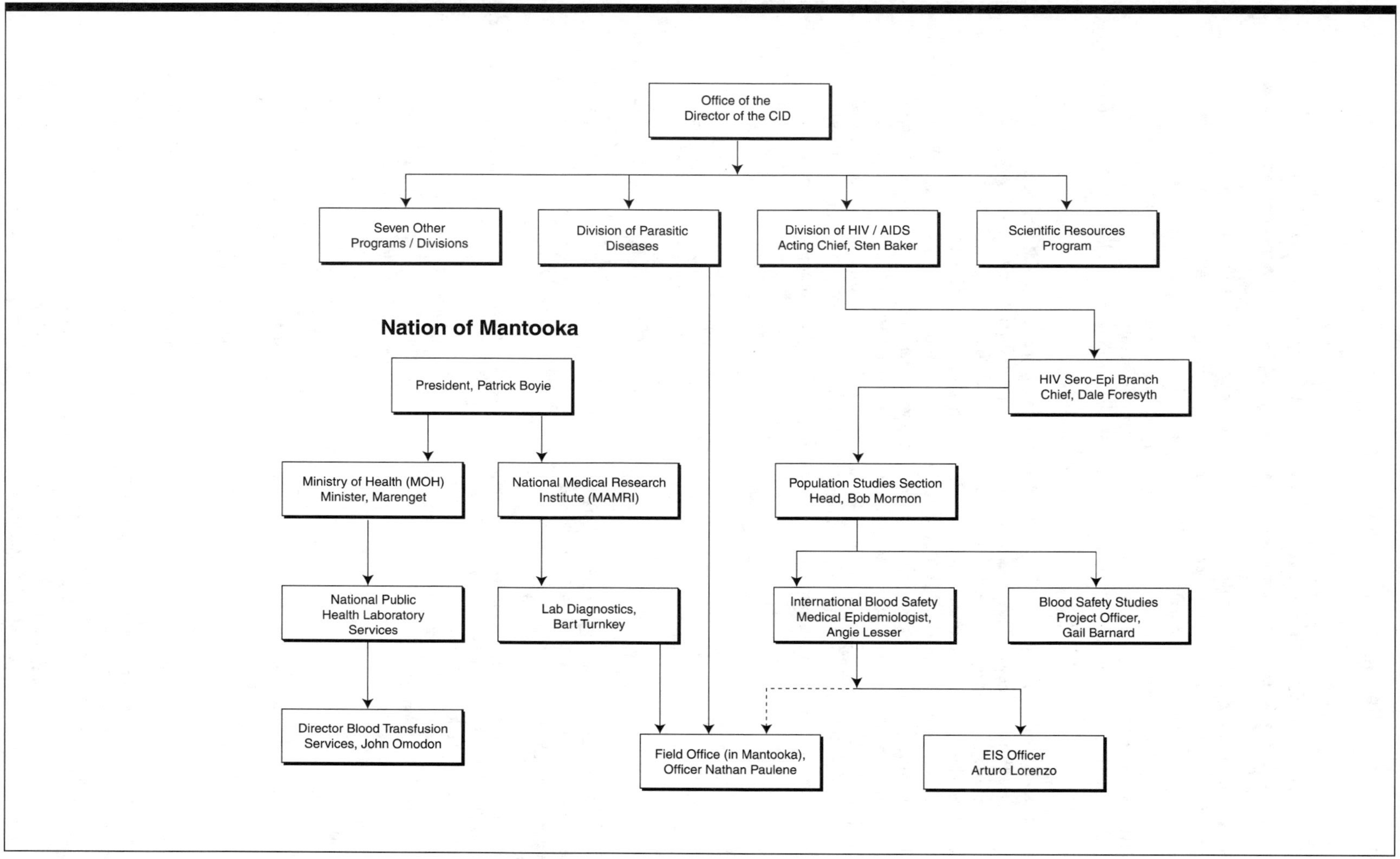

Exhibit 1-7. The CDC Preventive Medicine Residency (PMR)

Established in 1972, the CDC Preventive Medicine Residency Program, housed in the Epidemiology Program Office (EPO), had been fully accredited by the Accreditation Council for Graduate Medical Education since 1975. Its object was to prepare CDC clinicians for leadership roles in public health. The twelve-month program met the practicum year training requirements for certification by the American Board of Preventive Medicine in the General Preventive Medicine and Public Health specialty, one of the twenty-five recognized American Board of Medical Specialties. With a budget of about $1.2 million, the PMR program was one of the largest in the country.

Residents were typically drawn from the Epidemic Intelligence Service (EIS). Since its establishment in 1951, the EIS had trained health professionals in a two-year program for service in CDC, state, or local health departments as monitors and investigators of diseases of importance to the public, usually communicable diseases. The PMR program provided training beyond that given in the EIS. PMRs received both didactic and practical experience in epidemiology, statistics, behavioral and social sciences, leadership, administration, management, public health policy, and program development. Practical training was acquired at both CDC and at health departments; residents who were assigned to CDC as EIS officers were reassigned to a health department for training under the PMR program and vice versa. Most PMR graduates tended to work at CDC, many in positions of considerable authority and responsibility. Others went to state or local public health departments, or to academia. As of 1996, about 300 PMRs had completed the program.

Arturo,

I'm writing to request for a copy of your EIS presentation. Like I mentioned to you after your EIS talk, I would like to share your findings with some people in Mantooka who might not know what's going on but are in a position to move things much faster. When I was in Mantooka last summer, I initated a movement that is reforming healthcare as we speak. Your findings are a powerful testimony of what's wrong with the old system. I will keep you posted on what going on incase you are interested. Thanks

Jonathon

Arturo sent only the abstract, and Jonathon responded.

Arturo,

That's fine Arturo, the information on your abstract was good enough. I have just been wondering why the study was done in Western Mantooka and only in public hospitals. What is difficult to get the private hospitals to participate? Which hospitals did you do your study in and what's the hospital that didn't do tests despite the availability of kits? A friend of mine who was head of a district hospital in western Mantooka called me over the weekend from South Africa and said that he couldn't take it any more. He

decided that he was no longer ready to practice criminal medicine. Have the Mantookans received a copy of your report?

Jonathon

April 27, 1995: The first newspaper article appeared in Mantooka (Exhibit 1-11).

Tuesday, May 9, 1995: Dale Foresyth phoned Arturo Lorenzo to ask if additional information was given to Jonathon.

Wednesday, May 10, 1995: Dan Hatcher first became aware of the problem when he received e-mail from Dale Foresyth. Hatcher also received FAXed copies of newspaper articles and tried to contact Koeshi, who was in Washington, D.C., with the PMR residents.

Thursday, May 11, 1995: An e-mail was sent to Dan Hatcher and Stuart Koeshi, with copies to Baker, Foresyth, Mormon, and Lesser, concerning the impact of the articles in Mantooka.

From:	Barnard, Gail
To:	Hatcher, Dan; Koeshi, Stuart
CC:	Foresyth, Dale; Lesser, Angie; Mormon, Bob; Baker, Sten
Date:	Thursday, May 11, 1995 11:02 AM

Exhibit 1-8. CDC Policies on Outside Employment or Activity (relevant portions only)

1

DRAFT

CDC/ATSDR
Human Resources Management Manual
Chapter   , CDC Guide
Outside Employment or Activity

* Cover Note: In addition to guidance contained in this chapter, PHS Commissioned Officers
continue to be subject to the honoraria prohibition, 5 U.S.C. App. (Ethics in Government
Act of 1978), which prohibits an employee from receiving any compensation for an
appearance, speech or article, even if unrelated to official duties. Implementing regulations
are contained in 5 C.F.R. §§2636.201 through 2636.205.

* 3/1/96 - The Department of Justice will not be enforcing the Honoraria Ban against any
employee (including those in the Commissioned Corps). Therefore, all employees may now
receive honoraria for outside work, including any which had been in escrow.

DRAFT: 9/04/95

DRAFT

13

capacity and the views expressed are his/her own and do not necessarily represent the
views of the CDC, the Department, or the Federal Government.
b. Writing and Editing. Employees are encouraged to engage in outside writing and editing
whether or not done for compensation, when such activity is not otherwise prohibited.
The OGE Standards prohibit compensation for writing related to official duties, as
outlined in the NOTE in E.2. above.

In addition, to restrictions on all outside activities outlined in F.1. below, the following
conditions apply to writing and editing done as an outside activity:
– – Appearance of governmental sanction or official support must not be expressed or
implied in the material itself or advertising or promotional material (including
book jackets and covers), relating to the employee and the employee's
contribution to the publication.
– – The employee may use his/her official title or position with the Department
provided that the title is accompanied by a reasonably prominent disclaimer. The
disclaimer shall read as follows, unless an alternative is approved by the
Assistant General Counsel, Business and Administrative Law Division, Office of
the General Counsel:
* (This (article, book, etc.) was (written, edited) by (employee's name) in (his,
her) private capacity. No official support or endorsement by (name of
operating component of Department) is intended or should be inferred.

DRAFT: 9/04/95

Exhibit 1-9. The EIS Conference Abstract

Wednesday, March 29, 1995

2:15 Evaluation of HIV Testing of the Blood Supply in Mantooka

Arturo H. Lorenzo, A. Lesser, B. Mormon, J. Omodon, N. Paulene, S. Pound, M. Johnson, G. Barnard

Background: Blood transfusions account for an estimated 10 percent of all human immunodeficiency virus (HIV) infections in Africa. To identify ways to prevent transmission of HIV through blood transfusions, we evaluated current blood screening practices in Mantooka.

Methods: From April through September 1994, we collected demographic and laboratory data on all blood donors in five government hospitals in western Mantooka and one in the capital city of Port Mara. Blood donations were tested for HIV-1 by the hospitals in Mantooka and later by CDC. CDC supplied test kits when kits were unavailable.

Results: Of the 1,835 blood donations, 114 (6 percent) tested HIV positive at CDC. Because of the lack of HIV test kits at the national level, five hospitals used CDC test kits for 4 weeks of the study period. In the only hospital that had kits supplied by Mantooka throughout the study period, 44 (36 percent) of 121 donations were not screened; of these, 10 (23 percent) tested positive for HIV at CDC. Of the 114 donations testing positive at CDC, 86 (75 percent) were positive by screening in Mantooka. Overall, 28 (25 percent) of the 114 HIV-positive donations were transfused.

Conclusions: The unacceptably high risk of HIV transmission by transfusion in Mantooka would be decreased by (1) better procurement and distribution of test kits, (2) adherence by blood bank personnel to universal screening of donors, and (3) improved laboratory techniques.

We spoke with Dr. Nathan Paulene in Mantooka this morning, and I wanted to update you on issues related to the newspaper article that was written by Jonathon Myongo.

As you may know, the CDC field station is run in collaboration with the Mantooka Medical Research Institute (MAMRI). During a meeting of the MAMRI publications committee, the topic of the newspaper article was raised. MAMRI was concerned about the way CDC was disseminating information about their studies. MAMRI will be writing a letter of inquiry to Nathan Paulene, who is the director of the CDC field station.

We have not been able to contact our Mantookan collaborator today. He has been in meetings with the Ministry of Health, probably due to issues related to this article. We will continue to attempt to contact him to explain CDC's role in the article. We will also be calling individuals within MAMRI directly.

It is apparent that an official letter of explanation and apology by CDC will need to be written. This will also be important so that this issue does not undermine the upcoming visits to Mantooka by Drs. Satcher [the Director of CDC], Biggers, and Marksmann in June and July. Thank you for your attention to this matter.

Friday, May 12, 1995: The activity levels increased by this day, with almost all of the major players becoming more deeply involved. During the day, all of Stuart Koeshi's e-mails to Dan were forwarded to Dale.

Paula Davis, Stuart Koeshi's boss at CDC, and Joan Norton, the Chief Resident of the PMR Program, were alerted to the problem, and both women tried to get as much information about the situation as possible. Joan dug out all the CDC policies concerning outside publications that had been given to the PMR students at the beginning of their program. None of them seemed very clear to her (see Exhibits 1-8 and 1-12).

Jonathon was asked about the incident for the first time since his articles appeared.

The Mantookan government held a press conference, carried on the national media, denying the presence of HIV in the nation's blood supply

Exhibit 1-10.   Arturo Lorenzo

Arturo Lorenzo and Angie Lesser, both EIS officers, were the Principal Investigators on the GBS program in Mantooka. They had designed the study and had traveled to Mantooka to establish it; Arturo was first author and had presented the abstract at the EIS conference meetings. Arturo first spoke to Jonathon about Jonathon's interest in the findings on the day of the presentation, Wednesday, March 29. At that time, Jonathon had told Arturo that the information in his abstract might end up in a newspaper article.

On April 5, Arturo received an e-mail from Jonathon requesting a copy of the abstract. He thought Jonathon had asked for some information that might be confidential, and he knew the Mantookan government was concerned about complete confidentiality. However, the EIS abstract had been cleared by the Mantookan authorities: John Omodon was a Mantookan Ministry of Health official, and Nathan Paulene was the CDC Liaison Officer "on the ground" in Mantooka in charge of the CDC research station. So Arturo discussed the issue with Bob Mormon, the supervisor of the study group, who handled things such as personnel issues, and they had decided to tell Jonathon that they could give out only the information contained in the presentation and in the abstract.

(despite the CDC's findings) and naming the hospitals in which the studies were done.

Gail Barnard also communicated with Bart Turnkey at MAMRI in Mantooka.

From: Barnard, Gail
To: Foresyth, Dale; Lesser, Angie; Mormon, Bob;
         Lorenzo, Arturo
CC: Paulene, Nathan
Subject: Discussions with Dr. Turnkey
Date: Friday, May 12, 1995 9:52 AM

I talked with Dr. Turnkey this morning to explain what had happened regarding the article in the "Union." He recommended that we compose a letter of explanation to MAMRI about Arturo's presentation, along with a copy of his talk. He was concerned about the way that the information was presented. What seems to have happened is that people are reporting that 25 percent of all transfusions are infectious, instead of 25 percent of the positives. They are going to get a "science writer" to write a clarification of the article, and wanted more information. I asked if we could be involved in this response to ensure accuracy, but he didn't really respond to that request.

Angie, are you available to draft a letter of explanation? Turnkey recommended that the letter come from Angie, since she is viewed as Arturo's supervisor in-country. Let me know who you think this letter should be from.

I also told him that we wanted to eventually write a letter to the ministry. He said that was appropriate and that the letter should be sent to the Director of Medical Services. That

is another issue that we should bring up with John [Omodon] when we talk with him.

In general, I felt Turnkey understood what happened and didn't seem to be blaming us, and didn't feel this would jeopardize CDC's work with MAMRI, but that things needed to be dealt with.

Gail

* * * * * * * * * * * * * * * * * * * *

From: Mormon, Bob
To: Foresyth, Dale
CC: Lesser, Angie; Barnard, Gail; Lorenzo, Arturo
Subject: Blood transfusion related HIV in Mantooka
Date: Friday, May 12, 1995 11:43 AM

Dale,

Angie, Arturo and I spoke with John Omodon, Head of the [Mantookan] National Public Health Laboratory Service this morning. He is our collaborator on the blood safety study in Mantooka. John spent much of the last three days meeting with the Minister of Health, Hoshie Marenget, and his staff. The government held a press conference in Port Mara yesterday that was carried by TV, radio, and was published in the newspaper. I put a copy of the article about the press conference from the "Union" in your mailbox. You can see in the article that the Minister's response was that there was no HIV in the blood supply. The article goes on to give more detailed results from the study including releasing the names of the hospitals that participated in the study. Much of the data in the article seems to be incorrect but came from data we sent to John. John engineered the press conference. The issue is not rapidly

Exhibit 1-11.   Newspaper Article Submitted for Publication by Jonathon Myongo

---

Date: 27th April 1995
To: Tom Mashindi, "Nation Newspapers"
CC: Joseph Odino

By Dr. Jonathon Myongo, P.O. Box 00000, Atlanta, GA 30000
Tel: 404-123-4467 Fax: 404-123-5678

Although most scientists agree that the principal route of HIV transmission in sub-Saharan Africa is through heterosexual intercourse in the general population, between 10-15% of HIV infections are still acquired though blood transfusion. Whereas the behavioral risk factors for heterosexual HIV transmission continue to baffle scientists worldwide due to the complex factors associated with human behavior, the risk of acquiring HIV through blood transfusion has been virtually eliminated in other parts of the world since the discovery of an HIV test in March 1985. In Mantooka, where every ninth adult is HIV-infected in some urban areas according to the latest report from the National AIDS Control Program, and most politicians, including the head of state, agree that HIV prevention is a national priority, the easier options are still quite elusive.

Could Prince Charles, the heir to the British throne, have been right when he carried his own blood supply on a trip to Mantooka a few years ago? At the time, skeptics dismissed the matter as typical western arrogance and paranoia towards Africa. Maybe not. In a study done by Dr. Arturo Lorenzo and others of the Federal Centers for Disease Control and Prevention (CDC) in the United States and presented at the recent 44th Annual Epidemic Intelligence Service Conference at the CDC in Atlanta, the blood supply in Mantooka is very much contaminated. The findings of the study, which evaluated all the blood that was donated in five government hospitals in western Mantooka and the Mantookan National Hospitals between April and September 1994, are quite disturbing. Fifteen years into the Acquired Immunodeficiency Syndrome (AIDS) epidemic and ten years after a Human Immunodeficiency Virus (HIV) test was discovered, blood contaminated with HIV is still being transfused to the unsuspecting public in Mantooka.

When the blood samples were re-tested for HIV at the CDC laboratories using a similar test done in Mantooka and confirmed by a more advanced test, it was found that the Mantookan laboratory technicians missed one quarter of the infected blood which was all transfused as HIV-negative blood. In one hospital, 36% of the blood donations were not screened despite the availability of the HIV screening kits and, when these blood samples were re-tested at CDC, 23% carried the AIDS virus. For four weeks during the study period, there was a lack of HIV test kits nationwide, and emergency kits had to be flown from CDC to save the situation.

The high risk of HIV transmission through blood transfusion in Mantooka is unacceptable. Previous studies have estimated that blood transfusion accounts for up to 10% of all HIV infections in sub-Saharan Africa. In some areas where blood transfusion is more common due to malaria and other infection, the risk is much higher. The Ministry of Health should have learned from what happened in the United States, Germany and France several years ago.

When the HIV test was discovered in March of 1985, it took the U.S. Red Cross, the sole administrator of the blood supply in the United States, a few months to incorporate the new test as part of its screening program. This was a deadly mistake. The delay meant that some people were transfused infected blood when the Red Cross knew that a test was available and did nothing to protect the supply during that short period. The Red Cross was taken to court and ordered to pay millions of dollars in compensation to the victims. In France and Germany, where the delay was much longer than in the United States, the two governments took responsibility for the crimes committed against the public. Those in charge of the blood supply were sued for negligence, betrayal of public trust, and committing crimes against the public. As is typical in civilized societies, they paid dearly for their negligent actions. One wonders why, ten years later, HIV transmission through blood transfusion still occurs in Mantooka when it has been eliminated in most rich and poor countries. Since the blood bank serves both the government and the private hospitals nationwide, and due to constant exchange of blood between private and government hospitals, no hospital can be said to have a safe blood supply.

Exhibit 1-11.   Continued

These findings raise fundamental questions. Is the Government so poor that it cannot train laboratory technicians or improve laboratory techniques? Why is recordkeeping so poor that most records are torn, burnt, or simply missing? Why is the system so poor that children are often transfused their mother's blood which is not tested for HIV even in areas where previous studies have shown a 20-30% HIV infection rate among women of child bearing age? A mother who is infected with HIV has only a 20-25% chance of infecting her child during pregnancy, while if her blood is transfused to her child, the efficiency of HIV transmission is almost 100%. Don't these children who may not have been infected by the HIV-infected mothers deserve a chance in life? Why should a country go for one month without HIV test kits? Should the Mantookan hospitals be trusted? In simple economics, it's cost-effective for the health care system to invest M$ 100.00 to screen a unit of blood to eliminate HIV transmission through blood transfusion in the first place instead of spending M$ 27,200.00 to take care of one patient during the course of their AIDS illness. Prince Charles may have been right: when visiting Mantooka, don't take a risk; carry your own blood supply.

---

going away, since John had just finished meeting with journalists when we called today.

The major concern of the Minister was the premature release of data before he was made aware of it. In addition, the Minister questioned using the newspaper as a way to disseminate preliminary data. Finally, the Minister was very upset about the tone of the article. They want to know why Jonathon wrote the article. The Ministry of Health is planning on writing two letters. One letter which will be written next week will be drafted by the Director of Medical Services for Mantooka and, John thinks, signed by the Minister of Health. It is not clear who it will be sent to, but I think it will be sent to us since we conducted the study. The letter will primarily concern the avenue of release and want clarification from Jonathon as to why this happened. We will talk to John next week and get a little more explicit information before the letter comes. The second letter will go from the Mantooka Medical Research Institute to Nathan Paulene again inquiring about releasing data in this way. Nathan will fax us that letter when he receives it.

Finally, John suggested that we should write a letter to the Minister of Health explaining the circumstances of the data release, that this is not the way CDC operates. I agree with John, but it is unclear to me when such a letter should be sent to the Minister. It seems we should be proactive and respond to the article before we hear from the Minister. That would help demonstrate our good faith in this situation. On the other hand, if a letter is coming from the Minister, maybe we should wait. I don't know what is best. My feeling is that we should send a letter to the Minister of Health before we receive their letter. I don't feel that Jonathon's motives are our concern. What is our concern is the fact that preliminary CDC data were released to a newspaper by a person who did not conduct the study and who did not go through official clearance procedures. The newspaper article was not sanctioned by CDC. The final thing is who should sign such a letter. We certainly can

draft a letter, but it seems someone above us should be signing a letter to a Minister of Health.

Also take a look at Gail's e-mail about Bart Turnkey. He is a virologist at MAMRI.

Bob

* * * * * * * * * * * * * * * * * * * *

From: Foresyth, Dale
To: Hatcher, Dan; Baker, Sten
Subject: FW: Blood transfusion related HIV in Mantooka
Date: Friday, May 12, 1995 12:27 PM
Priority: High

Dan,

The newspaper article that we discussed seems to be creating an international incident that looks bad for CDC. The newspaper article was published in a newspaper that circulates in Uganda, Tanzania, and Mantooka. The article has had major repercussions in Mantooka with the Minister of Health having to hold a press conference. As you can see from the email [above], the Ministry is very upset with the way CDC has released these data. Our feeling is that some damage control by CDC needs to be done today. I will discuss this with Sten Baker in the next hour or so. I am faxing you more articles from the front page of "The Union."

Dale

* * * * * * * * * * * * * * * * * * * *

From: Hatcher, Dan
To: Foresyth, Dale
Subject: RE: Blood transfusion related HIV in Mantooka
Date: Friday, May 12, 1995 1:25 PM

Exhibit 1-12. Summary of Political Activity Restrictions (relevant portions only)

HRM BULLETIN

Human Resources Management Office   To all CDC & ATSDR Employees

SUMMARY OF POLITICAL ACTIVITY RESTRICTIONS

No. BN-96-2
March 25, 1996

SUMMARY OF POLITICAL ACTIVITY RESTRICTIONS
UNDER THE
HATCH ACT REFORM AMENDMENTS OF 1993
AND IMPLEMENTING REGULATIONS

Public Law 103-94, 107 Stat. 1001 (October 6, 1993)
Subchapter III of Chapter 73, Title 5, United States Code (5 U.S.C. §§7321-7326)
59 Fed. Reg. 5313 (February 3, 1994) (5 C.F.R. Part 733)
59 Fed. Reg. 48765 (September 23, 1994) (5 C.F.R. Part 734)

COVERED EMPLOYEES

The new law applies to all Department employees, including Senate confirmed Presidential appointees, non-career SES officials, Schedule C employees, career competitive and excepted service employees, and detailees under the Intergovernmental Personnel Act, submit to the following exceptions:

Career Senior Executive Service employees and Administrative Law Judges remain subject to the original version of the Act and to the additional prohibitions contained in the new law and part 734, subpart D of the implementing regulations. By Departmental regulation at 45 C.F.R. part 73, subpart F, Commissioned Corps officers are subject to standard equivalent to the old law.

U.S. Department of Health and Human Services
Centers of Disease Control & Prevention
Agency for Toxic Substances and Disease Registry

(Continued)

I got the fax. Stuart was to speak with Jonathon this morning but he did not appear to the PMR meeting [in Washington, D.C.]. Stuart is trying to find him. As you know, Darlene and I plan to see him on Monday. Mildred and OGC [Office of the General Council] have been notified. Let me know if Sten thinks we need to do more before Monday.

Dan

* *

From: Foresyth, Dale
To: Hatcher, Dan
Subject: Jonathon Myongo
Date: Friday, May 12, 1995 3:35 PM

Dan,

One of Jonathon's medical school class mates that works with the CDC field station in Mantooka informed our CDC personnel that Jonathon while still in Mantooka wrote inflammatory articles to the newspapers about other issues such as doctor's strikes and was viewed in Mantooka as a "loose cannon." They also thought he may have political ambitions with the opposition party. They said that he never finished his internship. I don't know if this latter information is true, but you may want to look into it. Please keep this information confidential

Dale

* *

Exhibit 1-12.   Continued

PAGE 3 - SUMMARY OF POLITICAL ACTIVITY RESTRICTIONS

- Join as an <u>active</u> member, or <u>serve as an officer</u>, of a political party, organization, or club. (If serving as an officer, particularly treasurer, an employee must not personally solicit, accept, or receive political contributions. Handling, disbursing, or accounting for funds duly received by others, however, is permitted.)

- <u>Initiate</u>, <u>circulate</u>, or sign nominating petitions.

- Campaign for or against referendum questions, constitutional amendments, and municipal ordinances.

- Distribute and display campaign literature, badges, buttons, stickers, signs, and other materials. (Bumper stickers may be displayed on autos parked at work, but must be covered if the vehicle is used on official duty.)

- <u>Stuff envelopes with campaign literature that includes an appeal for contributions</u>.

- <u>Make campaign speeches</u>.

- <u>Organize and participate in phone banks and voter preference surveys or opinion polls</u> (but no solicitation of funds even anonymously).

- <u>Solicit contributions from non-subordinate employees for the political action committee of a federal labor or employee organization to which the soliciting employee and donor both belong</u>.

- Run as a candidate for public office in nonpartisan elections.

- Run as an independent candidate only in local partisan races in areas designated by the Office of Personnel Management as partially-exempt communities based on a high concentration of federal employees.

(Continued)

From: Foresyth, Dale
To: Hatcher, Dan
CC: Baker, Sten; Mormon, Bob
Subject: Dr. Myongo, Mantooka
Date: Friday, May 12, 1995 5:43 PM

Dan,

We have spoken to John Ettinger and Wil Mann. Wil thinks a letter for Dr. Satcher explaining that this was an unauthorized article needs to be sent to the Minister of Health in Mantooka. We have drafted a letter and will send it through the proper channels on Monday. As soon as it clears with Dr. Ettinger, we will send you a copy.

Dale

* *

From: Koeshi, Stuart P.
To: Hatcher, Dan
CC: Norton, Joan; Davis, Paula A.
Subject: Monday mtg.
Date: Friday, May 12, 1995 11:11 PM
Priority: High

Jonathon and I spoke at length about the situation. Jonathon writes articles periodically for Mantookan newspapers, and he did write the articles in question. He said he wrote the articles in order to get the Ministry of Health to change the transfusion policies. Based on past experience, he felt that writing directly to the Ministry would have had no effect. According to Jonathon, he only reported the results that were in Arturo's abstract. He said he did not mention anything from his conversations with Arturo. He did not try to represent himself as a CDC employee in the article; and he did not identify hospitals or individuals. I indicated to him that his motivations were understandable,

Exhibit 1-12. Continued

- PAGE 5 - SUMMARY OF POLITICAL ACTIVITY RESTRICTIONS

- Solicit, accept, or receive political contributions from the general public. (Canvassing groups, businesses, or corporations to seek funds or contributions of paid or unpaid personal services for political purposes is prohibited. However, soliciting uncompensated volunteer services—as opposed to funds—from an individual who is not a subordinate is permitted, if done off-duty, off-premises, and without the specified indicators of a governmental connection.)

- Wear a partisan political button or display a partisan sticker or poster while on government premises or while engaged in official duty. (An employee's car with political bumper stickers affixed may be parked during the workday in an agency garage or a federally subsidized private parking lot. However, if the car is used for official travel, the sticker must be covered.)

- Participate in phone bank solicitations for political contributions, even if done anonymously. (However, stuffing envelopes with printed requests for political contributions is permitted.)

- Sign campaign letters that include solicitations for political contributions.

- Sell tickets or collect money for a fundraiser.

- Host a political fundraiser at home. (However, a spouse who is not a covered federal employee may organize such an event, and the employee may attend. Additionally, an employee may organize an at-home event not intended for fundraising purposes, such as an opportunity to "meet and greet" the candidate.)

- Permit the use of the employee's name as a sponsor, member of an inviting committee, or point of contact for a fundraising event. (An employee's name, though not official title, may appear on an invitation to a political fundraiser as a guest speaker, as long as the reference in no way suggests that the employee solicits or encourages contributions.)

but that he should have made it clear to Arturo that he was wearing the "journalist's hat," and that he had informed someone at CDC that he was intending to write an article as a "private" citizen. (If the EIS conference is open to the public, I guess he would have the right to "report" on what was presented?)

At any rate, I told him that the situation was serious and might result in some disciplinary action. He will be in your office at 4 o'clock on Monday.

A thought about disciplinary action, we need to think carefully about what should be done. It might be worse for CDC if the headlines read "Mantookan physician fired because of CDC blood transfusion cover-up."

Stuart

Saturday, May 13, 1995: Dan and Stuart corresponded via e-mail. Stuart also communicated with the Epidemiology scientists. He was very concerned that the whole situation could get out

of control both within CDC and between Mantooka and CDC. He also saw that a discrepancy existed between his impressions and the impressions of Bob and Dale as to who was the "injured party," if there was an injured party. How could it be a question of scientific integrity when Jonathon did not claim the scientific work as his own? Further, Jonathon had not even signed the articles as a CDC employee or member, and there did not appear to be any inaccuracies in the article. The more he thought about it, the more he thought that there were no "black hats" in the situation, only people wearing various shades of gray.

From:	Hatcher, Dan
To:	Koeshi, Stuart
Subject:	Monday Mtg.
Date:	05-13-95 07:38

Exhibit 1-13.   Stuart Koeshi

Stuart Koeshi, MD, MPH, the Director of the Preventive Medicine Residency Program, was in Washington, D.C., with the residents when his boss, Dan, first got the e-mail and the FAXed articles from Dale. He had missed the early e-mail correspondence, but by Friday morning he was well aware of the situation.

Stuart's responsibility was to oversee the residency program, a two-year training program which involved one year at CDC and one year at an internship position for each of the residents. He was deeply committed to providing a complete education for the PMR students, an education that would serve both the students and their countries and states well in the future, an education that would provide them both with the public health understanding and tools they would need, and with management skills to help implement programs in the public sector. Any disciplinary problems among the residents while they were at the CDC would be Stuart's responsibility, but after the first year, the residents officially reported to their internship supervisors.

Jonathon's class, now in its second year, had given Stuart many sleepless nights, but not because of discipline problems: the year they entered, the U.S. Government had enforced a hiring freeze. Residents, who were usually put on the CDC payroll, could not become CDC employees during this year because of the freeze. The incoming students who were not already on the CDC payroll had to be paid as "fellows" that year. That meant that Jonathon was not officially "employed" by the CDC, and that he, therefore, was not protected by the U.S. EEOC laws which made it impossible to summarily fire an individual without warning.

Stuart was also committed to complete scientific integrity. He wondered if scientific integrity only included doing the research or whether scientific integrity also included dissemination of findings. When should findings be made public? What did it mean when findings were "made public"? He wondered to whom the results of scientific inquiry "belonged." When the people doing the research were employees of the nation's central public health entity, did results "belong" to the public?

So what is your recommendation?

DH

* * * * * * * * * * * * * * * * * * * *

From: Koeshi, Stuart
To: Hatcher, Dan
Subject: Monday Mtg.
Date: Saturday, May 13, 1995 9:38 AM

Let me think about this more, but perhaps a letter of apology from Myongo to Dr. Satcher and perhaps one to Lorenzo for misrepresenting himself. We may also need to suspend with/without pay for two weeks or something else that we can report to the Ministry of Health. Let me think about this some more.

Stuart

* * * * * * * * * * * * * * * * * * * *

From: Koeshi, Stuart
To: Hatcher, Dan
Subject: Monday Mtg.
Date: Saturday, May 13, 1995 1:44 PM

Dan,

After re-reading the messages that you sent [Dan had sent all of the e-mail correspondence to Stuart] (I have not seen Jonathon's article or the MOH rebuttal), it seems to me that CDC has at least two problems. One is the relationship with the Mantookan government and the MOH, but the other is with the general public. HIV is such a hot issue, people could easily ask why did CDC wait so long to inform the MOH about the blood supply. "What did we know; and when did we know it?!" The public will not understand the notion of preliminary data and concern about future relations with Mantooka unless we explain it to them. In the current climate, we may be viewed as the typical plodding bureaucracy at best and covering up at worst. We don't want to be seen as being more concerned about our research or the bureaucracy than the people of Mantooka. I think CDC needs to be prepared to answer this question if anyone asks.

If this is getting so much press in Africa, we need to alert our public affairs people in case CNN or BBC international pick up on this (this is probably obvious and done already). Further, WHO and CDC needs to think about what it will do now that the MOH has denied there HIV in the blood

Exhibit 1-14. Jonathon Myongo

Jonathon, a native Mantookan, was one of the physicians chosen to be in the PMR Program from countries outside the United States. During his early days in the Program, he had told Joan Norton a bit about his family in Mantooka: his brother had died of AIDS, and he thought the Mantookan government was not taking the HIV virus seriously enough. While the government spent money on fruitless development projects, health care services in Mantooka had deteriorated over the past several years, he believed. He thought his training could help to ensure that health care in Mantooka would be upgraded in the future.

Jonathon was sorry to have caused problems, but he was also confused: he thought that part of his EIS training had been to tell and take action when he saw public health problems. After his Friday discussion with Stuart, Jonathon returned to Atlanta from Washington, D.C., and spent some time composing an e-mail to Dan Hatcher because he knew Dan would make the final decision.

---

supply. I am told the Mantooka government is known for its corruption. We don't want to be seen as being on their side. If they try to cover this up it will be a vindication of Jonathon's approach. It might not hurt to have some kind of action plan in place so that we maintain our credibility around our interest in people's health.

If Jonathon was operating as a private person and only reporting information in the public domain, I agree that CDC should not try to explain his motivations. We simply need to state that this was done without our knowledge or approval, outside the bounds of our policies and that disciplinary actions are being taken. If we write too early, it may seem like we knew all this was happening. It would be better for us to seem—as we were—out of the Myongo loop.

Finally, as to what to do about Jonathon, I think he needs to be impressed with all the ramifications of what he has done. It wouldn't hurt to show him all the e-mails at some point. In the end, he may get the blood supply cleaned up, but it will be at the cost of CDC and WHO's ability to do good in Mantooka in the future, not to mention the amount of staff he has tied up. Has HHS gotten hold of this? It will also be at some cost to him individually. He needs to make an apology to Arturo and Dr. Satcher, perhaps higher if this gets higher. Perhaps, he needs to be suspended "pending further investigation" if you think we need to say this the Mantookan officials. If we believe Jonathon has acted in good faith, but out of ignorance, I would stop with a reprimand and the letter of apologies. If we think we need to take stronger action, I would suspend him for some period of time. I would not dismiss him. He has the moral "high ground;" our major concerns are "bureaucratic;" we will lose if this gets into the press.

. . . I think he realizes now that there are consequences of this that he did not think about. A dismissal may alienate him from CDC. Right now, I think he is sorry and ready to work with us; and we might actually need some of his press contacts and cultural insights to help us get out of this situation. What do you think?

Stuart

* *

From: Hatcher, Dan
To: Koeshi, Stuart
Subject: Mantooka
Date: Saturday, May 13, 1995 3:02 PM

Tough to say. So far every one I have spoken to says we must dismiss him for a variety of reasons, most having little to do with the Mantookan government.
We can discuss.

DH

Also on May 13, Jonathon e-mailed Dan to explain his position.

From: Myongo, Jonathon
To: Hatcher, Dan
CC: Koeshi, Stuart
Subject: From Jonathon Myongo
Date: 05-13-95 04:00 EST
Priority: R

I met with Dr Koeshi last night and he informed me about the reactions to my article which appered in the Mantookan newspapers.

I would like to give my side of the story.

I'm a regular contributor to the "African Times" and the "Union" on medical issues. I wrote the article as part of my regular contribution and secondly because of the impact transfusion HIV has had on my family in western Mantooka where Dr Lorenzo did his study. One of my family members acquired HIV through blood transfusion two years ago. His hopes of becoming a lawyer were all shattered.

The article I wrote which I will show you at our scheduled meeting on Monday was not prompted by the EIS conference but it's something I have been planning for a while. Thus Dr Lorenzo's EIS abstract was only a reference material. Most of the article was based on my experience in Mantooka as a doctor. Since EIS conference is an open scientific conference, Dr Lorenzo paper became a public citable material immediately he presented it. Even reporters were present at the conference including some from Mantooka who wanted to write on Dr Lorenzo's paper. My experience at CDC is that no one can present at any conference any materials without approval from all the contributors. Given that one of the contributors is a top Mantooka government official (director of the National Public Health laboratories), I was under the impression that he had approved the information for public use. If this was not the case, then it was a gross oversight on the part of the principal investigator.

At all the scientific conferences I have attended, there is always sharing of information among scientists, reporters, and other interested parties. I have never heard of the issue of confidentiality after a paper has been presented to the larger audience and the public. Thus, asking Dr Lorenzo for more information did not mean I was using my position at CDC to get unauthorized information. I was surprised that he withheld information that concerned my family and was of great public interest in Mantooka.

Last night after our meeting with Dr Koeshi, I received several calls from the Mantookan press asking me to write a follow up story in response to the minister's remarks. I asked the newspapers to refrrain from publishing more articles. They then wanted to know whether I was being intimidated.

This matter is of great national importance to Mantooka and is likely to explode if pursued further. I hope that my intervention yesterday has laid the matter to rest.

I'm a proud member of the CDC family and a patriotic Mantookan. I have enjoyed my Atlanta family for the last three years, it's the best experience I have ever had. In no way can I ever come between CDC and the Mantooka government. I have been negotiating with GLOBAL EIS and the ministry of health to start a field epidemiology training center in Mantooka. I did not know that there was already a very cordial relations between CDC and the ministry of health. My intention was not to destroy the ties but to improve the public health knowledge in Mantooka. Over the years, we have learned to communicate important policy issues through the press.

The current furor is merely a result of misunderstanding of my intentions and actions. I shall forever be grateful for the opportunity to train at CDC.

I will try and see you very early Monday morning to answer any questions and to clarify and issues that you may have.

Thanks Dr Hatcher

Jonathon Myongo

* * * * * * * * * * * * * * * * * * * *

From: Baker, Sten
To: Hatcher, Dan
CC: Foresyth, Dale; Ettinger, John
Subject: RE: Monday Mtg.
Date: Saturday, May 13, 1995 4:51 PM

Dan—thanks for the update. I have forwarded your message to Dale. In going over this sequence of e-mails there are two points that were not clear but should be:

1. The paper presented at the EIS conference included Mantookan collaborators as co-authors, and the co-authors had approved the abstract before it was presented at the conference. The abstract included the key information presented in the talk.

2. The data in the newspaper article reflected the data in the talk. From that perspective, the article could theoretically have been written by any journalist in attendance. However, this does not alter our concerns about the important omissions in the article and our concerns about the impact the article may have on CDC's ability to assist Mantooka in its efforts to improve blood safety.

Sten

Sunday, May 14, 1995: Arturo became concerned that CDC might be blowing the incident out of proportion, and that Jonathon might suffer as a consequence. Arturo also felt that the findings reported in his abstract were not just numbers, but represented human lives, human lives that could have been saved with very simple solutions. "Every day of delay in adopting the solutions," he thought, "meant another human infected by HIV. Maybe, Jonathon's article might have speeded up the adoption of those solutions."

From: Lorenzo, Arturo
To: Mormon, Bob
Subject: Jonathon and Mantooka
Date: Sunday, May 14, 1995 4:36 PM
Bob,

I have been thinking about the problems created by Jonathon's article published in Mantooka. First of all, the first article appeared in the "African Times." We do not have a copy of that article and we have assumed that it is the same as the one that was published in the "The Union." It looks to me that the damage created by the publication of the article has been mainly to "Jonathon Myongo's" credibility. We do not know what were Jonathon's intentions by writing the article. We have to ask him. This is the first step before requesting an "investigation" into his EIS files. Lets not forget that he is a Mantookan national and maybe he did what he did with the best intentions. Can we tell the contrary for sure? I do not see in the article any reference of Jonathon speaking on behalf of CDC. I have the feeling that we (in our branch) are creating tidal waves of what is a natural reaction from a government that has been singled out for what it has failed to do regarding blood safety. Is Jonathon right? We (as CDC) have to make our position clear and distance from Jonathon's position. At the end this is an issue between Jonathon, the current government in his country, and whatever intentions he had when he wrote the article. This week we will be able to make a balance of the damages. I do not think CDC-MAMRI-Mantooka relationship has been damaged. We will have to politely clarify the situation without endorsing Mantookas government position. That will be a bigger mistake. This week lets sit down, cool down, and examine the issue with objectivity.

Arturo

* *

From: Foresyth, Dale
To: Hatcher, Dan
CC: Koeshi, Stuart
Subject: Jonathon and Mantooka
Date: Sunday, May 14, 1995 8:19 PM

Dan,

. . . I am seriously disturbed by the comments (contained in Stuart's email dated May 12, 11:11 PM) Dr. Myongo's intentions were not laudable. He never asked us what the Mantookan government was doing about transfusion safety. Obviously the government was enough concerned about it to have us come in and do a collaborative study (even at the risk of an incident like this). In fact, if he bothered to ask us, we would have told him that the government was using the data from the study to get external funds to improve the transfusion system in Mantooka. While the article had no factual errors, it did have serious omissions that were deliberate and deceitful. For example, he neglected to mention in the article that the Mantookan government was involved in the study (this was one of the first things mentioned in the Arturo's presentation). Furthermore, Dr. Myongo's claim that he wanted the government to do something about transfusion medicine by writing this article seems suspicious. As best we could tell, he had no previous interest in transfusion-related HIV infection. If he did, he certainly never contacted us about it. Finally, I think the most serious issue is that he deliberately misrepresented himself.

Dale

Monday, May 14, 1995: Stuart tried to make sure Dan had all available information before the meeting scheduled at 4:00. His experience with Dan had taught him that Dan would likely take a position based on policy until the actual people involved had spoken with him face-to-face. However, after talking personally with an individual, Stuart knew that Dan might change his position. He wanted to be sure that Jonathon would be at the meeting and would be heard, but he also wanted Dan to know what all the options were. Stuart, himself, became more convinced that there were no parties to the incident completely in the right, but also none completely in the wrong.

From: Koeshi, Stuart
To: Foresyth, Dale
Subject: Mantooka
Date: Monday, May 15, 1995 2:08 PM

Dale: I want to go on record that I am not a defender of Jonathon. I am a defender of CDC. You may be corrected that Jonathon's intentions were deceitful, but what we do to Jonathon is secondary to what we need to do to preserve CDC's reputation. We are all angered by the situation that Jonathon has put us in, but we need to manage the situation first. After we make sure that CDC will not be portrayed in the media as "dragging its feet" on an important issue to Mantookans, we can attend to Jonathon and his intentions. My concern is that in the public's eye, the blood supply is either safe of it isn't. If it is safe, then we don't need to worry about our role in this and can attend to sorting out Jonathon's intentions, laudable or not. If it is not safe, we need to make sure that CDC has been taking appropriate, timely actions with appropriate people/agencies. This may already have been done; if so, than we can focus on Jonathon.

I think we need to keep cool about this important issue. You may Jonathon much better than I, but I would not be surprised to find that Jonathon's agenda is a mix of personal, political, and public health concerns, both self-serving and selfless. But the issue is what is Jonathon guilty of. Is he guilty of medical, scientific, organizational misconduct, or all of the above? If his article reports results of an open meeting and reflects the truth, he is not guilty of medical or scientific misconduct (I realize I do not have all the info on this.). Violating CDC policy and misrepresenting himself to Arturo makes him clearly guilty of organizational misconduct. Most US journalists would find him guilty of a professional conflict of interest. All I am urging CDC to do is to suspend judgment until we have all the facts, Jonathon has had a chance to speak, and we can weigh the potential consequences of any CDC actions. You may have already spoken to him, but when I spoke with him on Friday, he told me that his 23 year-old brother is HIV-positive because of a blood transfusion he received in Mantooka. That would answer your question about his interest in transfusion-associated HIV in Mantooka. It might also answer your question about why he did not get in touch with you; right or wrong, he might think that he already knows a fair amount about this issue in Mantooka. What do you think?

Stuart

* * * * * * * * * * * * * * * * * * * *

From: Foresyth, Dale
To: Koeshi, Stuart
CC: Mormon, Bob

Subject: RE: Mantooka
Date: Monday, May 15, 1995 3:26 PM

Stuart,

I agree with your comments. We are disturbed mostly because of Jonathon's dishonesty and the fact that what he did, at a minimum, probably torpedoed our ability to continue to work with the Mantookans on improving transfusion safety. My own impression is that he is guilty of organizational misconduct and probably nothing more. As for what to do with him, we are not interested in revenge. If he is leaving CDC soon, the best thing may be to just let him finish his time here. We are interested, however, in demonstrating to our collaborators that we are serious about what was done. A letter to the Minister of Health from Dr. Satcher may be sufficient for that.

Dale

The Meeting: Making a Decision

By the time he went into the meeting Monday afternoon, Dan knew he had spoken to every person who should have any input except for Jonathon himself. Human Resources had outlined the options available. Almost every option was open because Jonathon was not officially an employee of the CDC or a U.S. citizen. The Legal Department concurred that there were few closed options given the situation. Dan agreed with Joan that the written policies were somewhat vague, but no one else in the PMR Program had written newspaper articles. He reviewed the whole series of e-mail messages in his mind as he waited for Jonathon,

Stuart, Paula, and Joan to appear for the meeting. He would have to make a decision based on what Jonathon said because Jonathon was the only person who had not been heard.

At the meeting, Dan let Jonathon do most of the talking. First, he asked Jonathon about his motivation in writing the article and if he knew that clearance was required to write articles. Jonathon replied that he thought, as a private person, he was allowed to write newspaper articles. HIV was an issue of ongoing interest in Mantooka, Jonathon told the group; he said that several Mantookan physicians had e-mailed or FAXed their support of what he had done, and that the Mantookan press was interested in what the outcome of their meeting today would be. Jonathon offered to write a letter to the Minster of Health explaining his motivation and distancing himself from CDC. As the others asked questions, Dan listened carefully to what Jonathon was saying. After the meeting was over and the others had gone back to their offices, Dan leaned back and rubbed his chin. He still didn't know what his decision should be.

Glossary of Acronyms Used at CDC

EPO—Epidemiology Program Office, directed by Dan Hatcher. One of the fourteen CDC programs and centers at the time of the case.

EIS—Epidemic Intelligence Service. Composed of scientists training at CDC in the Division of Field Epidemiology who designed and carried out scientific studies for CDC.

GBS—Global Blood Safety Project. Carried out by the CDC, in collaboration with the governments of several countries and other international health organizations such as the World Health Organization.

PMR—Preventive Medicine Residency and/or Resident(s). One of only twenty-five preventive medicine residencies recognized by the

American Board of Medical Specialties, the PMR accepted only a small number of residents each year out of the many applicants received from around the world.

MAMRI—National Medical Research Institute in Mantooka.

AIDSCAP Nepal

Background

It was September 1996, and Ravin Lama, Managing Director of Stimulus Advertizers, one of Nepal's larger advertising agencies, looked out of his Kathmandu office window pondering his future course of action. (See the appendix for an overview of Nepal.) He had just received a copy of a qualitative, quickly conducted, small sample study which had been developed by a research agency in order to assess the impact of *The AIDS Awareness and Condom Promotion Multimedia Campaign*, which his agency had helped develop and implement since mid-1995. The main focus of this campaign was to increase the accessibility of condoms, promote their correct and consistent use (particularly when engaging in high-risk behaviors), and communicate HIV/AIDS awareness messages. He had an upcoming meeting with Joy Pollock, Resident Advisor to the AIDSCAP (AIDS Control and Prevention) project, at which they had to both evaluate the impact of the current campaign, which was to conclude in April 1997, and develop a strategy for Phase II of their communication program. AIDSCAP was the primary sponsor of the campaign.

Launched in July, 1995, the campaign to reduce the rate of sexually transmitted HIV infection in AIDSCAP's project area—the Terai/Central region of the country—had been ongoing for more than a year. Lama was preparing for a meeting where he had to present a thorough evaluation of the progress made thus far in this phase, recommend any necessary changes, and develop his agency's plans for Phase II, which was to address issues of fear in the general public regarding people living with AIDS. Specifically, his task was to determine whether the results of the small sample study were sufficient to assess the effectiveness of the present campaign and, if not, to design an appropriate assessment tool. Phase II, the fear issue, had become important because the media were reporting that a large number of HIV-positive Nepalese commercial sex workers (CSWs) were returning home from brothels in India. Once Lama was satisfied that the current phase's objectives were being met, he had to set specific objectives for Phase II and design the promotion campaign.

Many Nepalese women worked as prostitutes in several large Indian cities such as Mumbai (formerly called Bombay) and Delhi. Mostly from rural areas where economic prospects were poor,

This case was prepared by Ven Sriram, University of Baltimore, and Franklyn Manu, Morgan State University. It is intended as a basis for classroom discussion rather than to illustrate effective or ineffective handling of an administrative situation. All rights reserved by the authors and the North American Case Research Association (NACRA). Copyright © 2000 by the *Case Research Journal* and Ven Sriram and Franklyn Manu. Used with permission from the *Case Research Journal*.

they were often part of an elaborate network where they were recruited, ostensibly for legitimate employment, and once in India were either coerced into or drifted into prostitution. Often abused and abandoned by their husbands and in-laws and having no means of financial support, many became CSWs. Although prostitution had not always been legal, attempts by Indian authorities to regulate it were sporadic and half-hearted. Once infected with HIV, the women were usually thrown out of the brothels, the only real "family" many of them had so far away from home. They generally returned home to Nepal in anticipation of receiving better care from their families than they would get in India. However, fear and rejection from society, frequently based on ignorance of the disease and how it spread, meant that they were often shunned.

AIDS: A Historical Perspective

Although AIDS was first recognized internationally in 1981, it was identified in Nepal in 1988. Data presented at a conference in Kathmandu in the mid-1990s indicated that although the HIV/AIDS epidemic in Nepal was at a relatively early stage compared with other countries, the incidence of HIV/AIDS was increasing. The total number of HIV/AIDS cases reported in the country was in the hundreds according to the National Centre for AIDS and STD Control (NCASC), but NCASC projected HIV cases at 15,000 by the turn of the century. His Majesty's Government of Nepal and national and international nongovernment organizations were actively participating in an attempt to control its spread. The NCASC chief stated that "the situation offers, therefore, a unique opportunity to support and undertake preventive activities before the disease reaches an epidemic stage in the country."

The evidence in the mid-1990s was that

- Extensive or epidemic spread of HIV had not been documented in Nepal

- A large proportion of HIV infections had been and would be acquired outside the country—Nepal had a long, open border with India and many Nepalese worked in India
- There would be an estimated 15,000 HIV cases and 1,000 AIDS cases and deaths annually by the year 2000
- HIV/AIDS surveillance needed to be strengthened and behavioral surveillance started as soon as possible, that is, more extensive screening and testing for infection and more detailed assessment of the extent of high-risk behaviors such as unprotected sex with CSWs
- STD services, condom distribution and promotion, and behavior change communications to high-risk groups needed to be strengthened

Additionally, epidemiological evidence indicated that the primary modes of transmission of HIV/AIDS in Nepal were heterosexual contact with CSWs followed by intravenous drug use. Some of the identified high-risk behaviors were premarital and extramarital sexual practices, wide availability of CSWs, and low condom use. Much of the pre- and extramarital sexual activity was with CSWs, given the taboos and social norms against such activity among "respectable" people, particularly for women. CSWs were a major medium of the spread of HIV/AIDS because once a client became infected, he could become the core transmitter of the virus as he traveled through Nepal and infected other CSWs, who in turn infected their other clients, if condoms were not used.

Despite the AIDS threat not being very immediate in Nepal, the issue was complicated by the close contacts between Nepal and India. A significant portion of Nepal's male population worked in India, and if they acquired the infection there, it could rapidly spread in Nepal when they had sexual contacts on their visits home. In addition, many Nepalese CSWs worked in brothels in large Indian cities such as New Delhi and Mumbai. Data from India indicated that the HIV infection rate among CSWs in Mumbai had increased from 0.5 percent in 1986 to 69 percent in 1995. Mumbai

Exhibit 2-1. Sociodemographics of CSWs and Clients: 1994 Baseline Study

	CSWs		Clients	
Variable	Project Area (n = 100)	Control Area (n = 62)	Project Area (n = 209)	Control Area (n = 103)
Age (in years)				
0–19	13.0%	24.2%	54.5 (15–24)%	41.7%
20–29	63.0%	45.2%	37.3 (25–34)%	50.5%
30–39	18.0%	27.4%	8.1 (35–44)%	7.8%
40+	6.0%	3.2%	0.0 (45+)	0.0
Mean age	26.0	26.0	24.9	25.8
Education				
Literate	44.0%	40.3%	90.5%	93.2%
Illiterate	56.0%	59.7%	10.5%	6.8%
Marital status				
Married	93.0%	83.9%	56.5%	66.0%
Unmarried	7.0%	16.1%	43.5%	34.0%
Presently living with husband/wife	(n = 93)	(n = 52)	(n = 118)	(n = 68)
Yes	43.0%	42.3%	83.9%	83.8%
No	57.0%	57.7%	16.1%	16.2%
Children	(n = 93)	(n = 52)	NA	NA
Yes	68.8%	19.4%	NA	NA
No	31.2%	80.6%	NA	NA

NOTE: The age ranges used for categorizing CSWs and their clients are different.

had an estimated 70,000 CSWs. India had almost 2.5 million CSWs out of a total population of more than 900 million.

Several studies had been conducted to measure awareness of, attitudes toward, and usage of condoms, oral and injectable contraceptives, brands and image, and general views about HIV/AIDS in Nepal. One such study was conducted in 1994 among CSWs and their clients along the highway route in AIDSCAP's project area and among similar groups in a control area where AIDSCAP did not have a campaign. This study interviewed 100 CSWs and 209 of their clients in the project area along with 62 CSWs and 103 clients in the control area. This study's key findings from the project and control areas are presented in Exhibits 2-1 to 2-5. This study reported on the general awareness

of AIDS along with condom use and purchase patterns. It also identified the main sources of information about AIDS and perceptions regarding means of prevention.

AIDSCAP

AIDSCAP, part of Family Health International (FHI), had its activities funded by the U.S. Agency for International Development (USAID). Futures Group International was appointed as the consultant for the project. For the initial phase, the activities of both Stimulus, which handled the communication program, and Contraceptive Retail Sales Company (CRS), which handled condom

Exhibit 2-2. Condom Use and Purchase Behavior of CSWs: 1994 Baseline Study

Condom Use/Purchase Behavior	Project Area (%)	Control Area (%)
Ever bought condoms for clients	($n = 100$)	($n = 62$)
Yes	26.0	24.2
No	74.0	75.8
Price of condom	($n = 26$)	($n = 15$)
Expensive	15.4	26.7
Reasonable	57.7	60.0
Cheap	26.9	13.3
Most convenient location to buy/get	($n = 96$)	($n = 57$)
Pharmacy	59.4	61.4
Retail store	50.0	66.7
Health worker/volunteer	29.2	0.0
Health post/center/hospital	25.0	1.8
Hotel/lodge	16.7	15.8
Public place	9.4	0.0
NGOs	0.0	14.0
Others	8.3	5.3
Clients using condoms	($n = 100$)	($n = 62$)
All of them	13.0	14.5
Most of them	16.0	29.0
Half of them	14.0	14.5
A few of them	13.0	19.4
None of them	44.0	22.6
Use by last client	($n = 100$)	($n = 62$)
Yes	35.0	48.4
No	65.0	51.6
Decision maker	($n = 35$)	($n = 30$)
Last client	42.9	50.0
CSW	57.1	50.0
Condom brought by	($n = 35$)	($n = 30$)
Client	57.1	56.7
CSW	42.9	43.3
Ever requested client to use condom	($n = 100$)	($n = 62$)
Yes	30.0	33.9
No	70.0	66.1
Any of those clients refused	($n = 30$)	($n = 21$)
Yes	60.0	47.6
No	40.0	52.4

distribution, were managed by Futures Group. For Phase II of the project, Stimulus would deal directly with AIDSCAP.

Given all the available evidence, AIDSCAP decided that its goal was to reduce the rate of sexually transmitted HIV infection in the Terai/Central region through the implementation of three major prevention and control strategies:

- Reduce sexually transmitted diseases
- Increase the use of condoms among the risk populations

Exhibit 2-3. Condom Use and Purchase Behavior of Clients: 1994 Baseline Study

Condom Use/Purchase Behavior	Project Area (%)	Control Area (%)
Ever used	(n = 209)	(n = 103)
Yes	52.6	55.3
No	47.4	44.7
Price of condom	(n = 108)	(n = 57)
Expensive	11.1	24.6
Reasonable	60.2	47.4
Cheap/inexpensive	28.7	28.1
Most convenient location to buy/get	(n = 209)	(n = 102)
Pharmacy	66.5	68.6
Retail store	49.8	40.2
Health worker/volunteer	7.7	10.2
Health post/center/hospital	17.2	9.8
Hotel/lodge	16.3	3.9
Public place	3.8	0.0
NGOs	8.1	4.9
Others/don't know	6.3	15.7
Frequency of condom use with CSWs	(n = 209)	(n = 103)
Always	22.0	6.8
Mostly	16.7	16.5
Sometimes	5.3	15.5
Rarely	5.7	14.6
Never	50.2	46.6
Reasons for not using condoms	(n = 63)	(n = 48)
Unavailability/no time	60.3	52.1
Complexity	34.9	12.5
Sexual dissatisfaction	27.0	64.6
Unreliability/others	6.3	22.9
Person who first mentioned condom	(n = 71)	(n = 22)
Myself	95.8	100.0
CSW	4.2	0.0

- Reduce risk behaviors through communications and outreach activities to targeted populations

It was decided to focus on the Terai/Central region because of the relatively high concentrations of CSWs working in these areas, the presence of major highways, and the movement of large numbers of people (including CSWs and their clients) across the border with India. Several studies had noted the pattern of Nepalese women working as CSWs in India, Indian clients crossing the border to patronize sex workers in Nepal, and Nepalese migrant workers returning occasionally from India to visit their families. The targets of the campaign were the individuals at highest risk: CSWs and their clients (e.g., transport workers, migrant laborers, military, and police). Transport workers—truck drivers and their helpers—were seen by AIDSCAP as a high-risk group because they tended to be away from home for long periods of time. In addition, because they traveled,

Exhibit 2-4. Knowledge of AIDS: 1994 Baseline Study

	CSWs		Clients	
Knowledge of AIDS	Project Area (%; n = 100)	Control Area (%; n = 62)	Project Area (%; n = 209)	Control Area (%; n = 103)
Ever heard of AIDS				
Yes	82.0	59.7	90.4	91.3
No	18.0	40.3	9.6	8.7
AIDS is				
A disease	79.0	54.8	88.5	70.9
Others	3.0	4.8	3.8	20.4
Not heard of AIDS	18.0	40.3	7.6	8.7
Is AIDS transmitted?				
Yes	53.0	38.7	75.1	80.6
No	47.0	61.3	15.3	10.7
Don't know	0.0	0.0	9.6	8.7
Modes of AIDS transmission				
Sex without condom	23.0	21.0	29.2	44.7
Multiple sex partners	29.0	24.2	51.2	47.6
Sexual intercourse	22.0	27.4	23.0	35.9
By blood	5.0	3.2	9.6	20.4
By syringe	1.0	3.2	5.3	7.8
Sex with AIDS-infected people	0.0	1.6	1.4	8.7
Sex with CSW	0.0	0.0	4.8	5.8
Other	1.0	1.6	0.5	1.0
Don't know	47.0	61.3	0.0	0.0
Consequences of AIDS				
Death	66.0	40.3	72.7	61.2
Remain sick for long	9.0	14.5	12.0	22.3
Others	4.0	3.2	4.8	5.8
Don't know	21.0	41.9	10.5	15.5
Preventive measures				
Use condom	34.0	27.4	54.5	51.5
Stop sex with multiple partners	25.0	22.6	30.1	45.6
Stop going to CSW	2.0	1.6	23.9	27.2
Use disposable syringe	1.0	0.0	1.9	2.9
Use tested blood	1.0	0.0	0.0	0.0
Don't use others' shaving material	0.0	0.0	2.4	2.9
Don't know	54.0	62.9	0.0	0.0
Knowledge of AIDS among those exposed to condom advertising				
Yes	50.0	44.4	79.4	85.4
No	50.0	55.6	20.6	14.6

Exhibit 2-5. Sources of Knowledge About HIV/AIDS: 1994 Baseline Study

| | CSWs | | Clients | |
| | Project Area | Control Area | Project Area | Control Area |
Source	(n = 82)	(n = 37)	(n = 189)	(n = 94)
Friends/neighbors	68.3%	54.1%	52.4%	42.6%
Radio	40.2	70.3	60.3	72.3
Health post/hospital	22.2	0.0	9.0	13.8
Newspapers/posters/magazines	13.4	18.9	43.9	46.8
Television	12.2	24.3	29.1	28.7
Health workers/volunteers	9.8	0.0	3.7	2.1
Pharmacy	7.3	16.2	16.4	9.6
Billboards	6.1	18.9	30.7	29.8
Clients	3.7	0.0	—	—
Street drama/theater	2.4	0.0	2.1	0.0
NGOs	1.2	18.9	5.3	7.4
Hotel/shop	0.0	0.0	2.1	0.0
Others/don't know	4.9	2.7	3.7	6.4

once infected they could easily spread the disease to the other CSWs they frequented along the highway. Military and police were targeted because the lower ranks usually were not provided family accommodations when posted away from home. They generally were housed in barracks while their families stayed behind in their home villages. This forced separation, along with peer pressure, made them high risks for HIV transmission. AIDSCAP felt that migrant workers were a high-risk group because they left their homes in search of construction jobs (e.g., road and bridge building) that were easier to find along the highway routes. Again, living away from home for long periods made them more likely to patronize CSWs.

Phase I

Condom Distribution

AIDSCAP recognized that in order for AIDS preventive communication strategies to work, increased accessibility of condoms was a vital element. To this end, it subcontracted with Futures Group International to conduct condom promotion and distribution activities in the target area. The issue was complicated by the fact that condom promotion in Nepal had traditionally focused primarily on its benefit as a family planning method, not so much as a means of disease prevention. In addition, AIDSCAP had to keep in mind that Nepalese society was very traditional and frowned on premarital and extramarital sexual activity. Any attempt to promote condom use for other than family planning activity had to be sensitive to this.

Futures Group worked with CRS to improve condom accessibility and availability through retail and nontraditional outlets in the AIDSCAP target region. A rapid assessment study conducted by AIDSCAP indicated that clients of CSWs wanted condoms to be easily available at all hours through nontraditional distribution outlets such as tea shops, *paan pasals* (small shops selling cigarettes and other frequently bought consumer products), hotels, and truck stops. Distribution efforts were toward these outlets, especially along major truck routes, so as to make access easy for the primary target market of the effort—clients of CSWs. Two brands of condoms, Panther and *Dhaal* ("shield" in Nepali), donated by USAID were marketed in Nepal. Panther was targeted primarily at the upper social class and *Dhaal* at the middle and lower classes.

Condom Promotion

The other major element in AIDSCAP's strategy was the communication program. This was where Lama's organization, Stimulus, entered the picture. The responsibility for communicating the goals of the project rested with him and his agency.

Objectives

Based on AIDSCAP's overall goals, three specific communication goals for the campaign were established:

- To increase the existing levels of awareness among the target audience that sexual transmission was the primary mode of acquiring HIV infection and AIDS
- To increase perception of individual risk of acquiring HIV/AIDS
- To promote consistent and correct condom use as a method of protection from HIV/ AIDS

These goals were expected to be achieved sequentially, following the traditional communication hierarchy of effects model, which suggested that consumer responses moved from the least

serious or involved through the most serious or complex. One classic approach, the AIDA model, proposed that a message's impact began with *attention*, moved to *interest*, then *desire*, and finally *action*. AIDSCAP wanted to develop awareness among the target audience about HIV/AIDS and its modes of transmission, then heighten attention and interest by communicating its risks, and finally, motivate action to take preventive measures.

Target Audiences

AIDSCAP identified clients of CSWs as the project's primary target audience. In order to reach the clients, the media proposed should match the target—defined as sexually active men aged 15–35 who engaged in commercial sex. CSWs were made the secondary target because of the difficulty in reaching them via mass media vehicles given their generally low levels of literacy, then high mobility along the transportation routes, and the limited reach of these media away from the major cities. Thus interpersonal counseling, peer counseling, and other such efforts conducted by AIDSCAP would be used to reach CSWs, in addition to the efforts of this communication campaign.

Creative

The first creative task for Stimulus was to develop a logo that would serve as the HIV/AIDS awareness campaign ID to be used in all communication and training material for the entire project. This logo was intended to communicate protection from HIV/AIDS and symbolize positive behavior change (i.e., use of condoms). Other considerations were that it represent positive feelings (no fear), represent positive outcomes of condom use, symbolize strength, and be easily understood. After initial focus groups and in-depth interviews with target group members, four logos were developed based on "structured brainstorming" (where participants were asked to suggest how best to visually communicate strength, lack

Exhibit 2.6. *Dhaaley Dai*

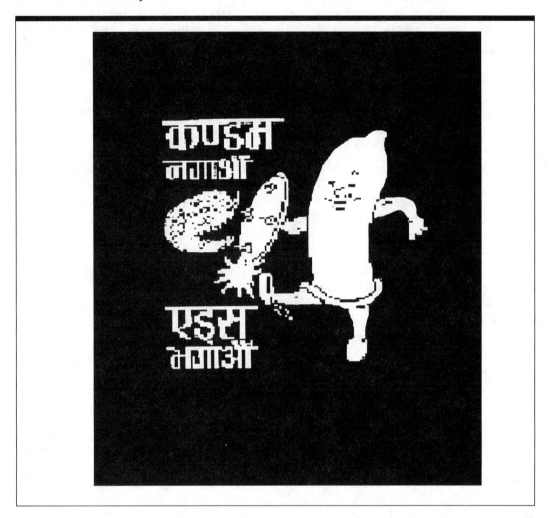

of fear, etc.) by a group of AIDSCAP implementing partners. Subsequently, a survey was conducted in early 1995 among the target group (bus/truck drivers and conductors) to test these logos. Based on this study, a logo showing an animated condom (named "Dhaaley Dai") holding a shield and kicking the AIDS virus (Exhibit 2-6) was selected as the one with the highest ranking in terms of overall liking; conveying the impression of strength, confidence, attractiveness, and protection against AIDS; and encouraging the use of condoms. This character was used in a message ("Dhaaley and Dhaal Bahadur") to communicate correct and consistent condom use.

To develop a slogan for the campaign, several condom benefit statements were tested. These revealed that protection and freedom from worry were the most strongly received concepts. As a result, the slogan "condom lagaon . . . AIDS bhagaon" (use a condom . . . drive away AIDS) was selected.

The creative strategy was developed around four primary ideas: (1) dispel myths regarding how HIV/AIDS was/was not transmitted (e.g., via dirty glasses and food, mosquitoes); (2) build awareness that anyone could become infected with AIDS even with one sexual contact in the same way as with sexually transmitted diseases (epidemiological studies suggest that the possibility of AIDS transmission per exposure increased substantially when the presence of STDs was high in a population); (3) create a general awareness about HIV/AIDS and the dangers of casual, unprotected sex; and (4) communicate the widespread availability of condoms and the lack of a need to feel fear or embarrassment about using them.

Media

A combination of media was used to communicate the key creative messages of the campaign. Billboards featuring the condom character *Dhale* along with the slogan "Use a Condom . . . Drive away AIDS" were placed at several points along the main highways in the project area. For radio, four 60-second spots and a jingle were developed. FM radio was used in Kathmandu; Radio Nepal, which had widespread reach across most of the country, was also used. The state-owned TV channel, Nepal TV, was used to telecast a 60-second animated spot of *Dhale* in Nepali.

The van that CRS used for its condom distribution activity was equipped with a video screen that was used to show a 45-minute soap opera–style film that was developed by Stimulus in mid-1996. This film's primary characters were a truck driver (named Guruji) and his assistant (Antare), and the main ideas—how to protect yourself from AIDS and other STDs, their means of transmission, the value of correct condom use, dangers of unprotected sex and other risk behaviors—were communicated in a conversational setting between these two characters. In addition, a film version of the TV spot and a shortened (19-minute) version of the *Guruji and Antare* video were screened at movie theaters in five towns in the target area.

The *Guruji and Antare* story was developed in the form of a comic book. Because of high visual content, comic books were seen as more interesting than text-heavy material. Given Nepal's high levels of illiteracy, particularly among truck drivers and laborers, comic books were an effective way to deliver the message. AIDSCAP contracted with a traveling group of street performers, who enacted the contents of the film at several villages along the highway. At these live performances and the video showings, copies of the comic book were distributed. A few days before these activities were scheduled for an area, project workers would put up posters and make public announcements in order to alert the residents about the upcoming arrival of the video van or the live performers. On these occasions as well, the project workers would distribute comic books. Other printed material, in Nepali, included brochures, stickers, and condom wallets. Metal signs, posters, and calendars were distributed to shops, pharmacies, health centers, and community buildings for display.

Details of the major media available in Nepal are presented in Exhibits 2-7 and 2-8.

Budget

Because of uncertain funding levels, Lama was not given a budget at the start of the Phase I campaign. He had to make periodic funding requests which, if approved after review, determined how much he had available to spend on different aspects of the campaign. Details of the media budget and schedule for Phase I are provided in Exhibit 2-9.

The Assessment

In May, 1996, AIDSCAP commissioned a market research agency to conduct a quick, small sample assessment of the impact of the program on behavior change among CSWs (with "CSW" defined as a woman who was involved in multiple sexual encounters for financial benefit) and their clients (with "client" defined as a person who had sexual contact with at least one CSW within three months from the date of the interview). A convenience sample of twenty-five CSWs and twenty-five clients from the AIDSCAP intervention area transportation routes was surveyed using personal interviews. The target sample was identified based on information supplied by hotels and tea-

Exhibit 2-7. Media Data: Broadcast

Medium	Broadcast Time	Content	General Rate (30 sec)	Sponsorship Rate (30 sec)
I. Radio: FM				
Hits FM	7:15 a.m.–3 p.m.	Nepali, English, Hindi songs	Rs. 300–800	Rs. 325–900
Image Plus	4 p.m.–5 p.m.	Nepali, English, Hindi songs	Rs. 600	n/a
Classic FM	6 p.m.–7 p.m.	Songs, phone-ins, business briefs	Rs. 300	Rs. 3,300 (30 min)
Kantipur FM	7 p.m.–10 p.m.	Songs, phone-ins, comedy	Rs. 275	n/a
Good Nite FM	10 p.m.–12 midnight	Music	Rs. 200–250	n/a
2. Radio: Medium wave (MW)				
Radio Nepal	7:45 a.m.–10:55 p.m.	News, music, educational, agriculture, health, sports, environment, etc.	Rs. 500–800	Rs. 6,700–9,000 (30 min)
II. Television				
Nepal TV	7 a.m.–7:40 a.m. daily 6 p.m.–10:15 p.m. daily 12 noon–5 p.m. (Saturday only)	News, English and Nepali educational and entertainment, Indian and Pakistani music and serials	Rs. 2,750–6,500	n/a

NOTE: Radio: 2,000,000 sets, 5 listeners/set, FM coverage in Kathmandu Valley only, MW coverage national and parts of neighboring countries.

TV: 250,000 sets, 6 viewers/set, coverage over most of the country, 60-second spot costs twice as much as a 30-second spot.

shops, bars, pimps, and local people, as well as through the CSWs and their clients themselves. The respondents were compensated for their participation in the interviews. The specific goals of this study were to

- Assess target groups' awareness and understanding of HIV/AIDS
- Assess target groups' awareness of AIDSCAP communication messages
- Assess target groups' self risk perception
- Collect information of target groups' recent condom use

The study concluded that the awareness of the campaign slogan ("condom lagaon . . . AIDS bhagaon") was high, with most respondents having been exposed to it via radio or through billboards. A sizable number had heard some of the other campaign messages as well. It appeared that

Exhibit 2-8. Media Data: Print

Publication	Language and Frequency	Content	Circulation	Cost		
				Black and White	Color	
				Column/cm	Column/cm	
Newspapers						
Kantipur	Nepali, daily	Domestic and international news, business reports, sports, etc.	45,000–50,000	Rs. 90	Rs. 250	
Gorkhapatra	Nepali, daily	Domestic and international news, business reports, sports, etc.	40,000	Rs. 90	n/a	
Aajo Samacharpatra	Nepali, daily	Domestic and international news, business reports, sports, etc.	10,000	Rs. 75	n/a	
Himalaya Times	Nepali, daily	Domestic and international news, business reports, sports, etc.	10,000	Rs. 59	n/a	
Sagarmatha	Nepali, daily	Domestic and international news, business reports, sports, etc.	5,000	Rs. 75	Rs. 250	
Kathmandu Post	English, daily	Domestic and international news, business reports, sports, etc.	12,000	Rs. 90	n/a	
Rising Nepal	English, daily	Domestic and international news, business reports, sports, etc.	8,000	Rs. 90	n/a	
Independent	English, weekly	Domestic and international news, business reports, sports, etc.	5,000		Rs. 55 (1 color) Rs. 69 (2 colors)	
Saptahik	Nepali, weekly	Domestic and international news, business reports, sports, etc.		Rs. 40	Rs. 200	

Exhibit 2-8. Continued

Publication	Language and Frequency	Content	Circulation	Cost Black and White Full Page (black and white)	Color Full Page (Color)
Magazines					
Kamana	Nepali, monthly	Movie news	30,000	Rs. 4,000	Rs. 11,000
Sadhana	Nepali, monthly	General interest, family	25,000–35,000	Rs. 3,000	Rs. 6,500
Asmita	Nepali, monthly	Women's issues	15,000	Rs. 4,000	Rs. 15,000–20,000 (cover)
Yuva Manch	Nepali, monthly	Children and youth, 8–21	n/a	Rs. 4,000	n/a
Wave	English, monthly	Youth, 12–22	15,000	n/a	n/a
Spotlight	English, monthly	Political, news, sports, business, leisure, South Asian focus, tourism	5,000	n/a	n/a
Himal	English and Nepali, monthly		10,000	US$ 1,000	US$ 1,200

NOTE: Average number of readers per copy: 5.

Exhibit 2-9. Phase I Media Schedule: 1995–97

Medium	Period	Number of Spots, Performances, Shows	Cost
I. Radio			
Radio Nepal	July 1995–April 1997	1,096	Rs. 1,982,700
FM	November 1995–February 1996	151	121,400
	May 1996	8	5,040
	September 1996–April 1997	80	53,700
II. NTV	February 1996–April 1997	128	902,840
III. Cinema	February 1996–August 1996	3,125	17,005
(in 5 towns)	October 1996–April 1997	3,155	19,058
IV. Street drama	August 1995–July 1996	60	300,000
	October 1996–April 1997	64	355,840
V. Video van	September 1996–March 1997	61	5,000,000
Total media cost			4,257,583

the AIDSCAP promotional campaign did have a positive impact on AIDS awareness levels; however, perceptions of risk from AIDS were low. Details of the study are provided in Exhibits 2-10 through 2-13.

The Future

As Lama contemplated his upcoming meeting with Pollock, two sets of issues confronted him. The first, and more immediate, was to determine whether the results of the small sample study gave him sufficient information with which to evaluate the impact of the communication campaign thus far. His initial reaction was that because these results were based on a limited sample of CSWs and their clients, perhaps a more detailed follow-up was necessary, using a larger sample from the intervention area along with a sample from the control area. This was especially significant because a successful execution of this phase's communica-

tions goals was essential before Phase II could be launched; without successful execution, the effectiveness of Phase II would be limited. Specifically, Lama had to determine, if he decided to initiate a detailed assessment, the methodology he should employ (i.e., research design, measures, data collection) to evaluate the current phase. Was the methodology used in the small sample study adequate, or were more comprehensive data necessary?

The second issue was to start thinking about the Phase II, due to be launched in mid-1997. His task was to address issues of fear in the general public regarding people living with AIDS. This was of particular concern in Nepal given the large number of HIV-positive women who had returned from brothels in Mumbai and elsewhere in India and the resulting fear among many sections of the Nepalese population. Lama wondered whether launching Phase II was the correct decision at this point in time. Was it timely to move ahead with these new issues, or should he focus on

Exhibit 2-10. Sociodemographics of CSWs and Clients: 1996 Study

Variable	CSWs (n = 25)	Clients (n = 25)
Age		
0–20	16.0%	20.0%
21–25	40.0	28.0
26–30	16.0	16.0
Over 30	24.0	36.0
Not known	4.0	—
Education		
Literate	48.0	96.0
Illiterate	52.0	4.0
Marital status		
Ever been married	88.0	72.0
Unmarried	12.0	28.0
Children		
Yes	36.0	44.0
No	64.0	56.0

Exhibit 2-11. Condom Use Behavior: 1996 Study

Condom Usage	CSWs (n = 25)	Clients (n = 25)
Ever use condom		
Yes	76.0%	68.0%
No	24.0	32.0
Used condom with last CSW/client		
Yes	60.0	44.0
No	16.0	24.0
Not applicable	24.0	32.0
First to initiate use of condom		
CSW	28.0	20.0
Client	32.0	24.0
Not applicable	40.0	56.0
Condom provided by		
CSW	24.0	16.0
Client	36.0	28.0
Not applicable	40.0	56.0
Always use condoms with CSWs	Not applicable	
Yes		28.0
No		16.0
Not applicable		56.0
Condoms used by		Not applicable
All the clients	12.0	
Most of the clients	48.0	
Few of the clients	16.0	
None of the clients	24.0	

Exhibit 2-12. Knowledge of AIDS: 1996 Study

Knowledge of AIDS	CSWs (n = 25)	Clients (n = 25)
Ever heard of AIDS		
Yes	96.0%	100.0%
No	4.0	0.0
AIDS is		
A disease	88.0	100.0
A fatal disease	8.0	0.0
Not heard of AIDS	4.0	0.0
Is AIDS transmitted		
Yes	76.0	96.0
No	20.0	4.0
Don't know	4.0	0.0
Modes of AIDS transmission		
Sex without condom	52.0	44.0
Multiple sex partners	36.0	56.0
Sexual intercourse	32.0	24.0
By blood	—	20.0
By syringe	—	16.0
Other	4.0	4.0
Don't know	24.0	—
Consequences of AIDS		
Death	60.0	76.0
Remain sick for long	20.0	28.0
Don't know	20.0	8.0
Preventive measures		
Use condom	64.0	84.0
Stop sex with multiple partners	44.0	64.0
Stop going to CSWs	—	4.0
Use disposable syringes	—	8.0
Avoid blood transfusions from AIDS patients	—	8.0
Don't know	24.0	4.0

strengthening the current prevention campaign? If he decided to tackle the fear issue, Lama had to design the entire communications strategy for Phase II of the campaign. He had to develop specific objectives, generate the creative and media strategies, and identify appropriate measures to assess the communications effectiveness of this phase of the AIDSCAP project.

APPENDIX
Nepal: A Brief Overview

Topography and Climate

Nepal was a landlocked country with a total land area of 147,181 sq. km. It was roughly rectangular in shape and extended approximately 885 km east-west and between 145 km and 241 km north-

Exhibit 2-13. Awareness of AIDSCAP Messages: 1996 Study

	Heard/Seen Condom Ad in Past 3 Months		Heard/Seen "Condom Lagaon AIDS Bhagaon"		Heard/Seen "Dhaaley and Dhaal Bahadur"		Heard/Seen Guruji and Antare	
	CSWs (n = 25)	Clients (n = 25)	CSWs (n = 25)	Clients (n = 25)	CSWs (n = 25)	Clients (n = 25)	CSWs (n = 25)	Clients (n = 25)
Radio	18	18	16	19	5	10	1	0
Billboards	15	12	13	8	1	3	0	1
Pharmacy	8	9	8	4	1	2	0	0
Cinema hall	8	6	8	4	1	2	7	6
Outreach workers	8	5	8	7	4	5	0	0
Print material	7	8	6	11	5	9	3	8
Video van film	3	4	2	5	0	5	3	6
Television	2	4	3	2	2	0	2	0
Street drama	2	1	2	1	0	1	0	2
Friends	—	1	2	8	1	7	0	0
Health centers	—	2	1	3	0	1	0	0
Not seen/heard	0	3	2	2	18	11	14	9

south. It was bordered by China on the north and by India on the south, east, and west. The topography ranged from the mountainous high Himalayas in the north; to the mid-Himalayas in the middle, with their terraced slopes and fertile valleys; to the flat, subtropical Terai region along the country's southern border with India. Many of the world's tallest peaks, including Mount Everest, lay within Nepal.

The climate varied from subtropical in the Terai to alpine in the mountains. Kathmandu, the capital, was located in a valley and had a pleasant climate, with none of the extremes of the north or the south. The southwest monsoon brought rainfall during the period from June to August, mostly in the Kathmandu valley and the east. The western portion of the country received most of its rainfall in the winter.

History and Political System

Nepal, which had never been under foreign domination, consisted of several small autonomous kingdoms that were unified by King Prithvi Narayan Shah in 1769. The powerful Rana line of hereditary prime ministers ruled the country from the early 19th century until their overthrow in 1951 after a popular revolution led by King Tribhuvan. In 1959, when a people's movement ushered in democracy again, the country was governed by the monarchy with the assistance of a *Rashtriya Panchayat* (National Parliament). The members of this parliament were not affiliated with any party and were initially indirectly elected. Later, from the early 1980s, the people directly elected parliamentary representatives, but it was still a party-less system. In 1990, the country adopted a new constitution with a parliamentary system of government based on multiparty democracy with a constitutional monarchy.

Social and Cultural Environment

Nepal was a highly diverse country ethnically, linguistically, and culturally. The people were mostly of either Indo-Aryan or Tibeto-Burmese stock. Although almost 90 percent of the population was Hindu, there were a significant number of Buddhists and a small number of Muslims and Christians. Nepali was the *lingua franca* of the country, although several other languages were spoken as well, such as Newari, Tamang, Gurung, Maithili, and Magar. English was spoken and understood by the educated people and in most urban centers.

The country was very rich culturally, finding expression in art, music, and dance as well as in the exquisite and intricate wood, stone, and bronze images found in the many temples, pagodas, and palaces.

Economic System

Nepal was classified as a least developed country on the basis of several macroeconomic indicators. Per capita income was around $200 annually, and the country was primarily agrarian, with less than 10 percent of GDP coming from the manufacturing sector. The population was nearly 19 million, with a growth rate of a little over 2 percent annually. As was the case in many developing countries, the birth rate and infant mortality rates were very high. Average life expectancy was only 56.5 years. Although the overall literacy rate was almost 40 percent, it was 54 percent for males and only 25 percent for females.

The country's major trading partners were India, the United States, Japan, and Germany. The bulk of industrial, consumer, and durable products were imported from India, a country on which Nepal was very reliant. The country had been running a trade deficit; it had 1994 exports of $363 million and imports of $1,176 million. Its primary exports were carpets and garments, and its primary imports were petroleum products, raw wool, and manufactured products. The currency was the rupee (Rs.) with an exchange rate of US$ 1 = Rs. 56.75 in 1996.

The Indiana State Department of Health

Managing Strategically

John C. Bailey, MD, was appointed by Governor Bayh to the Executive Board of the Indiana State Department of Health (ISDH) in 1989 and became State Health Commissioner in November, 1990. He was responsible for agency operations and served as secretary of the eleven-member executive board of ISDH. After being appointed commissioner, Dr. Bailey carefully reviewed the plans and organization of the Department of Health and decided that a major strategic planning effort was required. He was convinced that this organization had not dealt with change very well in the past and over the years had grown far too bureaucratic to be effective in the rapidly changing environment that the Department now faced.

To a meeting of his management team, Dr. Bailey said,

> I believe that strategic management will provide an understanding of the trends and issues that the Department of Health has to address in the next several years and that the process can be instrumental in developing a course of action for us. I feel that we need to better establish the role of the public health department in the State of Indiana.
>
> Because I believe that everyone should be a part of strategic management, I am inviting employees from throughout the department and from all organizational levels to participate. I've appointed Joe Hunt and Nancy Blough to manage the process that I expect to take about a year to complete.

Joe D. Hunt, the director of the Office for Policy Coordination, became responsible for coordination of the various strategic management activities, development of the written strategic plan, and future strategic management activities. Because of Dr. Bailey's commitment to include employees from throughout the organization, a task force structure with five working groups was adopted to carry out the strategic management process (see Exhibit 3-1). Each group had about twenty members. Thus, at the outset, approximately 100 employees were involved. Nancy C. Blough, an attorney appointed as deputy state health commissioner of the Indiana State Depart-

This case was prepared by Peter M. Ginter, University of Alabama at Birmingham; Linda E. Swayne, University of North Carolina at Charlotte; and W. Jack Duncan, University of Alabama at Birmingham. It is intended as a basis for classroom discussion rather than to illustrate effective or ineffective handling of an administrative situation. Used with permission from Peter M. Ginter.

Exhibit 3-1. Indiana State Department of Health Strategic Management Organization

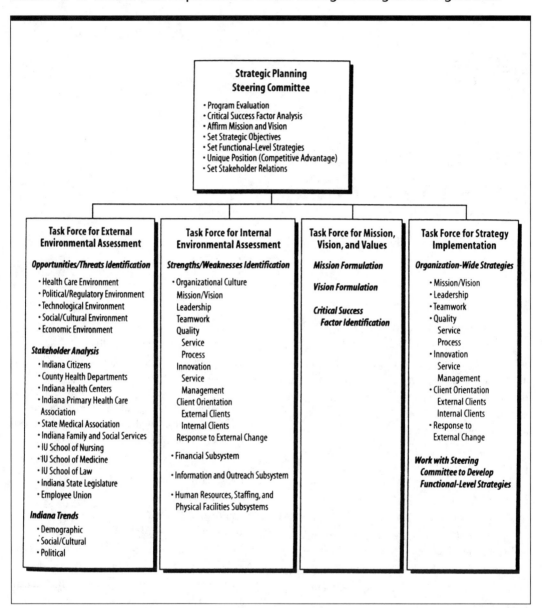

ment of Health in 1992, was committed to the process and ensured that the project remained on schedule.

Joe Hunt stated,

We realized early on that every organization is unique and no one method or approach can be applied blindly. The strategic management process and tools used to implement it must be understood in terms of the objectives of our organization and the logic of our situation. As an aid, we developed a milestone chart [see Exhibit 3-2] that helped the more than 100 people involved visualize the entire process and the interrelationships of the work of the different groups. The milestone chart highlighted specific priorities and the appropriate se-

Exhibit 3-2. Indiana State Department of Health Strategic Management Milestone Chart

TASKS	Timeframe (Months, Weeks 1–4)
Months	May · June · July · August · September · October · November · December · January · February · March · April
• Organization of the Process	May (weeks 1–3)
• External Environmental Assessment	
Opportunities and Threats Identification	June–September
Stakeholder Analysis	June–September
Indiana Trends Identification	June–September
• Internal Environmental Assessment	
Strengths and Weaknesses Identification	June–September
Financial Subsystem	June–September
Information and Outreach Subsystem	June–September
Human Resources, Staffing, and Physical Facilities Subsystem	June–September
• Mission, Vision, and Values	
Mission Formulation	June–September
Vision Formulation	June–September
Critical Success Factor Identification	June–September
• Steering Committee	
Critical Success Factor Analysis	September–November
Affirm Mission and Vision	September–November
Set Strategic Objectives	September–November
Program Evaluation	November–December
Formulate Statement of Strategy	
Set Functional-Level Strategies	January–February
Set Organization-Wide Strategies	February–March
• Implementation	
Organization-Wide Strategies	March–April
Coordinate Functional Strategies	March–April

quence for accomplishing the required tasks. And it helped keep us on schedule.

Situational Analysis

The first months of the process were spent developing the situational analysis. The ISDH's unique situation was brought into perspective by a thorough examination of the external environment, the internal environment, and the mission, vision, values, and critical success factors.

General Situation and Background

The citizens of Indiana were independent and generally did not favor government "interference." They considered themselves to be "typically American." In 1990, Indiana's population was approximately 5.5 million; however, in more recent years the growth had slowed to 1 percent per year. The state ranked as thirty-fifth in population. In addition, the citizens of the state were getting older. In 1990, about 13 percent of the population was 65 years or older, as compared with 12 percent in 1986. About 9 percent of the population was nonwhite. In 1990, about 76 percent of the population aged 25 years and older had graduated from high school; 16 percent had earned a bachelor's degree or higher.

Of the land in Indiana, 70 percent was devoted to agriculture. Corn and soybeans were the state's primary cash crops. The northwestern portion of the state was a major industrial area fostered by the close proximity to industrial centers in Chicago, Detroit, and Toledo. Iron, steel, and petroleum products were major manufacturing outputs. Other manufactured products included aluminum, chemicals, clay products, furniture, and automotive parts. On a national basis, Indiana was a major producer of pharmaceuticals, manufactured housing, and musical instruments; however, service industries accounted for 60 percent of the gross state product.

In 1988, Indiana's total general expenditures of $8.4 billion ranked it as thirty-seventh among the states on a per capita basis. The major categories of state expenditure included $3.66 billion for education, $1.48 billion for public welfare, $903 million for highways, $604 million for health and hospitals, and $117 million for the management of natural resources.

High-priority statewide health needs that had been identified and were being actively addressed included high-risk pregnancies, child abuse/neglect, unintentional injuries, older adults, environmental health, and the medically underserved. The ten leading causes of death in 1990 were diseases of the heart, cancer, cerebrovascular diseases, pneumonia, other chronic obstructive pulmonary diseases, diseases of the arteries, diabetes mellitus, motor vehicle accidents, accidents excluding motor vehicle accidents, and suicide.

County Governance

The population's "home rule" attitude limited the influence of state and federal government and created an unusual operating environment in In-

diana. Marion County (which included the capital city of Indianapolis) was governed by a mayor/council form of government. All other counties in the state had two governing bodies, a board of commissioners and a county council. Generally, the board of commissioners performed the executive and legislative functions of county government, and the county council served as the fiscal body. Counties in Indiana followed this home rule authority as granted in Title 36 of the Indiana code, which specified that counties had the powers granted by law and other powers necessary or desirable to conduct county affairs.

The Indiana State Department of Health

The Indiana State Department of Health was a freestanding, independent state agency. The commissioner was appointed by and served at the pleasure of the governor. As chief executive officer, the commissioner was responsible for overall management of the ISDH. The governor appointed eleven individuals who served on the executive board of the state board of health as well. The executive board was responsible for providing policy advice and guidance for the ISDH. An organization chart for the agency is presented in Exhibit 3-3.

An important role of the ISDH staff was to function as consultants to staff members of local (county) health departments within the state. In addition, there existed a division for local support services; these staff were assigned on a geographical basis to work directly with local health departments to provide both technical and management consulting services.

Interaction between state and local public health agencies in Indiana was highly decentralized. Under this arrangement, local governments somewhat independently operated and financed their own local health departments. The state had ninety-six local health departments: ninety county, one multicounty, and five city health departments. According to state law, the ISDH was the "superior agency" to each of the local health de-

Exhibit 3-3. Indiana State Department of Health Organizational Chart

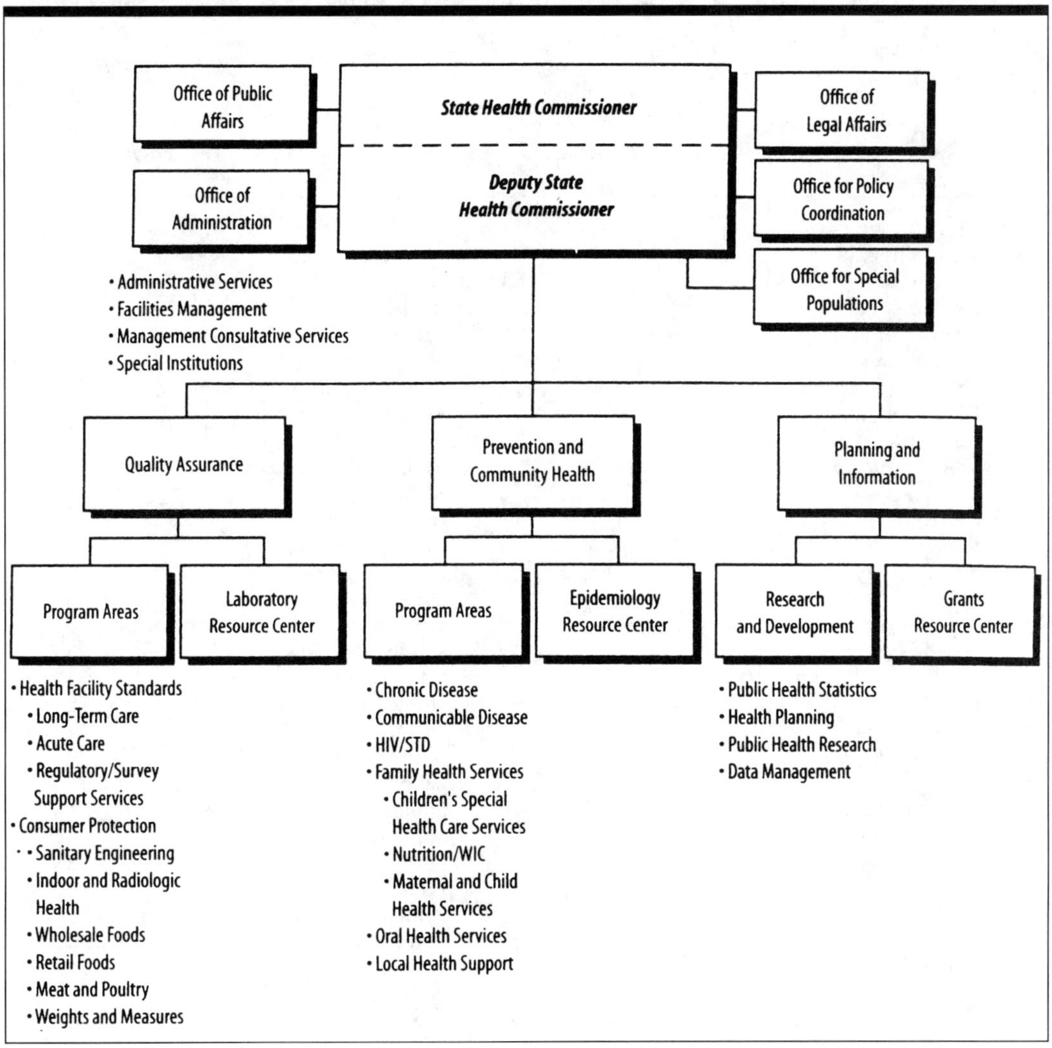

partments. In this capacity, the ISDH was charged with the responsibility for recording the appointments of local health officers and overseeing the programs and activities of the local health departments. Staff members of local health departments, however, were employed and supervised by the local jurisdiction. The number of staff members for a local health department ranged from 1 to 550.

Because of the quasi-autonomy of the local health departments, public health services varied widely from county to county depending on local funding and the decisions of the local commission and county council. Services provided in one county, therefore, might not be provided in a contiguous county, or these services might be carried out in a different manner or with varying levels of enthusiasm. In general, the services offered by the local health departments were classified as (1) assessment, (2) policy development, and (3) assurance activities. Exhibit 3-4 provides a list of these services and identifies the number of local health departments that provided each service within the state.

Exhibit 3-4. Services Provided by Local Health Departments

Services	Number of Departments Providing Each Service	Services	Number of Departments Providing Each Service
Assessment activities			
Data collection/analysis			
Behavioral risk assessment	13	Environmental (Continued)	
Morbidity data	38	Radiation control	17
Reportable diseases	71	Sewage disposal systems	87
Vital records and statistics	89	Solid waste management	61
Epidemiology/surveillance		Vector and animal control	76
Chronic diseases	38	Water pollution	65
Communicable diseases	85	Personal health services	
Policy development		AIDS testing and counseling	22
Health code development and		Alcohol abuse	3
enforcement	51	Child health	61
Health planning	49	Chronic diseases	50
Priority setting	21	Dental health	9
		Drug abuse	6
Assurance activities		Emergency medical services	4
Inspection		Family planning	16
Food and milk control	67	Handicapped children	53
Health facility safety/quality	21	Home health care	45
Recreation facility safety/quality	30	Hospitals	2
Other facility safety/quality	8	Immunizations	89
Licensing		Laboratory services	17
Health facilities	6	Long-term-care facilities	1
Other facilities	63	Mental health	4
Health education	56	Obstetrical care	11
Environmental		Prenatal care	29
Air quality	41	Primary care	5
Hazardous waste management	50	Sexually transmitted diseases	26
Individual water supply safety	76	Tuberculosis	75
Noise pollution	9	WIC (women, infant, children)	
Occupational health and safety	12	program	30
Public water safety	51		

SOURCE: Public Health Practice Program Office, Division of Public Health Systems, Centers for Disease Control, *Profile of State and Territorial Public Health Systems: United States, 1990* (Atlanta: U.S. Department of Health and Human Services, Public Health Service, Centers for Disease Control, 1991), pp. 121-122.

NOTE: Ninety-four of ninety-six local health departments reported.

External Environmental Analysis

External analysis for the ISDH was carried out in two phases. First, stakeholder analysis was used to identify the relationships of the ISDH with other organizations. Second, the department used trend/ issue identification and analysis to identify and focus on the issues considered most important.

Stakeholder Analysis

The task force identified more than 250 stakeholder groups and organizations, 12 of which were considered to be central to the department's mission. Stakeholder analysis was selected because of the belief that these outside organizations would be in a good position to suggest areas of excellence within the ISDH as well as areas for improvement. Furthermore, the stakeholders had important perspectives on the changing economic, social, and political environment of Indiana and the future role that the ISDH should play.

The conclusions of the stakeholder analysis were that relations with stakeholders were generally positive, although relations were sometimes strained between the ISDH and the local health departments (Exhibit 3-5). There was a high level of cooperation with other agencies, and the members generally understood the reciprocal relationship between their agency and the ISDH. Most of the agencies desired an even closer working relationship with the ISDH.

The major deficiency in stakeholder relations was with the county health departments. As indicated in the section "General Situation and Background," the quasi-autonomous county health departments delivered most public health services. That is, the county health departments actually provided the services such as food inspections, immunizations, and health code enforcement. The ISDH created policy and supported the activities of the counties. Often counties saw the ISDH as bureaucratic, unresponsive, and inappropriately staffed to serve the needs of the counties.

Trend/Issue Analysis

In an effort to identify the major trends and issues, the External Environmental Assessment Task Force was divided into five subcommittees that the ISDH believed represented the major classifications of the public health environment in Indiana:

- Health care
- Political/regulatory
- Technological
- Social/cultural
- Economic

Each subcommittee was given the responsibility for gathering information, using internal/external and personal/nonpersonal sources of data to identify key trends and issues within its category. After the initial data-gathering activity, the External Environmental Assessment Task Force decided that the trends and issues identified by the various subcommittees should be classified by (1) scope—national, state, or county issues and (2) strength—current, emerging, or speculative issues. Using this approach, each subcommittee identified more than fifty issues. Because only the most important issues ultimately could be addressed by the strategic plan, each subcommittee reduced the list to ten or fewer trends/issues by assessing the importance of the impact of the trends and issues on the ISDH.

Subsequent discussions and the combination of some issues resulted in a total of thirty-four environmental issues. To verify the validity of the trends and issues identified by the subcommittees of the External Environmental Assessment Task Force, 317 external stakeholders (including the administrators of the ninety-six local health departments) were surveyed. The stakeholders were asked to evaluate each of the thirty-four trends and issues as being very important, important, less important, or not important. Mean scores for each trend were calculated, and stakeholder and task force results were compared. The trends and issues rated as very important (mean scores above 3.38) for both groups are presented in Exhibit 3-6.

After considerable discussion concerning the survey results, the task force decided that the views of the stakeholders and the task force should be considered by combining several of the important individual trends and issues under broader headings. By collapsing the trends and issues, fewer areas could be highlighted, allowing the ISDH to focus on the most important trends and issues. It was the belief of the task force that each of the major trends and issues represented both opportunities and threats for the ISDH. To highlight this belief, the task force agreed to identify the implications of the opportunities and threats for each of the most important issues (Exhibit 3-7).

Exhibit 3-5. Indiana State Department of Health Stakeholder Relationships

Stakeholder	General Purpose/Mission	Nature of the Relationship
Indiana citizens	To achieve health and happiness	The medically underserved depend on ISDH for clinical services; entire community depends on department for prevention and protection
County health departments	To deliver public health services such as clinical services, permits, inspections, birth and death certificates, and so on, at the county level	Provide for the direct delivery of public health in Indiana; policy guidance from the state-level organization; rely on state expertise and advice; little financial dependence; semi-autonomous, county departments prefer to stay independent (home rule) but also need the expertise of the state
Indiana Health Centers	To provide health services to those who, because of poverty or location in rural areas, do not have access to affordable health care; emphasis is on farmworkers	ISDH provides many important regulatory functions and contracting opportunities for Indiana Health Centers
Indiana Primary Health Care Association	To provide family care to the underserved through health centers/clinics, advocacy, data analysis, and so on	Cooperative agreement with ISDH; have a similar mission, want to maintain a close relationship
Indiana Medical Association	Professional association to represent state physicians; provides licensure services as well as lobbying activities	ISDH has important regulatory functions and collects useful epidemiology and vital statistical data; the two organizations tend to be on the same side of lobbying issues; Indiana Medical Association would like to see more mutual efforts to communicate with ISDH
Indiana Family and Social Services	To protect and serve families in need of human services resources or support, including family and children, mental health, Medicaid, aging, and rehabilitative services	Similar mission to serve the public; clients overlap; would prefer more communication with ISDH
ISDH Executive Board	To provide advice from different perspectives to facilitate the highest quality of strategic decision making in ISDH	Board composed of a panel of relevant experts willing to volunteer time and assistance to ISDH

(continued)

Exhibit 3-5. Continued

Stakeholder	General Purpose/Mission	Nature of the Relationship
Indiana University School of Nursing	To provide undergraduate and graduate education; the largest nursing school in the United States.	ISDH is seen as a key player in the debates concerning nursing practice and licensure; School of Nursing wants statutes changed to allow independent nursing practices
Indiana University School of Medicine	To ensure the highest quality of medical education, contribute to medical research, and provide health services	Participation in joint research ventures; reciprocal assistance to ISDH when mutually beneficial
Indiana University School of Law	To provide high levels of teaching, research, and service to the legal community and citizens of Indiana	Some limited participation in mutually beneficial joint activities
Indiana State Legislature	To provide informed governance to citizens of Indiana through enlightened and responsive legislation	Primary funding agency of ISDH; ISDH directly assists through contribution to the legislature's health care agenda
Employee union	To represent department employees	Membership of approximately 20 percent of department employees

Internal Environmental Analysis

The specific objective of the Internal Environmental Assessment Task Force was to provide the steering committee with an assessment of the strengths and weaknesses of the major operating systems within the organization. It decided to form four groups to investigate organizational culture, finance, information systems, and human resources. At the first meeting, the information systems group was redefined as the information and outreach group to highlight the importance and uniqueness of the department's communication with external organizations and the public. In addition, the human resources group became the human resources, staffing, and physical facilities group.

Assessing the Organizational Culture

The organizational culture group assessed the culture of the ISDH with the aid of a sixty-one–item, self-administered questionnaire. The questionnaire was designed to obtain the opinions of the department's 900 employees regarding seven different areas: mission/vision, service and managerial innovation, leadership and employee orientation, responsiveness to external change, teamwork, external and internal customer/client orientation, and quality. In addition to the response scales ranging from *strongly disagree* to *strongly agree* for each question, respondents were provided an opportunity to elaborate on any responses through open-ended comments. More than 500 usable questionnaires were returned.

Results indicated that although most of the employees were familiar with the mandated pur-

Exhibit 3-6. Trends/Issues Rated as Important by Stakeholders and Task Force Members

	Code
Trends With Means Greater Than 3.38 for Stakeholders but Not External Task Force	
No growth in total economy with less tax revenue	E-1
Fewer health insurance benefits offered by employers	E-3
Increasing amount of substance abuse	S-7
Increasing number of federal and state mandates	PR-3
Increasing need for collaboration between public and private providers	HC-2
Trends With Means Greater Than 3.38 for Both Stakeholders and External Task Force	
Limited funding for public health	E-7
Increasing amount of violence (child abuse, rape, etc.)	S-5
Increasing need for emphasis on prevention (communicable diseases, smoking, substance abuse, etc.)	HC-4
Medicaid reform	HC-5
Impact of health care reform	PR-1
Increasing demand for community-based services	PR-6
Increasing need for cooperation among community, state, and federal agencies	PR-7
Trends With Means Greater Than 3.38 for External Task Force but Not Stakeholders	
Inadequate access to health care within the state	HC-3
Inadequate support by ISDH in some technical areas	T-1
Low budget allocations for the procurement of technology	T-4

pose or mission of the ISDH, they were not sure about the department's vision or its direction over the next five years. The respondents did not believe that the department was a highly creative organization; they perceived innovation to be severely limited due to regulatory mandates and excessive policies and procedures imposed on all state agencies. Respondents believed, however, that department leadership valued new ways of doing things and that individuals were allowed to experiment with new procedures without excessive fear of punishment for failure.

Leadership and employee orientation were particularly troublesome areas as reported on the questionnaire. There was widespread belief that top leadership was excessively distant from the operational level of the department, that leaders were not as concerned as they should be about the welfare of employees, and that management was too concerned with political pressures, to the detriment of key public health priorities. Without a doubt, much of the discontent came about because the employees had not had a wage increase in three years and the recently enacted state budget virtually assured no raises for two more years.

The department's ability to deal with external change was ranked highly, although it was perceived as needing some improvement. Open-ended comments indicated that most employees believed that the ISDH was aware of changing forces in the external environment, had some means of monitoring and forecasting trends, and generally responded to environmental changes.

Teamwork was not ranked very highly by employees. Many of the questionnaire respondents believed that most employees were more concerned with their individual jobs and the welfare of their work units than with the overall success of

Exhibit 3-7. Opportunities and Threats for Significant Trends/Issues

Trend/Issue	Opportunities for Action	Threats From No Action
Impact of health care reform	More emphasis placed on core public health—assurance, policy development, and assessment	Major populations remain without access to health care; no meaningful provisions for rural populations
Need for cooperation-based strategies	Integrated health care initiatives; public and private partnerships; state and counties share common goals; higher level of community-based services	Health care remains fragmented and inconsistent throughout the state
Limited funding for public health	Emphasis on efficiency and essential services	Decline in community health; provision of fewer services; lag in technology; lower level of cooperation between state and counties
Increasing amount of violence	New programs directed toward vulnerable populations; education; counseling safety; etc.	Continued increase in violence; fewer intervention services
Increasing need for emphasis on prevention	More emphasis on core public health; improved community health	Breakdown in disease control, epidemiology
Access/care for special populations	Special population programs designed to meet specialized needs	Increasingly large segments of the population without access; inadequate health care
External technological advancements	Upgrade of technology—laboratories, computers, etc.	Low image of ISDH remains; inefficiency; public turns to other organizations for technology-based services
Increasing amount of substance abuse	New programs for substance abuse—education, etc.	Continued rise in substance abuse among more populations

the department. As a result, people sometimes protected rather than shared information, made decisions based on the welfare of their unit rather than the ISDH, and did not work effectively as teams. Competition among work groups was perceived to be more common than cooperation.

The items on the customer/client orientation section of the questionnaire were designed to assess employee responses to both internal and external customers. Considerable agreement existed that employees respected and responded to external and internal customer needs. On the other hand, there was a belief that rules and regulations were more important to many employees than was a true devotion to serving customers. Additionally, it was thought that many people attempted to make their own jobs easier by hiding behind rules and regulations rather than trying in every practical way to facilitate responsiveness to all customers. A consensus was clear that everyone could do more to improve customer orientation.

Finally, concern for quality was widespread in the department. It was generally agreed that employees were professional, well trained for what they did, and committed to public service. Respondents often indicated, however, that high levels of service quality were not adequately emphasized or rewarded; that the hiring, retention, and promotion policies were not based on the quality of services provided; and that the general work environment made high levels of quality difficult to ensure.

The results of the questionnaire indicated a perceived need for improvement in all seven areas. There was a need to more clearly state and communicate the future direction of the department to all employees and reduce as much as possible the excessive policies that frustrated many managers and nonmanagerial employees in performing their jobs in the most effective manner. In addition, more managers needed to exercise leadership and encourage teamwork.

Assessing Finances

Finance was a particularly serious problem for the ISDH (as well as other Indiana state agencies). State employees had not been able to maintain their incomes, and programs and facilities reflected the deteriorating financial situation. In an attempt to isolate the most important strategic considerations, the financial assessment group examined the present, past, and projected future financial resources; interviewed financial personnel at other Midwestern state health departments; and conducted internal interviews and surveys.

Before beginning the specific analysis, the financial situation of the ISDH was put in perspective based on what was happening in other states in the region. In the year immediately prior to the beginning of the strategic planning process, Illinois and Michigan reduced their public health

workforce, and Ohio endured about an 11 percent decrease in public health funding.

During the five years prior to the initiation of the strategic planning process, the ISDH's proportion of annual state appropriations was relatively fixed at less than 1 percent of the state general fund. According to the Public Health Foundation, this level of funding placed Indiana as forty-ninth (of the fifty states) in per capita funding for public health. As illustrated by Exhibit 3-8, state general funds for all purposes increased about 9 percent in 1990; the rate of increase gradually declined to an increase of a little more than 3 percent by 1993. It was clear that increases in state general funds had declined significantly over the past five years and that, of the smaller increases, public health received increasingly smaller shares.

There was one bright spot in the ISDH funding picture. During the five-year period immediately preceding the initiation of the strategic planning process and during a period when state funding was almost level, federal funds increased by 45 percent. In 1989, for example, the ISDH received approximately $63 million in federal funds. This amount increased to more than $90 million in 1993 (Exhibit 3-9).

The Finance Division had developed a strong internal customer orientation. A survey of internal users conducted by the division indicated that virtually everyone who responded was satisfied with the manner in which the payroll, travel reimbursements, and similar services were accomplished.

Although industry, state governments, and health care were moving toward increased automation and computerization, the Finance Division had not "kept up" technologically. Only a few personal computers were available to do the work of the division. Moreover, the capability for on-line assistance with financial services was extremely limited, representing a significant restriction on the staff's ability to provide needed services, particularly in the area of budget development and administration.

In addition, the decline in funding for the department over the past five years had not reduced public expectations and demands for public

Exhibit 3-8. Percentage Increase in State General Funds Versus Indiana State Department of Health Appropriations

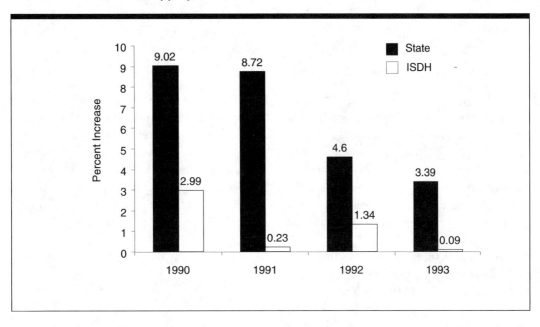

Exhibit 3-9. State and Federal Budget Receipts

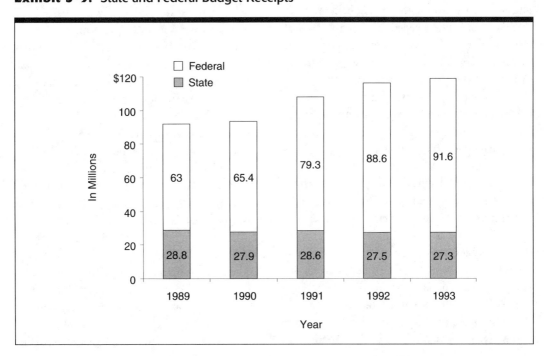

health services. As a result, despite a period of extremely limited funding, services had increased, making the financial plight of the ISDH even more critical.

Assessing Information and Outreach

The analysis of the information and outreach subsystems indicated that the individuals in Management Information Systems (MIS) and the Office of Communications were resourceful and able to accomplish a great deal despite limited resources. The department was fortunate to have found the resources that enabled it to interface with a large number of useful electronic databases. In addition, a "satellite feed" made it possible to communicate electronically with locations throughout the nation and the world. Internally, it was perceived that the MIS staff understood the problems of the overall system and the department was considered to be well prepared to ensure the security of confidential information.

The Office of Communications was thought to have used the power of the "public health message." That is, external communications focused on those issues that captured the interest of the citizens relative to public health issues in Indiana.

A weakness that needed attention was a lack of consistently effective communication up and down the organization as well as with external groups. Substantial confusion existed concerning the protocol for contact and communication with the media. Some of this was attributable to the lack of external and internal customer/client orientation on the part of both MIS and the Office of Communications. It was agreed that the human resources information system was nonfunctioning and did little, if anything, to help managers and employees with personnel matters. There was no parity in the internal distribution of information processing resources, and the internal telecommunications infrastructure—telephone system, e-mail, and fax—was inadequate and unreliable. MIS could not afford to employ the human resources necessary to keep all the hardware and software operating on a timely basis, and

computer expertise to temporarily "fix" things until help arrived was inadequate. There was inadequate physical space for effective hardware operations not only for centralized MIS but also for individual work units.

Overall, the picture of the information and outreach systems was consistent. The devotion and hard work of the individuals at all levels had made the systems work adequately despite severely limited resources. In the process, however, the staff of both the Management Information Systems and the Office of Communications processing units had become internally oriented and had lost sight of the importance of identifying and serving all their relevant customers/clients.

Assessing Human Resources, Staffing, and Physical Facilities

The basic human resources, staffing, and physical facilities infrastructure were primary concerns of the employees of the department. Again, it was perceived that colleagues—managerial and nonmanagerial—were committed to the success of the department and to public health in Indiana. Because of this devotion, loyalty, and hard work, the department was able to accomplish a great deal with relatively little in terms of resources. From a physical facilities perspective, a significant strength was the department's location adjacent to Indiana's primary academic medical center.

There were, however, a number of weaknesses. As was the case with many high-technology organizations, people were promoted to management positions based on their technical expertise rather than their existing or potential management skills, and little management training was provided. As a result, there were many good public health technicians and scientists who became frustrated and unremarkable managers.

There was widespread concern over the inadequacy of the physical facilities. Air quality, ventilation, storage space, and power supply were not adequate for the quality of work expected of employees. More than a few employees suggested that the department would probably "fail" its own health inspections. Finally, as with MIS and the Office of Communications, it was believed that the human resources staff was not properly oriented to serve either external or internal customers/clients.

Mission, Vision, and Values

The objective of this task force was to address the formulation of the departmental mission and vision, to suggest the values that would become the basis for decision making, and to develop an initial list of critical success factors for the department. The group decided not to develop a separate value statement for the department because values such as respect for all individuals, quality, trust, concern, ethical standards, and so on were integral parts of both the mission and vision statements (see Exhibit 3-10).

From Mission and Vision to Critical Success Factors

Having achieved some consensus concerning what should be the ISDH's mission and its vision for the future, the task force proceeded to determine critical success factors. The task force members drafted six factors that they believed were critical to the success of the department:

1. Public health workforce: Become the employer of choice for public health professionals and support staff rather than the employer of last resort.
2. Communications: Improve expertise with internal communication as well as with external stakeholders.
3. Funding: Secure adequate and stable funding.
4. Collaboration: Expand and improve the network of collaborative relationships with local health departments and other relevant public and private agencies.

5. Service quality: Improve quality of services from the viewpoint of external clients and internal clients.
6. Organizational focus: Concentrate on professionalism and scientifically identified causes of disease, prevention, disability, and premature death.

Similar to the mission and vision statements, the draft of critical success factors was regarded as a starting point for organization-wide discussion and forwarded to the steering committee for revision and finalizing.

Strategy Formulation

Based on the results of the situational analysis, the ISDH began the process of finalizing the directional strategies that would set the future course of the ISDH.

The Directional Strategies

The steering committee reviewed the external environmental issues, the internal capabilities, and the draft of the directional strategies that were developed, analyzed, and summarized by the three task forces. Directional strategies such as mission, vision, goals, and values provide "direction" for the entire organization to follow. The mission, vision, and values task force was to develop a final mission statement, develop a vision statement, and set the overarching goals for the organization; however, the steering committee felt that it could proceed given the tentative points that had been outlined by the task force.

Finalizing the Critical Success Factors

Input and discussion concerning the critical success factors were solicited from all divisions and levels of the ISDH. There was a great deal of agreement that the critical success factors generated by the mission, vision, and values task force were important, but the committee believed that one factor (organizational focus) should be

Exhibit 3-10. Components of the Indiana State Department of Health Mission and Vision Statements

	Descriptions (Key Words)
Mission statement components	
1. Target customer/clients and markets	People in Indiana—especially those in need, as identified by measures of health and economic status
2. Principal services delivered	Training and technical assistance, prevention and health education programs, surveillance and analysis of health data, policy development, and planning and evaluation
3. Geographical domain of operations	Borders of Indiana
4. Commitment of specific values	Respect for the individual, quality services, innovation, personal integrity, trust, concern, and high ethical standards
5. Explicit philosophy	Proactive leadership through the application of public health sciences and epidemiology and the quest for efficiency of operations
6. Other important components	Recognition of interdependence with the larger world
Vision statement components	
1. A clear hope for the future	A future in which communities, local health agencies, and the private sector cooperate to increase the span of healthy life for all Hoosiers, reduce the disparities among segments of the population, and ensure access to preventive services for all people
2. Challenging and excellence concerns	Strive for excellence, display initiative, and demonstrate achievement
3. Inspirational and emotional	Forging alliances with public and private sectors to ensure timely, cost-effective public health interventions with primary commitment to local health departments
4. Empowers employees first and clients/customers second	Value employees
5. Prepares for the future	Catalyst for progress that will result in healthier people and a healthful environment
6. Memorable and provides guidance	Memorable terms—catalyst for progress, public health leader in the Hoosier state, core values integral to public health, innovation, and so on

Exhibit 3-11. Critical Success Factors and Rationale

Workforce: The Indiana State Department of Health (ISDH) must provide a working environment and resources that will attract and retain qualified staff members and empower them to achieve or exceed agency goals. The working environment will support responsive personnel policies, competitive salaries/ wages, adequate training, advancement opportunities, trust, and sensitivity to diversity, as well as efficiency, innovation, and excellence.

Communication: The ISDH must communicate effectively both internally with employees and externally with local, state, and federal public health agencies and other stakeholders. Communication must accurately and consistently reflect the mission, vision, and activities of the agency.

Funding: The ISDH must establish funding priorities; pursue innovative strategies to obtain adequate, stable financial resources for ensuring that fundamental public health services are available; and monitor use of funds to achieve established objectives.

Collaboration: The ISDH must expand and improve internal teamwork and external partnerships with local health departments and other local, state, and federal public and private organizations to promote public health.

Service: The ISDH must maintain a client orientation and ensure the quality of all services for internal and external clients.

Leadership: The ISDH must be a visible, active, and persistent advocate on behalf of its employees and public health. This leadership must be based on efficiency, innovation, respect for the individual, and science. Leadership qualities will be recognized and promoted at all levels of the agency.

Management: The ISDH must implement a process that plans and sets priorities within the constraints of available resources and in the context of strategic thinking. Management processes must promote interprogram coordination and cooperation to achieve agency goals.

Data and Information: The ISDH must acquire and use timely and accurate data to assess needs, develop policy, and ensure quality services. The data and information acquired must be shared with all people who need it to carry out their responsibilities.

expanded and that further rationale or explanation of each factor would help clarify and provide focus for subsequently setting organizational objectives. The revised critical success factors and rationale are presented in Exhibit 3-11.

Developing Agency Goals
(Strategic Objectives)

Strategic objectives (called agency goals by the ISDH) needed to be developed for each of the critical success factors. The steering committee be-

lieved that it was better to have a few well-defined goals rather than a long list of objectives that would be impossible to accomplish in view of resource limitations. It was decided, therefore, that one agency goal relative to each critical success factor would be developed. For each goal, specific activities were to be outlined to guide the various programs toward the achievement of the agency goals. Individual programs could then develop their own set of objectives, using the ISDH goals and actions as models.

The Adaptive Strategies

On completion of the directional strategies (mission, vision, and objectives), the steering committee began to develop the adaptive strategies (the basic strategies for the organization that enabled it to "adapt" to its environment). After reviewing the evaluative tools available for analyzing the adaptive strategies, the steering committee decided that program evaluation would provide the best results. Because of the not-for-profit nature of the agency, funding from state appropriations and grants, and the program orientation of the ISDH, the steering committee was somewhat concerned about how to determine which of the department's seventy-three programs should be slated for expansion, stabilization, or contraction (see Exhibit 3-12 for a listing of the programs). There was never an easy answer in public health because all programs were important.

The committee determined that both approaches to program evaluation—program priority setting and needs/capacity assessment—would facilitate strategic thinking within the agency. In addition, because the prospect of health care reform (both industry evolution and legislation) was such a dominant environmental theme, three possible scenarios for health care reform were developed as a backdrop for assessing the various programs. The scenarios are presented in Exhibit 3-13.

Program Priority Setting

The steering committee decided to use the Q-sort method to set priorities because all programs were important. (See the appendix to this case for a detailed discussion of the Q-sort method.) The seventy-three identified programs were to be sorted, with four programs being labeled most important, five programs next most important, and so on, with each column of programs being "next most important." The Q-sort would have four, five, nine, eleven, fifteen, eleven, nine, five, and four programs in the columns, progressing from the first four being the most important programs to the last four being the next most important (rather than the least important). Exhibit 3-14 provides a Q-sort worksheet that various groups were to use.

Needs/Capacity Assessment

Another tool used by not-for-profits was a needs/capacity assessment. The agency's seventy-three programs would be evaluated based on perceptions of the community need for the program and the capacity of the agency to meet that need. The programs would be rated as very high, high, low, or very low for both community need and organizational capacity. Exhibit 3-15 was used by the executive staff and various program managers within ISDH for the needs/capacity assessment.

Developing the Adaptive Strategies

Using the results of the program priority setting and needs/capacity assessment, the committee would develop an adaptive strategy. The adaptive strategy was viewed as a process of evolving the agency toward a desired profile or portfolio of programs. The makeup of that profile was influenced by the strategic assumptions (external issues, internal issues, and the mission, vision, and goals). Dominant in the strategic assumptions was the belief that, in the long term, health care reform would be successful and that the agency would move toward more community or core public health (Scenario I) activities. However, it was the belief of the steering committee and executive staff that, in the short term, special populations and certain medical treatments would not be "covered" by insurance or government programs and that the health department would have to remain in (or enter) those segments (Scenario II).

Based on these evaluative tools (program priority setting, needs/capacity assessment, and scenario analysis), the executive staff began discussions on programs that needed to be expanded, stabilized, or contracted. For example, programs with high community need but low organization

Exhibit 3-12. Indiana State Department of Health Programs

1. MCH: Indiana Family Helpline
2. MCH: Genetic Diseases/Newborn Screening
3. MCH: Childhood Lead Poisoning Prevention Program
4. MCH: Prenatal Substance Use Prevention Program
5. MCH: Adolescent Health
6. Children's Special Health Care Services
7. Nutrition/WIC Program
8. Oral Health Services (includes fluoridation and sealants)
9. Epidemiology Resource Center
10. Management Information Systems
11. Health Planning
12. Health Planning: Certificate of Need
13. Health Planning: Hospital Financial Disclosure
14. Public Health Research
15. Public Health Research: County Needs Assessment
16. Public Health Statistics
17. Public Health Statistics: Vital Records
18. Public Health Statistics: Birth Problems Registry
19. Grants Resource Center
20. Office of Legal Affairs
21. Local Health Support: Local Health Department Coordination and Liaison Activities
22. MCH: Family Planning Program
23. Office for Policy Coordination
24. Office for Special Populations: Disability Concerns
25. Office for Special Populations: Interagency Council for Black and Minority Health
26. Office of Public Affairs: Health Education
27. Health Education: Film Library
28. Health Education: Library
29. Office of Public Affairs: Media Relations
30. Office of Public Affairs: Photographer
31. Office of Public Affairs: Print Shop
32. Office of Administration: Administrative Services
33. Office of Administration: Correspondence Center
34. Office of Administration: Finance
35. Office of Administration: Purchasing
36. Office of Administration: Human Resources
37. Facilities Management: Safety Programs Coordination
38. Facilities Management: Environmental Services
39. Facilities Management: Physical Plant
40. Facilities Management: Security
41. Facilities Management: Asset Service Center
42. Office of Administration: Management Consultative Services
43. MCH: Breastfeeding Promotion Program
44. Health Facility Standards: Long-Term Care Program
45. Health Facility Standards: Regulatory/Survey Support Services
46. Acute Care Services: Hospital, Lab, ASC, Home Health Inspections
47. Laboratory Support Services
48. HIV/STD Program: CTS/STD Program (sexually transmitted disease control)
49. HIV/STD Program: HIV Prevention Activities
50. HIV/STD Program: Clinical Data and Research
51. Communicable Disease Program: Immunization, TB Control, General Communicable Disease Control
52. Chronic Disease Program: Injury Control Program
53. Chronic Disease Program: Renal Program, Cancer Registry, PHBG Activities, Antitobacco Activities
54. MCH: Pregnancy Risk Assessment Monitoring System (PRAMS)
55. Family Health Services: Women's Health
56. MCH: Prenatal Care, Primary Care/Managed Care, School-Based Clinics
57. Consumer Services: Retail Food Division
58. Consumer Services: Meat and Poultry
59. Manufactured Food Section
60. Consumer Services: Weights and Measures
61. Wholesale Food Division
62. Wholesale Food Division: Milk
63. Sanitary Engineering: Residential Sewage Disposal Section
64. Sanitary Engineering: Vector Control Group
65. Environmental Health Laboratory
66. Sanitary Engineering: Plan Review Section
67. Disease Control Laboratory
68. Indoor and Radiologic Health
69. Consumer Health Laboratory
70. Office for Special Populations: Rural Health Initiative
71. Sanitary Engineering: Environmental Health Section
72. MCH: Healthy Pregnancy/Healthy Baby Campaign
73. MCH: Sudden Infant Death Syndrome Project (SIDS)

Exhibit 3-13. Health Care Reform Scenarios

Scenario I: Return to Core Public Health. In this scenario, comprehensive health care reform legislation is passed that provides some form of health insurance for everyone. Thus, individuals who formerly relied on public health agencies and emergency rooms for primary care now have access (through their insurance) to private providers. In addition, providers have found it advantageous to serve this population. Under this assumption, the private sector would assume virtually all the personal primary-care responsibilities. The health department would emphasize data collection, monitoring, health promotion, education, regulation, assessment, environmental health, disease control, research, and policy leadership. In this situation, the department's focus would be almost exclusively on community health issues rather than the provision of personal primary care.

Scenario II: Core Public Health Plus Special Care Needs. In this scenario, health care reform is passed; however, because of high costs, major gaps in coverage remain. Under this assumption, most treatments and special populations would be covered by the private sector; however, significant "gaps" in coverage will continue. The only source of care for these populations will be in the public sector. In this scenario, the department would emphasize community health (core public health) but would continue to provide primary health care for special populations and treatments not covered under any type of (revolutionary or evolutionary) health care reform.

Scenario III: Health Care Reform Bogs Down. In this scenario, no significant health care reform legislation is passed. Even the evolutionary restructuring of the health care industry has left major "gaps" for significant populations and treatments. Under this assumption, any type of health care reform fails to change significantly the ratio of people without access to primary care. Primary care may even be expanded under this assumption as the health department plays a larger role in ensuring access. In this scenario, the department would emphasize community health and the provision of primary care about equally.

---

capacity and a "high" Q-sort ranking might be marked for expansion. Programs with low community need, high capacity, and a "low" Q-sort ranking could be considered for contraction.

In addition to understanding services and service population decisions concerning expansion, stabilization, or contraction, the executive staff believed that program managers should understand the agency's resource commitment to the various programs. For each program, the executive staff would allocate funding and staffing based on its designation as "expand," "stable," or "contract."

What's Next?

The task force groups met to report on progress to the Steering Committee. The work of the External

Environmental Assessment Task Force, the Internal Environmental Assessment Task Force, and the Mission, Vision, and Objectives Task Force were completed or nearing final stages. The Steering Committee's objectives included the following:

- Review and confirm the external opportunities and threats and internal strengths and weaknesses
- Finalize the mission, vision, and critical success factors
- Specify the set of programs and services that will achieve the mission and vision
- Operationalize the critical success factors with clean and concise strategic objectives (later called agency goals) to provide direction for departmental operations
- Coordinate the development of adaptive, market entry, and positioning strategies

Exhibit 3-14. Q-Sort Worksheet for Seventy-Three Programs

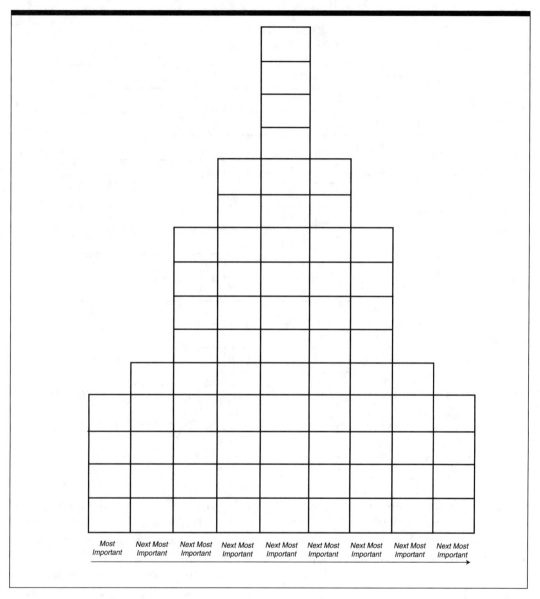

Most Important | Next Most Important | Next Most Important | Next Most Important | Next Most Important | Next Most Important | Next Most Important | Next Most Important | Next Most Important

- Coordinate the development of program implementation work plans
- Foster strategic thinking throughout the organization

Joe Hunt was satisfied with the progress to date. He commented, "Each task force did its job better than I anticipated. There was a real com-

mitment to do the assigned task well and in a timely manner."

It was time to involve the Implementation Strategy Task Force. He scheduled a meeting for Monday of the following week. The major work for this task force would be to develop implementation plans. He knew this was where strategic management sometimes bogged down. He would

Exhibit 3-15. Needs/Capacity Assessment Program Plot

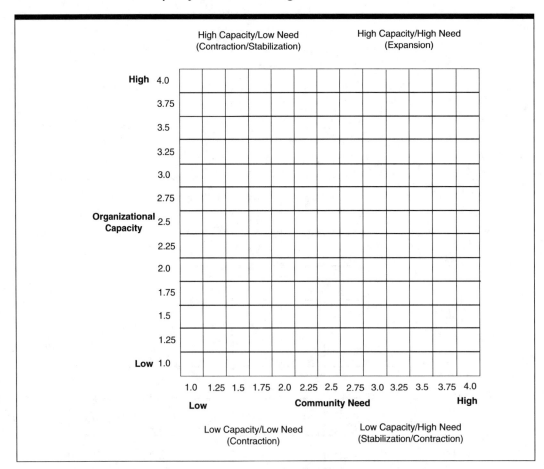

ask the task force, "Are you prepared to set the strategies that will constitute the work of ISDH for the next two years? Is there any more information that you need from any of the other groups?"

APPENDIX:
Program Evaluation Primer

Program evaluation was especially useful in organizations in which market share, industry strength, and competitive advantage were not particularly important or were not relevant. Such organizations were typically not-for-profit, state and federally funded institutions such as state and county public health departments, state mental health departments, Medicaid agencies, community health centers, and public community hospitals. Despite the fact that these organizations were public and not-for-profit, they needed to develop explicit strategies and evaluate the adaptive strategic alternatives open to them. Although SWOT (strengths, weaknesses, opportunities, and threats) and a form of portfolio analysis could be used to evaluate public health programs, evaluation methods that considered increasing revenue and market share were inappropriate or difficult to use.

Public and not-for-profit institutions typically maintained any number of programs funded through such sources as state appropriations, federal grants, private donations, and fee for service. In a public health department, such programs might include HIV/AIDS education, disease surveillance, disease control, immunizations, food sanitation inspection, on-site sewage inspection, and many more. Usually, these programs were initiated to fill a health care need within the community that had not been addressed through the private sector. These "health care gaps" occurred because of federal or state requirements for coordination and control of community health and because of the large number of individuals without adequate health care insurance or means to pay for services.

Within the context provided by an understanding of the external environment, internal environment, and directional strategies, these not-for-profit institutions charted a future through a set of externally and internally funded programs. The set of programs maintained and emphasized by the organization constituted its adaptive strategy. The degree to which they were changed (expansion, contraction, stabilization) represented a modification of the adaptive strategy. The fundamental question therefore was "Does our current set of programs effectively and efficiently fulfill our mission and our vision for the future?" This question was addressed through a process of program evaluation. Two program evaluation methods that have been used successfully are needs/capacity assessment and program priority setting.

Needs/Capacity Assessment

The set of programs in not-for-profit organizations such as public health departments essentially were determined by (1) community need and (2) the organization's capacity to deliver the program to that community. Of course, some programs were mandated by law, such as disease control, disease surveillance, and the maintenance of vital records (birth and death records). However, the assumption was that the legislation was a result of an important need and, typically, the mandate was supported by nondiscretionary or categorical funding (funding that may be used for

only one purpose). Therefore, in developing a strategy for a public health organization or not-for-profit organization serving the community, community needs must be assessed, as well as the organization's ability (capacity) to address the needs.

Community need was a function of (1) clear community requirements (environmental, sanitation, disease control, and so on) and personal health care (primary care) gaps, (2) the degree to which other institutions (private and public) filled the identified health care gaps, and (3) public/community health objectives. Most not-for-profit institutions entered the health care market to provide services to those who otherwise would be left out of the system. Despite efforts to reform health care, these gaps were likely to remain for some time. Health care gaps were identified through community involvement, political pressure, and community assessments such as those carried out by the Centers for Disease Control and Prevention (CDC). These gaps existed because there were few private or public institutions positioned to fill the need. Where existing institutions were willing and able to fill these gaps, public and not-for-profit organizations should probably have resisted entering the market. In addition, public and community health objectives must be considered when developing strategy.

Organization capacity was the organization's ability to initiate, maintain, and enhance its set of adaptive strategy programs. Organization capacity was composed of (1) funding to support programs, (2) other organizational resources and skills, and (3) the program's fit with the mission and vision of the organization. Availability of funding was an important part of organization capacity. Many programs were supported with categorical funding and accompanying mandates (program requirements dictated by a higher authority, usually federal or state government). Often, however, local moneys supplemented federal- and state-funded programs. For other programs, only community funding was available. Thus, funding availability was a major consideration in developing strategy for public and not-for-profit organizations. In addition, the organization needed the skills, resources, facilities, management, and so on to initiate and effectively administer the program. Finally, program strategy depended on the program's fit with the organization's mission and vision for the future. Programs outside the mission and vision would be viewed as luxuries, superfluous, or wasteful.

Where the community need was assessed as high (significant health care gaps, few or no other institutions addressing the need, and the program was a part of the community's objectives) and the organization's capacity was assessed as high (adequate funding, appropriate skills and resources, and fit with mission/vision), then the organization could expand. When the community need assessment was low (no real need, the need had abated, need was now being addressed by another institution, or the need did not fit with community objectives) but organization capacity was high (adequate funding, appropriate skills and resources, and fit with mission/vision), there could be an orderly redistribution of resources, suggesting contraction or stabilization. Contraction strategies should be given priority as the community need diminished; however, phasing out a program might take some time, or the uncertainty concerning the changing community needs might dictate stabilization in the short term.

Where community needs were assessed as low (no real need, the need had abated, need was now being addressed by another institution, or the need did not fit with community objectives) and the organization had few financial or other resources to commit to programs (low organization capacity), contraction strategies should occur. When community needs were assessed as high but organizational capacity was low, stabilization or contraction was appropriate. Stabilization strategies should be given priority because of the high community need, but if resources dwindled or funding was reduced, contraction might be required. As resources became available and organization capacity increased, programs could be expanded.

Program Priority Setting

The second method of developing adaptive strategies for public programs involved ranking programs and setting priorities. This process was significant because community needs (both the need itself and the severity of the need) were constantly changing and organizational resources, in terms of funding and organization capacity, were almost always limited. Invariably, programs with high community need outstripped resources available; therefore, the most important programs (and perhaps those with categorical funding) might be expanded or stabilized. The organization must have an understanding of which programs were the most important, which should be provided incremental funding, and which should be the first to be scaled back if funding was reduced or eliminated.

The nature of and emphasis on programs was the central part of strategy formulation in many public and not-for-profit organizations. A problem in ranking these programs was that typically all of them were viewed as "very important" or "essential." This was particularly true when using Likert-type or semantic differential scales to evaluate the programs. It was necessary, therefore, to develop evaluation methods that further differentiated the programs. One method that could be used was to list all the programs of the agency or clinic, each on a separate paper posted in different areas of a room. Three different colors or types of stickers could be provided, one for each of the alternatives—expansion, contraction, or stabilization. Each member of the management team would be asked to sort the organization's programs into categories—those that should be expanded, reduced, or remain the same—based on their perceived importance to the organization's mission and vision. The group might agree on several programs. Discussions could then be focused on those programs where there was disagreement. After points were raised and discussed, the programs could be ranked again, with the hope of discussion leading to greater consensus from the group.

The Q-sort method provided a more formal means for differentiating the importance of programs and setting priorities. Q-sort was a ranking procedure that forced choices along a continuum in situations in which the difference between the choices might be quite small. The program Q-sort evaluation was particularly useful when experts differed on what made one choice preferable over another. By ranking the choices using a Q-sort procedure, participants saw where there was wide consensus (for whatever reasons used by the experts) and had an opportunity to discuss the choices for which there was disagreement (and, if discussion went well, develop greater consensus).

The Q-sort was a part of Q-methodology, a set of philosophical, psychological, statistical, and psychometric ideas oriented to research on the individual. Q-sort evaluation helped overcome the problem of ranking all programs as "very important" by forcing a ranking based on some set of assumptions. The Q-sort was a way of rank-ordering objects (programs) and then assigning numerals to subsets of the objects for statistical purposes. Fred N. Kerlinger characterized the Q-sort as "a sophisticated way of rank-ordering objects."[1]

Q-sort focused particularly in sorting decks of cards (in this case, each card representing a program) and in the correlations among the responses of different individuals to the Q-sorts. Kerlinger reported good results with as few as forty items (programs) that were culled from a larger list, but usually greater statistical stability and reliability resulted from at least sixty items but not more than one hundred.

For ranking an organization's programs, only the first step in using Q-methodology was used—the Q-sort. In the Q-sort procedure, each member of the management team was asked to sort the organization's programs into categories based on the programs' perceived importance to the organization's mission and vision. To facilitate the task, the programs were printed on small cards that could be arranged (sorted) on a table. To force

ranking of programs, managers were asked to arrange the programs in piles from most important to least important. The best approach was that the number of categories be limited to nine and that the number of programs to be assigned to each category be determined in such a manner as to ensure a normal distribution. Therefore, if a public health department had forty-nine separate programs that management wished to rank (culled from a larger list of programs), they might be sorted in a manner similar to that shown in Exhibit 3-15 (on page 194). Notice that to create a normal distribution (or quasi-normal), about 5 percent of the programs were placed in the first pile or group, 7.5 percent in the second group, 12.5 percent in the third, and so on. In this example, there were two programs in the first group, four programs in the second group, six in the third, and so on.

Depending on the group where it was placed, each program was assigned a score ranging from 1 to 9, where 1 was for the lowest-ranked and 9 was for the highest-ranked programs. The score indicated an individual's perception of that program's importance to the mission and vision of the organization. A program profile was developed by averaging individual member's scores for each program. Based on the results of the Q-sort, programs were designated for expansion, contraction, or stabilization.

The Q-sort procedure worked well using several different sets of strategic assumptions. For example, the programs might be sorted several times, each based on a different scenario or set of assumptions. Then the group could determine which of the scenarios was most likely and make decisions accordingly.

Note

1. Fred N. Kerlinger, *Foundations of Behavioral Research* (New York: Holt Rinehart and Winston, 1973), p. 582.

Cooper Green Hospital and the Community Care Plan

An Overworked CEO

There were certain days when life seemed unbearable. For Max Michael, MD, it had been one of those days. He had the difficult responsibility of balancing costs with access to care, of rationing procedures with policy, and of juggling personnel with budgets, performance, and demand. Dr. Michael, a former chief of staff at the hospital and now its chief executive officer (CEO), had spent the better part of his day fighting a losing battle in an understaffed, understocked, overflowing outpatient clinic. It was there, on the front lines, where he had first encountered the nature of the health care problem and developed his vision for its solution. As Dr. Michael left the clinic that evening, he mulled over a decision he was going to have to make. It was his last patient who reminded him of the importance of that decision.

Martha James Spent Her Day at Cooper Green Hospital

It was the second day in a row that Martha James missed work because she was running a fe-

ver and ached all over. She dared not miss another day for fear of losing the job she had with a small local business that paid above minimum wage but offered no health insurance. Her husband also was employed full-time but did not receive any insurance benefits. Money was very tight for the couple and their two children, yet, based on federal guidelines, they were not eligible for financial assistance from the Aid to Families With Dependent Children (AFDC) welfare program, nor were they eligible for state Medicaid benefits. With no money to spare, the cost of a visit to a physician's office was a luxury Martha felt she could not afford. She did the only thing she knew to do: she headed for the emergency room at Cooper Green Hospital.

It was nearly 9:00 a.m. when Martha arrived, after a forty-five-minute bus ride. She waited for more than two hours before her name finally was called. The nurse asked her about her symptoms. Barely even looking up, the nurse said Martha would have to be seen over at the Outpatient Clinic because her case was not truly an "emergency." She was told to sign in at the clinic desk, and they would try to "work her in."

This case was prepared by Alice M. Adams and Peter M. Ginter, University of Alabama at Birmingham, and Linda E. Swayne, University of North Carolina at Charlotte. It is intended as a basis for classroom discussion rather than to illustrate effective or ineffective handling of an administrative situation. Used with permission from Alice M. Adams.

After more than four hours of sitting in the overcrowded waiting room, Martha finally heard her name called again. The doctor who took her case was a silver-haired man with sharp eyes and a concerned demeanor. Dr. Michael quickly determined the problem: a respiratory tract infection that had been "going around" for weeks. When asked, Martha admitted she had been coughing for more than a week but had hoped the severe cough would go away on its own. "Besides," she said, "I can't afford to take a day off work to go to the doctor for just a cold."

"The problem," Dr. Michael explained, "is the infection is now affecting your lungs, which requires more intensive treatment than if you had come for help a week ago."

Glancing at her chart, he realized she lived near Lawson State College, the location of one of the hospital's Community Care Plan (CCP) clinics. He asked, "Martha, are you aware of the Community Care Plan clinics and the services they offer? They have medical office visits with much shorter waiting times."

She replied, "I have heard something about them, but don't really know what it is about or how it could help me."

Martha still had to stop by the hospital pharmacy to pick up two medications, and it was nearly 5:30 p.m. She knew she could get them much faster at a local drugstore, but they would be several times as expensive. Instead, she settled in for another wait. By the time she headed back to the bus stop—some nine hours after she left home—Dr. Michael was wrapping up his afternoon in the clinic.

Dr. Michael's Day

As Dr. Michael entered his office, Martha James was still on his mind. It had been nearly four years since he launched the Community Care Plan, but in many ways it was still struggling. In his heart, he still believed it was a good model to provide access to preventive and routine medical services to the population traditionally served by Cooper Green Hospital: the poor and uninsured of Jefferson County. It placed small outpatient clinics within local neighborhoods. They were staffed by physician assistants or nurse practitioners, who were supervised by a physician. For a quarterly fee, members could receive routine medical care at the CCP clinics. When needed, they also received care from specialists and even inpatient hospital care at Cooper Green. To Dr. Michael, it made perfect sense; CCP offered better access to services, less waiting time, less travel time, and a better atmosphere.

But the numbers didn't agree. Although some of the CCP clinics established a reasonably sized patient base, others were struggling to attract members. If Martha James had been a CCP member, she could have been seen and received treatment before the infection had migrated to her lungs, and she would not have had such a long waiting time. "For her, and thousands more like her," he thought, "it's important to keep CCP running—if at all possible." Few people knew about CCP, though, and even fewer had joined.

The five-year funding that enabled the hospital to launch CCP was about to run out. Dr. Michael knew he was facing a critical decision: Should he push forward with expansion plans for CCP, maintain the clinics that existed, or fold the program altogether?

Cooper Green Hospital

In 1998, Cooper Green Hospital (CGH) was the current incarnation of Mercy Hospital. Built in 1972 with Alabama State and Hill-Burton funding, Mercy Hospital served the vision of the Alabama legislature to provide care for the indigent population of Jefferson County. Despite numerous organizational, structure, and name changes, the mission of the facility remained essentially the same: to provide quality medical care to the residents of Jefferson County, regardless of their ability to pay.

Mercy Hospital opened with 319 inpatient beds—a number based on an epidemiological study using the number of indigent cases reported

Exhibit 4-1. Inpatient Statistics for Cooper Green Hospital, Fiscal Year 1998

Location	Admissions	Discharges	Average Length of Stay (days)
4 West	1,464	1,518	4.1
7 West	1,742	2,197	4.6
MSICU	673	145	3.8
5 East	303	1,827	2.3
Labor and delivery	1,596	75	1.0
Nursery	1,444	1,441	2.1
Total	7,222	7,203	3.0

in county hospitals during the mid-1960s. The study projected that the hospital would operate near 80 percent capacity. Occupancy never reached the initial projections. The highest average census for the hospital was 186.3, in fiscal year 1974. The numbers of inpatient admissions and discharges and the average length of stay for 1998 are shown in Exhibit 4-1.

The role CGH played in the community faced constant scrutiny from a county commission with increasing budget pressures. Media and public challenges about the quality of care provided by CGH limited its ability to attract patients with private insurance. For the first two decades of the hospital's operations, cost overruns were common as the county's indigent population grew and medical costs soared. Facing increasing costs, Dr. Michael and the administrative staff initiated a stringent budget-cutting program that included personnel layoffs, taking beds out of service, postponing most capital improvements, and eliminating some services. The hospital's financial statements for the fiscal years 1994-1998 are included in Exhibits 4-2 and 4-3.

Early in his tenure as CEO, Dr. Michael initiated a strategic planning program for the hospital. Mission, vision, and value statements were developed (Exhibit 4-4), strategic objectives were outlined, and plans for meeting those objectives were created. Each year, the strategic objectives for the upcoming fiscal year were developed by the "man-

agement group"—consisting of the CEO, COO (Chief Operating Officer), CFO (Chief Financial Officer), Medical Chief of Staff, and Nursing Administrator—and distributed to all departmental supervisors.

As a result of ongoing strategic planning, Dr. Michael took the initial steps to transform Cooper Green Hospital into the Jefferson Health System (JHS) in 1998. JHS consisted of CGH (the inpatient facility) and Jefferson Outpatient Care (comprising the outpatient clinics located in the hospital and six satellite clinics of CCP). JHS provided services to patients through two plans: HealthFirst, a traditional fee-for-service plan, and the Community Care Plan (CCP), a prepaid membership plan.

Part of the motive for the transformation and expansion of CGH was to enhance its ability to generate external revenue, including attracting patients with private insurance. If CGH could attract paying patients on the basis of quality and satisfaction, it could mold itself from a provider of last resort into a true competitor in the market.

HealthFirst

Charges for services under the HealthFirst plan were determined by a sliding-fee scale that was based on federal poverty guidelines. Depending on the number of people in the family and the family's income, patients were assigned to one of

Exhibit 4-2. Cooper Green Hospital/Jefferson Health System Sources of Revenue

	1994	1995	1996	1997	1998
Indigent care fund	$13,126,249	$23,168,333	$31,638,294	$34,824,238	$36,199,381
Disproportionate Share Fund	4,419,644	8,854,308	3,329,871	3,5966,076	3,238,323
Medicare (total payments)	10,566,183	9,566,505	9,974,860	10,033,547	7,056,823
Medicaid	7,107,137	11,442,428	8,934,432	7,900,835	15,604,803
Blue Cross	449,653	262,415	258,808	296,152	264,792
Commercial insurance	350,978	307,604	925,646	458,266	362,785
Self-pay (payments from patients)	915,047	914,589	1,129,513	1,067,686	1,015,164

eight financial support categories. At the lowest level, patients paid as little as $2 for an office visit. At the highest level, patients paid full price for services (approximately $50 for an office visit). The HealthFirst financial support categories are shown in Exhibit 4-5. Initially, HealthFirst patients could be seen only at the Outpatient Clinic located at the hospital. In 1998, these regulations were relaxed, allowing HealthFirst patients to be seen at any of the satellite (CCP) clinics.

Community Care Plan

An important part of Dr. Michael's vision for JHS was CCP. His initial approach to developing the plan was best described as a "Field of Dreams" strategy: If you build it, they will come. "I envisioned offices filled with patients who were appreciative of the opportunity to receive quality medical care for a fair and affordable price—with less time waiting," Dr. Michael remembered.

CCP was developed around the ideas that catastrophic care was more expensive, patients waited until their conditions worsened, and they were treated in the more costly CGH Emergency Department. Dr. Michael asked himself, "Why not avoid these unanticipated high health care costs by allowing patients to pay a low monthly pre-

mium for unlimited services?" This would require that CGH, as well as the patients, change the way they thought about health care. Furthermore, for the system to survive, Dr. Michael and his executive staff would have to understand and respond to the rapidly changing health care environment.

The Health Care Environment

Change in the U.S. health care system was occurring dramatically and pervasively. Managed care was altering how providers interacted with patients, funding for care was being restricted, and many health care systems were using nonphysician providers to cut costs.

The Changing U.S. Health Care System

Because of its mission to provide medical care to the poor and uninsured, Cooper Green Hospital was considered one of the "safety net providers" across the United States. Safety net providers had large Medicaid and indigent care caseloads relative to other providers and were willing to provide services regardless of a person's ability to pay. Although safety net providers were the primary source of care for the poor and uninsured, they

Exhibit 4-3. Cooper Green Hospital/Jefferson Health System Statements of Revenue and Expense

	1994	1995	1996	1997	1998
Operating Revenue					
Inpatient revenue	$ 37,288,811	$ 34,529,493	$ 33,248,117	$ 32,217,566	$ 35,830,206
Outpatient revenue	12,097,455	13,791,112	14,568,700	15,197,207	16,470,205
Total patient revenue	49,386,266	48,320,605	47,816,817	47,414,773	52,300,411
Deductions from revenue (bad debt, subsidized care)	28,956,540	25,313,448	26,224,910	28,682,168	33,024,781
Net patient revenue	20,429,726	23,007,157	21,591,907	18,732,605	19,275,630
Other operating revenue	2,256,812	2,719,377	3,111,157	2,845,788	3,792,735
Total operating revenue	22,686,538	25,726,534	24,703,064	21,578,393	23,068,365
Operating Expenses					
Salaries and wages	19,390,676	20,547,467	20,976,332	21,275,798	23,017,889
Fringe benefits	4,681,390	4,680,937	4,607,439	4,731,080	4,976,824
Contract services	1,690,145	1,833,616	1,443,654	1,558,705	2,416,836
Utilities	986,035	921,191	866,758	844,867	911,943
Outside services	1,489,785	1,132,401	826,958	975,837	1,229,699
Services from other hospitals	2,567,655	2,447,907	1,881,087	2,129,683	1,915,322
Jefferson County Department of Health	2,003,193	1,861,591	1,933,874	2,040,062	1,800,396
Physician services	9,843,577	10,068,571	10,200,031	10,681,650	11,370,273
County maintenance	1,059,678	1,094,720	1,045,600	1,032,207	1,619,744
Indirect county appropriation	3,693,500	1,281,983	1,281,983	1,278,006	1,558,907
All other	10,134,544	11,095,892	12,248,708	11,399,367	11,378,434
Total operating expense	57,540,178	56,966,276	57,312,424	57,947,262	62,196,267
Gain/(Loss) from Operations	(34,853,640)	(31,239,742)	(32,609,360)	(36,368,869)	(39,127,902)
Non-Operating Revenue					
Indigent care fund	13,126,249	23,168,333	31,638,294	34,824,238	36,199,381
Disproportionate share fund	4,419,644	8,854,308	3,501,061	3,565,485	3,238,323
County appropriation	19,581,071				
Transfer from County General Fund	579,179				
Interest and other income	70,244	124,406	117,249	90,577	144,192
Total non-operating revenue	37,776,387	32,147,047	35,256,604	38,480,300	39,581,896
Gain/(Loss) Before Depreciation	2,922,747	907,305	2,647,244	2,111,431	453,994
Depreciation	1,581,901	1,615,024	2,098,569	1,833,237	2,040,682
Net Gain/(Loss)	$ 1,340,846	$ (707,719)	$ 548,675	$ 278,194	$(1,586,688)

Exhibit 4-4. Mission, Vision, and Value Statements of Cooper Green Hospital

Mission Statement
Cooper Green Hospital is committed to serve Jefferson County residents with quality health care regardless of ability to pay. We strive to attract and maintain a dedicated and compassionate staff of professionals who believe in the worth of our services. We seek to continuously improve our services and adapt to meet the changing health needs of the communities we serve.

Vision Statement
Cooper Green Hospital is the leader of an equitable and just health care system through excellence, quality, compassion, and trust.

Values Statements
We are committed to the health and well-being of those we serve.
We expect from ourselves the highest levels of excellence.
We know the vital importance of advocacy for those we serve.
We are committed to our staff having opportunities for personal and professional growth.
We expect for ourselves the highest ethical standards.
We understand that creativity and innovation are essential.
We recognize the importance of working with the patient and the community.
We are dedicated to all levels of education for health professionals.

Exhibit 4-5. HealthFirst Membership Categories

Total income per Year ($)[a]	Membership Fee per Year ($)	Copayment per Visit ($)	Copayment per Prescription or Refill ($)
Family plan			
Up to 1,850	35	2	0.50
1,851 to 3,700	65	2	0.50
3,701 to 5,500	95	2	1
5,501 to 7,400	130	2	1
7,401 to 11,000	195	2	2
11,001 to 14,800	260	2	2
Individual plan			
Up to 920	15	2	0.50
921 to 1,840	25	2	0.50
1,841 to 2,760	40	2	1
2,761 to 3,680	65	2	1
3,681 to 5,520	100	2	2
5,521 to 7,360	150	2	2

a. Income is per family for the family plan and per individual for the individual plan.

also provided critical access to health services in areas where health care was difficult to obtain.

Safety net providers faced many challenges in covering the cost of uncompensated care because they relied on Medicaid and fee-for-service reimbursement from other patients as major sources of revenue. Because of increased interest in Medicaid patients by for-profit Medicaid managed care programs, there was a decrease in the number of Medicaid patients using safety net providers, resulting in a financial drain and necessitating cuts in service levels.

Experts agreed that because of health care reform and cutbacks in funding, increased demand for uncompensated care and decreased capacity of the health care delivery system to meet this need would continue. This forced safety net providers to focus on improving operational efficiency as well as on utilizing financial and staffing resources more effectively. Flexibility in the rapidly changing health care environment was essential to future survival; however, many safety net providers were unable to adapt quickly to changing market conditions, in part because of restrictions imposed by local regulations, labor relations, and dependence on politically driven funding mechanisms.

Managed Care

Health care costs rose at twice the rate of inflation from the mid-1980s to the mid-1990s, creating a $1 trillion industry that accounted for 14 percent of the United States' gross domestic product (GDP). By the end of the century, the health care industry had grown to more than $1.5 trillion, or 18 percent of GDP. Health care purchasers (insurors, employers, government, and individuals) were seeking ways to curb this growing burden. Increasingly, they turned to managed care as a solution. In 1995, nearly three quarters of American workers were insured by health maintenance organizations (HMOs), preferred provider organizations (PPOs), and point-of-service plans (POSs), up from only 27 percent in 1987. By 1998, managed care was the dominant form of insur-

ance in the United States, and enrollment was expected to increase.

The central concept underlying managed care was the attempt to control health care costs by reducing inappropriate utilization of services through utilization review, gatekeeper functions such as referral requirements, and case management.

In 1999, health maintenance organizations (HMOs) were regulated in the state of Alabama by the Alabama Department of Public Health under Title 27 Chapter 21A (27-21A). The State Board of Health worked in conjunction with the Alabama Department of Insurance to license and regulate HMOs operating within the state.

Medicare and Medicaid Funding

Medicare was a provision of Title XVIII of the Social Security Act. The Medicare program was established in 1965 to ensure medical coverage for the aged and disabled. In the years following, Medicare expanded to encompass other population groups, including persons entitled to Social Security or Railroad Retirement disability benefits for at least twenty-four months and persons with end-stage renal disease (ESRD) who required continuing dialysis or kidney transplant. Another provision allowed noncovered, aged individuals to buy into the plan.

Medicare benefits were broken into two separate programs: Part A-Hospital Insurance and Part B-Supplemental Medical Insurance. Medicare Part A provided coverage for medical expenses incurred from hospital admissions, skilled nursing facilities, home health services, and hospice care. Part A was free of charge for qualified Medicare beneficiaries. Medicare Part B, a supplemental coverage purchased by the Medicare beneficiary at a monthly fee, covered ancillary medical expenses such as non-inpatient lab fees, physician fees, outpatient services, and medical equipment and supplies. In 1997, Medicare as a whole covered 38 million people. Utilization of Part A, Part B, or both was 87 percent of enrollees. Medicare enrollment statistics for 1995 for the United States and Alabama are shown in Exhibit 4-6.

Exhibit 4-6. Medicare Enrollment Statistics, 1997 (in thousands)

Category	National	Alabama
Aged (Part A and/or B)	33,630	544
Disabled (Part A and/or B)	4,815	113
Total enrolled (Part A and/or B)	38,445	657

Exhibit 4-7. Population and Medicaid Eligibles as a Percentage of Population

Year	Population	Eligibles	Percentage
1996	4,127,562	635,568	15.4
1997	4,141,341	632,472	15.3
1998	4,155,080	637,489	15.3

In 1996, Medicare was the largest health coverage program in the nation. Benefits were estimated to be $191 billion that year; 6,273 hospitals nationwide were Medicare certified. The Health Care Financing Administration (HCFA), a federal agency under the Department of Health and Human Services, was responsible for formulating Medicare policies and managing the Medicare program.

Title XIX of the Social Security Act of 1965 gave rise to Medicaid as part of the federal-state welfare structure to aid America's poor population. Title XIX allowed federal funding for state-run programs. To receive funding, the state programs were required to make provisions for basic health services, including hospital inpatient care, outpatient services, laboratory and X-ray services, and physician services, among others. If funding allowed, states could offer additional services, including medicine, eyeglasses, and dental care.

Providers of services for Medicaid recipients received payment directly from the state Medicaid agency. Providers were required to accept the Medicaid reimbursement as payment in full. Medicaid agencies could require cost sharing by the recipient in the form of copayments, but the recipient's inability to meet the copay could not be used to deny services.

In 1998, the Alabama Medicaid program provided some benefits for a variety of populations, but the majority of expenses were for indigent women and children, indigent elderly persons in nursing homes, and the disabled. Exhibit 4-7 shows the percentage of Alabama residents who were eligible for the Medicaid program from 1996 through 1998. In fiscal year 1998, 15.3 percent of Alabama's population was eligible for Medicaid services, up nearly 5 percentage points from FY 1990 (10.4 percent). Medicaid expansion to cover more populations (particularly children) and the increase in the elderly population increased the budget.

The population actually enrolled in the Medicaid program averaged 267,258 recipients per month in FY 1998. Of the 637,489 individual Medicaid eligibles in FY 1998, approximately 83 percent actually utilized services.

Balanced Budget Act

The Balanced Budget Act of 1997 was labeled the most significant change to the Medicare and Medicaid programs since their inception. A significant change for Alabama hospitals was the CHIPs (Children's Health Insurance Plans) initiative that infused an additional $23 million into Alabama's health care reimbursement for children under the age of 19. Phase I of the Alabama plan was a Medicaid expansion that funded Medicaid coverage of children from ages 16 through 18 whose family income was less than 100 percent of the poverty level. Phase II, known as the ALLKIDS program, provided payments for insurance coverage of Alabama children through age 18 if the family income was under 200 percent of the poverty level and the child was not eligible for any other Medicaid program. The ALLKIDS program was a little different in coverage because a third-party payor was responsible for provider reimbursement, not Medicaid. ALLKIDS was not an entitlement program like Medicaid or the CHIPs Medicaid expansion; coverage was on a first come, first served basis. Therefore, if funding ran out to pay the insurance premiums for the ALLKIDS program, applicants were put on a waiting list.

Nonphysician Providers

Nonphysician providers (NPPs) such as physician's assistants, nurse practitioners, certified nurse midwives, nurse anesthetists, and clinical nurse specialists were health care professionals licensed to practice medicine with physician supervision. Nurse practitioners were registered nurses who received additional education and clinical

training in the "nursing model." Physician's assistants were trained by physicians in the "medical model." Physician assistant programs were structured similar to—but were shorter in duration than—medical school programs.

Although the scope of services that they could legally perform varied by state, most NPPs provided primary care services such as well-care physical examinations, tests, and diagnosis of and treatment for acute illnesses, as well as diagnosis, treatment, and monitoring of chronic conditions (such as diabetes and hypertension). In addition, in most states they were licensed to write prescriptions (with some limitations that varied by state). For more complex tasks and cases, NPPs sought consultation from their supervising physician or referred patients to a specialist.

Nurse practitioners and physician's assistants were often viewed as more appropriate for primary care services because these professionals tended to take a more holistic view of patient care, focused on health care prevention and education, and spent more time with their patients than most physicians. It was estimated that NPPs could perform 60 to 80 percent of services traditionally rendered by physicians in family practice settings. In addition, NPPs were viewed as good economic alternatives for primary care physicians because their salaries were usually 50 to 65 percent of those earned by physicians. Although they were required to be "supervised" by a physician, one physician could supervise three to four NPPs. Thus, NPPs were often referred to as "physician extenders." In 1998, there were estimated to be more than 48,000 nurse practitioners and more than 34,000 physician's assistants in clinical practice in the United States.

The Local Environment

Once known as a center of the steel-making industry, Jefferson County, Alabama, boasted a diversified economy by the 1990s. Biotechnology, health care, research, engineering, and a vast array of financial and service industries had supplanted much of the industrial core that had built the city in the early part of the century. As of 1998, the Birmingham metropolitan statistical area (MSA) population was approximately 875,000; Jefferson County's population was approximately 652,000.

According to a 1993 survey conducted by CGH's Center for Community Care, more than one-third of Jefferson County residents were uninsured. Many poor residents delayed seeking necessary medical care because they had no health insurance, and an estimated 48,000 residents had been denied care within the past twelve months because they lacked health insurance. When asked what issues were most important to their community, low-income residents overwhelmingly listed crime, violence, housing, and drugs as the highest priority issues. On average, health care was listed as the sixth most important issue, despite the fact that more than 64,000 residents reported their health status as fair or poor.

Exhibit 4-8 provides additional demographic and socioeconomic data for Jefferson County.

Other Health Care Providers in Birmingham, Jefferson County

Twelve acute care hospitals were located in Birmingham, the largest city in Jefferson County. In 1998, eight of the twelve hospitals reported a decline in admissions; inpatient capacity in the area exceeded demand. As a result, many Jefferson County hospitals were scrambling to earn a share of the rapidly developing outpatient market. In their efforts to reposition themselves to respond to these and other changes in the health care environment, several hospitals had entered into alliances with other hospitals. For instance, Brookwood Medical Center, Medical Center East, and Lloyd Noland Hospital formed an alliance in 1995.

Exhibit 4-9 provides a brief description of each of the other acute care hospitals in Jefferson County. Exhibit 4-10 contains selected operating statistics for each of them. Exhibit 4-11 provides

enrollment and ownership information for each of the managed care organizations that were operating in Jefferson County in 1998.

Jefferson County Health Department

CGH and the Jefferson County Department of Health (JCDH) established a working alliance to improve continuity of care for the county's indigent patients. JCDH physicians were accorded staff privileges at CGH, and JCDH agreed to refer to CGH its patients who needed diagnostic testing or acute care. Although CGH and JCDH maintained a close working relationship, at times partnering on individual projects and exploring the idea of a more comprehensive alliance, no such plans had come to fruition by 1999.

JCDH operated an extensive health care network, providing pediatric and adult health care services to approximately 80,000 people every year. The JCDH network consisted of eight community-based health centers and nineteen school health programs. Health care services were available to any resident of Jefferson County, with the cost of services based on the patient's ability to pay. Services available at the centers included maternity care; family planning; well- and sick-child care; adult primary care; the Women, Infants, and Children (WIC) nutritional program; social services; dental care; pharmacy; and sexually transmitted disease testing and treatment. In addition, health centers sponsored seminars on disease prevention and health promotion topics. The locations of the JCDH clinics are shown on the map in Exhibit 4-12.

County Government/Authority for CGH

The Alabama state legislature granted county governments the authority to develop, own, and operate hospitals and other health care facilities for the benefit of county residents. Jefferson County was governed by a five-member county commission that was elected for four-year terms.

Exhibit 4-8. Selected Jefferson County Statistics

Total Population (1997)		659,524
Births (1997)		9,352
Deaths (1997)		7,096
Urban and Rural		
	Urban	581,973
	Rural	69,552
Sex		
	Male	303,713
	Female	347,812
Race		
	White	417,881
	Black	228,187
	American Indian	1,242
	Asian	3,643
	Other	572
Household income		
	Less than $5,000	22,749
	$ 5,000–$10,000	27,477
	$10,000–$15,000	24,802
	$15,000–$20,000	24,294
	$20,000–$30,000	42,879
	$30,000–$40,000	34,373
	$40,000–$50,000	25,108
	$50,000–$60,000	17,124
	$60,000+	32,488
Median household income		$32,632
Per capita income (1994)		$21,915
People of all ages in poverty		105,779
People under age 18 in poverty		40,006
Medicare beneficiaries		
	Aged	93,443
	Disabled	32,503

The commission was responsible for administering finances, collecting taxes, allocating resources, and providing for the delivery of services such as law enforcement, sewer services, and health care.

In 1998, the commission oversaw the reorganization of Cooper Green Hospital into the Jefferson Health System (JHS). County Commissioner Jeff Germany assumed responsibility for governmental oversight of JHS as its Commissioner of Health and Human Services, a position he had held for Cooper Green Hospital during the past twelve years.

Whereas some county hospitals operated as independent organizations or under the auspices of independent "health authorities," JHS was an operational department of the county government. Although Dr. Michael, as the CEO, had operational and administrative control over the hospi-

Exhibit 4-9. Descriptions of Other Jefferson County Hospitals

Princeton Baptist Medical Center: As part of the Baptist Health System (http://www.BHSALA.com), Baptist Princeton serves primarily those citizens located on the west side of the Birmingham MSA.

Montclair Baptist Medical Center: As one of thirteen tertiary care and acute care hospitals in the Baptist Health System, Montclair serves those residing on the east side of the Birmingham MSA.

Brookwood: The medical center (http://www.brookwood-medical.com) is part of the Tenet Healthcare System (http://www.tenethealth.com) and has a staff of more than 300 physicians, representing every major specialty. Brookwood also has a Women's Medical Center, specializing in OB/GYN and other health services for women.

Carraway Methodist: As the flagship of the Carraway system (http://carraway.org), Carraway Methodist places special emphasis on emergency medicine, laser surgery, cardiology and cardiac surgery, cancer treatment, diabetes care, hyperbaric medicine, and other high-tech services.

Children's Hospital: Children's Hospital (http://www.chsys.org) is the leading provider of comprehensive pediatric services in Alabama.

Healthsouth Medical Center: Home of the corporate headquarters, Healthsouth (http://www.healthsouth.com) is the nation's leading provider of comprehensive outpatient and rehabilitative health care services.

Lloyd Noland Hospital: Affiliated with Tenet Healthcare System, this hospital became the South's first industrial medical experiment. As one of the state's first teaching hospitals, Lloyd Noland continues to provide excellent disease control and health care maintenance.

Medical Center East: This hospital is Birmingham's most modern medical center. As the flagship of Eastern Health System (http://www.medicalcentereast.com), it has more than 300 physicians on staff, representing nearly seventy medical specialties.

Saint Vincent's Hospital: As a member of the Daughters of Charity National Health System, St. Vincent's (http://www.stv.org) is dedicated to providing quality health care to the public by offering patient-centered, economical services, with a special emphasis on the sick and poor. It focuses on cardiology, maternal and pediatric, neurological, oncology, and occupational health services.

University Hospital of Alabama: As a major teaching and research institution, University Hospital (http://www.health.uab.edu) provides patients with the most advanced health care available. University Hospital offers a comprehensive range of primary care and specialty services.

Bessemer Carraway Medical Center: As part of the Carraway Medical System, Carraway Bessemer is the principal provider of tertiary care services to the residents of the city of Bessemer.

---

tal, it remained very closely tied to the county government system. The most restrictive aspects of this relationship were regulations that mandated the hospital's use of the county's personnel system as well as its financial services system.

Hospital Operations

Prior to the 1998 reorganization, the hospital was broadly organized into outpatient and inpatient divisions. All department managers reported to then-COO Antoinette Smith-Epps. The 1998

Exhibit 4-10. Selected Operating Statistics for Jefferson County Hospitals

Hospital	Number of Beds	Admissions in 1996	Status
Baptist Medical Center–Princeton	499	14,103	Not-for-profit Church affiliated
Baptist Medical Center–Montclair	534	19,650	Not-for-profit Church affiliated
Brookwood Medical Center	586	20,651	For profit
Carraway Methodist Medical Center	617	13,449	Not-for-profit Church affiliated
The Children's Hospital of Alabama	225	10,727	Not-for-profit
Cooper Green Hospital	*319*	*5,938*	*Not-for-profit County-owned*
Healthsouth Medical Center	219	6,615	For profit
Lloyd Noland Hospital	319	5,095	For profit
Medical Center East	282	11,467	Not-for-profit
Saint Vincent's Hospital	338	14,540	Not-for-profit Church affiliated
University Hospital	908	37,226	Not-for-profit State-owned
Bessemer Carraway Medical Center	300	6,452	Not-for-profit

SOURCE: Compiled from SMG Marketing Group Inc. data for 1998.

reorganization into the JHS structure created distinct inpatient and outpatient divisions. Ms. Smith-Epps was named Hospital Administrator and remained in charge of inpatient services and most of the support and administrative services. Responsibility for outpatient services was assigned to Jerome Calhoun, who was named Administrator of Jefferson Outpatient Care. The organizational chart for the JHS (reflecting changes made in the 1998 restructuring) is shown in Exhibit 4-13.

Throughout the 1990s, the number of outpatient visits continued to increase at CGH. This fol-

lowed the national trend, in which there was an increasing emphasis on outpatient care driven by the need to reduce costs, coupled with new technology that enabled more types of care to be delivered on an outpatient basis. Exhibit 4-14 shows outpatient visits, by specialty, for fiscal years 1993 to 1998.

According to Ms. Smith-Epps, JHS faced several problems. The first was one that most health care providers confronted in the late 1990s, the problem of tight revenue. The Balanced Budget Act of 1997 had reduced the revenue of most providers and had affected CGH significantly because

Exhibit 4-11. Jefferson County Managed Care Organizations

Managed Care Organization	Commercial Enrollment[a]	Ownership
UnitedHealthcare of Alabama	82,485	UnitedHealthcare, Inc.
Health Partners of Alabama	80,386	Baptist Health System
CACH HMO	36,562	Children's Hospital
Viva Health	25,610	University of Alabama at Birmingham
Apex Healthcare	5,855	DirectCare, Inc.

SOURCE: Compiled using data from *Health Maintenance Organizations* (Harkey Associates, March, 1999) Managed Care Research and Publishing.

a. Commercial enrollment includes self-insured covered lives under HMO-style medical management by region. The Birmingham region includes Blount, Calhoun, Etowah, Jefferson, Shelby, St. Clair, and Tuscaloosa counties.

Exhibit 4-12. Jefferson County Department of Health Primary Care Center Locations

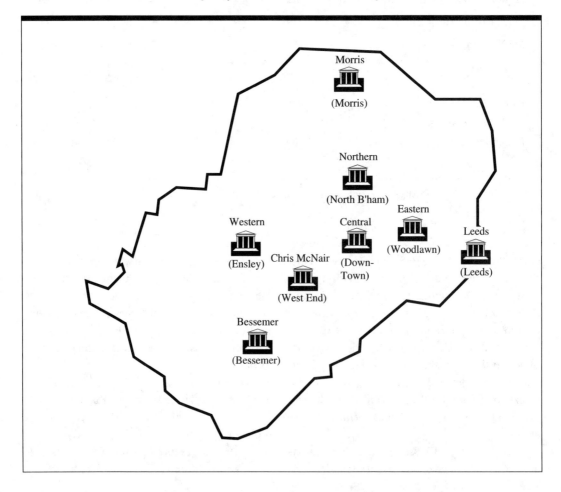

Exhibit 4-13. Organizational Chart for the Jefferson Health System

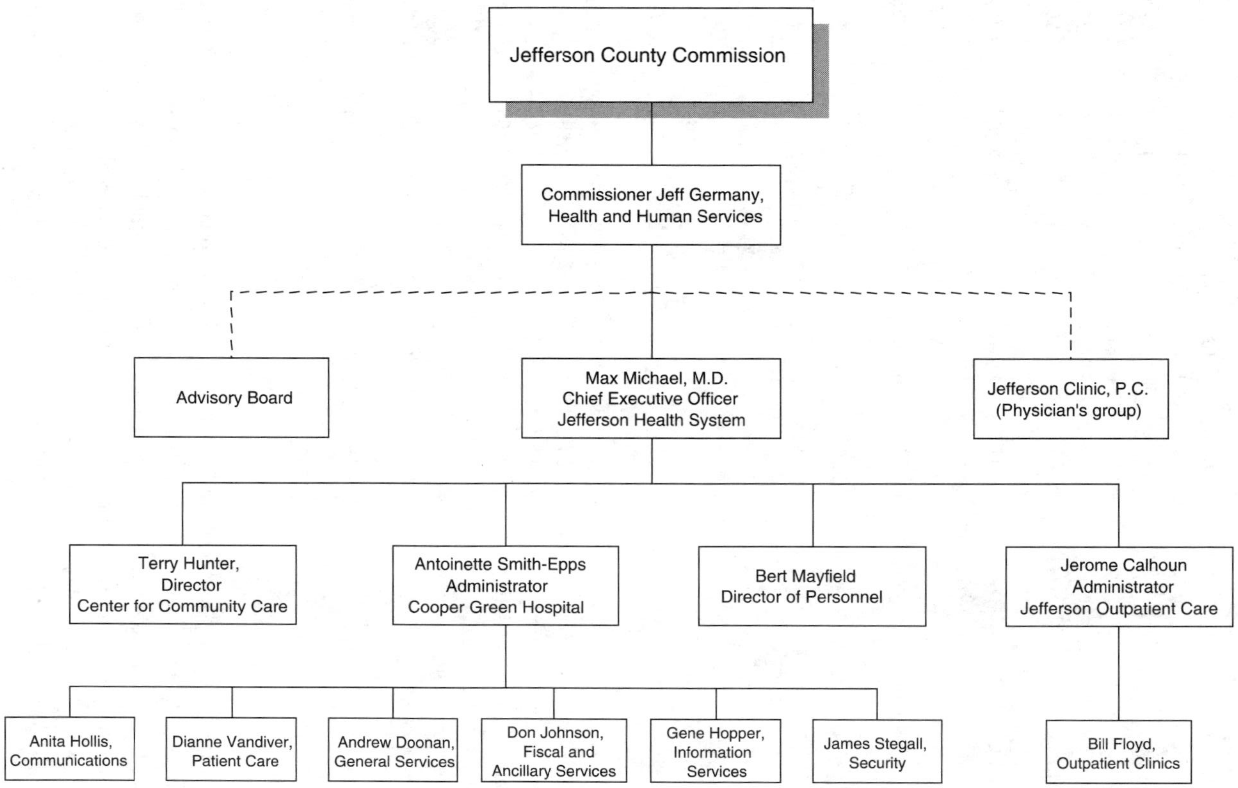

Exhibit 4-14. Outpatient Visits for Cooper Green Hospital

	FY 93	FY 94	FY 95	FY 96	FY 97	FY 98
Cardiac	1,164	603	795	846	670	0
Medicine	21,723	23,361	25,340	24,690	23,903	22,873
Neurology	1,239	1,300	1,488	1,260	1,182	1,273
Pulmonary	828	1,081	1,242	1,221	1,155	1,033
Renal	431	443	593	659	861	907
Rheumatology	1,183	1,160	1,286	1,295	1,206	1,415
Dermatology	1,713	1,791	1,677	1,666	1,562	1,678
Ear, nose, throat	2,991	2,760	2,726	2,469	2,402	2,474
Ophthalmology	5,812	5,368	6,120	7,148	7,110	6,561
Coagulation	422	581	669	820	831	683
Gynecology	6,472	6,756	8,015	9,453	9,965	10,128
Chemotherapy	361	279	353	518	558	867
St. George (AIDS clinic)	1,332	1,331	1,904	2,124	2,566	2,505
Genitourinary	1,495	1,563	1,764	1,616	1,414	1,558
Hematology/oncology	1,453	1,508	1,828	2,048	2,425	2,364
Surgery	9,193	8,999	8,716	8,017	8,609	8,196
Orthopedics	4,932	4,748	4,706	4,207	3,813	4,108
Teens First	0	0	0	28	28	15
Total clinics	62,744	63,632	69,222	70,085	70,260	68,638
Emergency	39,262	37,982	36,959	33,736	34,124	34,671
Labor and delivery	3,420	3,997	3,169	2,903	3,018	3,228
Same day surgery	2,147	2,106	2,199	2,045	2,169	2,195
Referred testing (from JCDH)	14,103	14,680	17,994	14,155	13,745	15,127
Physical therapy	0	0	0	3,914	3,968	5,251
Community care clinics	0	0	0	1,706	3,025	4,997
Total non clinics	58,932	58,765	60,321	58,459	60,049	65,469
Grand Total	121,676	122,397	129,543	128,544	130,309	134,107

CGH served the indigent population and had few sources of revenue. Fortunately, during the late 1990s losses had been somewhat offset by an increase in the county's indigent care fund (ICF). Funded by county tax revenues split among several organizations, including CGH, Children's Hospital, and JCDH, ICF revenues were distributed on a straight percentage basis, so when the economy was good (and therefore tax revenues high), the hospital received more income.

A second issue was the lack of resources to invest in capital projects such as upgrades and enhancements to the information system, new medical equipment, or renovations to improve patient flow and access. Because the facilities were constructed in the late 1960s, when the focus was on inpatient services, the physical layout of the hospital and the outpatient clinics was not conducive to providing outpatient services efficiently. The shortage of examination rooms, work space for nurses and clerks, and waiting room space was particularly acute in the outpatient clinics. This resulted in very long waiting times to get an appointment as well as very long waiting times to be seen by a health care provider on the day of the appointment.

The frustration experienced by patients was sometimes compounded by discourteous staff members. JHS employed more than 600 staff, all part of the "civil service" structure of the county personnel system. Compared to other health care providers, staff turnover at JHS was low. There were many very dedicated, talented staff members who could have easily worked elsewhere, in better working conditions and for more money. They chose to work at JHS because they believed in its mission and enjoyed serving those in need. The hospital, however, had its share of employees who were attracted primarily by the job security of the civil service system. Some of these employees tended to perform at minimally acceptable levels and display negative attitudes to patients and others. The administration had made several efforts to improve the morale and customer service orientation of the staff, although with limited success. Annual employee satisfaction surveys indicated there had been a slight improvement from 1993 to 1998, but there seemed to remain a core of "negative" individuals whose attitudes demoralized other staff members and angered patients.

Patients at Jefferson Health System had widely varying views about the service and quality of care received. Overall patient satisfaction with JHS, as measured by patient surveys, averaged about 90 percent. Patients recorded the most satisfaction with aspects related to the health care providers; they recorded the least satisfaction with issues related to making appointments, waiting times, and the facility. On the surveys, many patients expressed gratitude for the care they received at the hospital and had high praise for various staff members. They often remarked that without JHS, they would have no way of obtaining health care. One of the most common phrases seen on the written responses was "God Bless Cooper Green Hospital."

Some patients, however, expressed frustration over long waiting times and poor customer service. Some complained about specific staff members, often citing a lack of respect or a lack of caring about patients. Other complaints involved poor coordination between departments that sometimes resulted in patients experiencing long waits in two or three different departments and difficulty in scheduling appointments in a timely manner. Many patients had to wait three weeks to see a doctor, and when they arrived at the hospital on the appointment date, they experienced long waits before being seen. Patients also cited the small, uncomfortable waiting rooms and the overall layout of the hospital as sources of frustration.

The Community Care Plan

When Dr. Michael assumed the position of CEO of Cooper Green Hospital in 1992, managed care was growing nationwide. Through coordinating health care and creating an organized system for receiving medical care, "managing care" was supposed to reduce costs. Managed care reached into every sector of health care—investor-owned health plans, not-for-profit organizations, Medicare plans, and state-run Medicaid projects.

It was within that context that Dr. Michael began to formulate his idea for a means of providing affordable, quality care to the poor, underserved residents of Jefferson County. Just as other managed care plans were using primary care physicians as gatekeepers to monitor the health of their patients on a long-term basis, the local CCP clinics would serve as the members' first stop for receiving health care and preventive services. Specialists at Cooper Green Hospital would serve their needs for services that extended beyond the capacity of the clinics. Dr. Michael envisioned this concept as a coordinated hub-and-spoke configuration for the provision of more effective and efficient health care.

Funding

Given the financial pressures facing the hospital, Dr. Michael had known that funding CCP would be a challenge. With pledges of $250,000 from funding partners, including local businesses, foundations, and government agencies, CGH was

Exhibit 4-15. Community Care Plan Membership Fees and Copayments

Total Income per Year ($)[a]	Membership Fee per Year ($)	Copay per Visit ($)	Copay per Prescription or Refill ($)
Family plan			
Up to 1,850	35	2	0.50
1,851 to 3,700	65	2	0.50
3,701 to 5,500	95	2	1
5,501 to 7,400	130	2	1
7,401 to 11,000	195	2	2
11,101 to 14,800	260	2	2
Individual plan			
Up to 920	15	2	0.50
921 to 1,840	25	2	0.50
1,841 to 2,760	40	2	1
2,761 to 3,680	65	2	1
3,681 to 5,520	100	2	2
5,521 to 7,360	150	2	2

a. Income is per family for the family plan and per individual for the individual plan.

awarded a matching grant from the Robert Wood Johnson Foundation (RWJF) for $500,000 for the development of six clinics over the four-year project period.

In 1995, the first CCP clinic opened. It was located in the public housing community of Cooper Green Homes (neither affiliated with nor located next to the hospital). The second clinic opened shortly thereafter in Pratt City (approximately ten miles southwest of the hospital). The Cooper Green Homes site was chosen for the first clinic for three reasons: (1) as a public housing community, its residents clearly had a need for affordable health care; (2) the housing community's Resident Advisory Board was very active and supported the placement of the CCP clinic; and (3) the Birmingham Housing Authority had pledged to provide and renovate space for the clinic. The third and fourth clinics, Southtown (two miles northeast of the hospital) and Bessemer (fifteen miles southwest of the hospital), were opened in the fourth quarter of 1997. In early

1998, the Cooper Green Homes clinic was closed because of continuing problems with vandalism, gang violence, and low enrollment; it was relocated to the Lawson area.

CCP Member Services

To receive services, patients were required to enroll in CCP. Only residents of Jefferson County were eligible for membership. Members paid an enrollment fee at the beginning of each year that could be paid in four installments. Copayments were required to receive services (Exhibit 4-15). Similar to the HealthFirst program, copayments and membership fees were based on a sliding-fee scale determined by family income. Those covered by Medicaid, Medicare, or certain qualified insurance plans did not have to pay a membership fee.

Membership began with a complete physical (at no extra charge) that served as a health assessment. In addition, the CCP wellness program, HealthPoints, was an incentive plan to keep members healthy. It provided participants with discounts on their copayments and membership fees. The program's motto was "With HealthPoints, it pays to improve your health." To participate in the HealthPoints program, members set quarterly goals and visited their health care provider every three months to monitor progress. Members received "points" for met goals. Examples of HealthPoints goals included getting regular checkups, obtaining referrals before visiting the emergency room, exercising 20 minutes three times per week, eating a balanced diet, following the "well baby" schedule, quitting smoking, and losing weight.

CCP membership included both outpatient and inpatient services. Satellite health clinics provided primary care outpatient services such as immediate treatment of illnesses and minor injuries, lab tests, care for chronic illnesses (diabetes, arthritis, high blood pressure), yearly checkups, immunizations, family planning services, special health classes, and prescription drugs from the JHS pharmacy (located at the hospital). Members were referred to specialists when nécessary. With a written referral, members were also eligible to receive home care services, hearing tests, eye exams, and glaucoma screenings. Additionally, social services and other programs were provided through JHS, JCDH, and other local agencies.

Staffing

Each clinic had at least three full-time staff members: a nurse practitioner or a physician's assistant, a registered nurse, and a receptionist/licensed practical nurse. The RN and LPN were employed by the county and reported directly to Bill Floyd, manager of outpatient services at JHS. The nurse practitioners and physician's assistants were employed by Jefferson Clinic (the physician practice group affiliated with CGH through a contract with the Jefferson County Commission) and reported to Mark Wilson, MD, Medical Director of Outpatient Services (Jefferson Clinic). As medical director and supervisor for the non-physician

providers, Dr. Wilson rotated throughout all the clinics.

Turnover rates for employees at each of the outpatient clinics were extremely low, and morale was generally high. Staff members at the clinics tended to be satisfied with their work and remained employed at CCP for extended periods. When new positions opened up at a CCP site, many employees from JHS applied to work there.

For the first three years, CCP did not have any full-time administrative staff; administrative duties were handled by a team of JHS staff and interns who each devoted part of their time to CCP. As manager of the JHS Outpatient Clinic and the CCP clinics, Bill Floyd spent approximately 25 percent of his time on CCP matters. In mid-1997, Jerome Calhoun was hired to oversee all outpatient operations and could devote approximately 30 percent of his time to CCP.

Costs

Each CCP site required approximately $225,000 for start-up and general operating expenses during its first year. The estimated ongoing operating costs for one clinic with 1,000 patients was $170,000. During the initial years of CCP, approximately 30 percent of costs was provided through the RWJF grant. The remaining 70 percent was provided through local matching funds (30 percent), in-kind support from JHS (34 percent), and operating revenues (6 percent). The program was designed so that as individual sites increased enrollments, a greater percentage of operating expenses would be covered by operating revenue. The break-even point for a given clinic was estimated to be 1,000 members, although that number was somewhat low because the calculation did not include in-kind support or subsidies from JHS in the form of administrative resources and specialist physician services. It was expected that each clinic would reach the break-even point by its third year of operation; however, by mid-1999, none of the Community Care Plan Clinics had done so.

Exhibit 4-16. CCP Enrollment

Site (opening date)	October, 1995	October, 1996	October, 1997	October, 1998	As of March, 1999
Lawson (4/95)	143	262	323	560	700
Pratt City (10/95)	N/A	242	498	728	852
Southtown (9/97)	N/A	N/A	N/A	219	350
Bessemer (9/97)	N/A	N/A	N/A	355	424
Total	143	504	821	1,862	2,326

Enrollment and Utilization

Enrollment for CCP generally fell below expectations, although the experiences of the clinics were varied. The first clinic, initially located in a public housing community, experienced the slowest growth. Although slow growth was somewhat expected because of its "pioneering" role, this clinic's growth continued to be slow even after other clinics opened. The clinic and administrative staff felt that growth at that site had been limited by the problems with gang violence and vandalism. The other clinic located within a public housing community, Southtown, experienced somewhat slower growth as well. The clinics in Pratt City and Bessemer appeared to be on track to reach 1,000 members by their fourth year of operation. Enrollment for each of the clinics is shown in Exhibit 4-16.

According to Bill Floyd, members tended to readily use the services available to them. As of March 1999, the average patient load per day at Lawson was fifteen patients, at Pratt City twenty patients, at Southtown ten patients, and at Bessemer thirteen patients. One nurse practitioner or one physician's assistant was located at each site and could handle seeing between twenty-two and twenty-five patients per day. Mr. Floyd expected patient loads to increase as HealthFirst members became aware of the option to receive services at the CCP clinics.

Marketing and Market Research

Marketing for CCP was still largely a work in progress. In an effort to publicize the first clinic, a health fair was scheduled at the site approximately two months before opening. However, because of construction delays, the clinic did not open for several months after the fair, nullifying the impact of the publicity efforts. The primary approaches to marketing during the first two years were appearances by Dr. Michael, Mr. Floyd, and staff members at community organizations, church groups, and schools, along with promotional materials placed within the hospital.

A more formal marketing effort began in 1997. The intention was to educate the staff of Cooper Green Hospital, neighboring communities, county health departments, Social Services, uninsured populations, small businesses, and other hospitals in the area regarding CCP and how to access the services. Clinic staff members, interns, and administrative staff made appearances at schools, churches, neighborhoods, and local shelters, and held or attended twelve to fifteen health fairs each year. Additionally, promotional materials were placed more prominently at Cooper Green Hospital in hopes of raising awareness among patients. Printed materials were often used because they could be produced at low cost, but CCP staff members realized they were beyond the reading level of many of the patients and potential patients. Word of mouth had proven to be the most promising and reliable avenue of enrolling and retaining patients.

Because of limited administrative staff, no single person was responsible for coordinating the marketing effort. Although Floyd, as manager, set the tone for the marketing activities, specific duties were handled by a number of different people. Radio spots were placed sporadically with stations serving a predominantly African American audience. In late 1995, eight billboards were placed in the western side of town, in the general vicinity of the first two clinics; they remained for approximately two months. Later, in conjunction with St. Vincent's Hospital, a television advertisement was developed that aired once a week for eight weeks. According to Floyd, such promotions generated a great deal of interest, but it was not clear how effective they were in recruiting members.

Prior to opening of the first clinic, focus groups were used to assess the printed membership information packet, but there were no surveys to assess patient awareness, attitudes, or understanding about CGH or CCP specifically, or about prepaid health plans generally. Additionally, although some information from the 1993 HealthWatch needs assessment survey was available to guide placement of CCP clinics, that process was driven more by long-standing political promises and community lobbying than systematic data analysis.

Coordination Efforts Between CCP and CGH

Coordination efforts between CCP and CGH developed slowly. The first challenge was staff education and training for all hospital employees regarding the purpose and function of CCP. Although progress was slow during the initial years of CCP, Ms. Smith-Epps believed that by 1999, most hospital employees were aware of CCP and had a basic understanding of its purpose.

A second challenge involved coordinating the administrative functions of CCP with those of CGH. For example, billing functions were carried out both at CCP and in the business office of

CGH, resulting in overlapping systems and confusion about patients' accounts. As CCP grew, communication of employee concerns, issues, and suggestions became more complex. Whereas the staff members of the first clinic had been part of a tightly knit team that included both clinical and administrative staff members from CGH and CCP, each new clinic presented the challenge of developing effective channels of communication.

CCP experienced "growing pains" in the area of information services. It outgrew current hardware capacities, and enhanced software was needed to link the clinics and CGH. Because CGH and CCP shared the same computer and medical records system, this modernization was vital to the success of the project. Another complication was the need for compatibility with the information system of Jefferson County.

HMO License

Alabama state law required any organization operating a health maintenance organization (HMO) or similar health plan to have an HMO license. The CCP development team did not consider the plan to be a true HMO or insurance product because it was essentially just a different way of offering the same health services to the same population for which the county had always provided services. Nonetheless, preferring to err on the side of caution and prior to opening the first CCP clinic, Dr. Michael inquired with the appropriate agency. Because of the uniqueness of the CCP model in a public hospital, the agency was not able to determine immediately whether CCP would be required to obtain an HMO license and essentially "tabled" the matter indefinitely. The first CCP clinic opened shortly thereafter.

Following favorable press coverage of the first CCP clinic, the state agency received a complaint from a Birmingham health plan alleging that Cooper Green Hospital was operating an HMO without a license. Although the agency previously had declined to make a ruling on whether a license was required, following the complaint it informed CGH that CCP would be required to obtain an

HMO license or shut down within ninety days. Unable to complete the complex and expensive application process within the allotted time frame, Dr. Michael instead entered into an agreement with United Healthcare of Alabama to operate CCP under its HMO license. JHS paid United Healthcare approximately $20,000 each year to operate the plan under its HMO license, but JHS retained all operational control over the plan. The affiliation with United was not marketed, so members were not aware of any affiliation. Although United Healthcare underwent several leadership changes that created some administrative delays in processing renewal applications for CCP, Dr. Michael described the situation as "a good working relationship and a bargain for JHS. If we tried to obtain our own HMO license, I estimate that it would cost JHS between $750,000 and $1,000,000."

Issues for the Future

As Dr. Michael left his office that evening, he glanced at his calendar—May 1999. He thought,

In less than a year, the RWJF funding will run out and the CCP clinics will have to make it on their own. There isn't enough excess in the JHS budget to subsidize their operations to any greater extent. Yet, I believe that CCP represents the system's best chance to improve the delivery of care for the underserved population, as well as ease the strain of overcrowded waiting rooms at CGH.

The original plan, as funded by RWJF and the local funding partners, had called for six clinics to be opened within five years. "We only have four now," he mused. "Should we forge ahead with expansion plans to try to achieve a critical mass, hold steady until we work out the 'growing pains,' or give up on the plan altogether?"

As he pulled out of the parking lot, he noticed that the crowd from the ER waiting room had spilled out onto the sidewalk.

InterMark

Designing UNICEF's Oral Rehydration Program in Zambia

The setting sun gave a pink tone to the Washington skyline across the Potomac River as the jet glided over the river to National Airport in early August, 1991. Allison Boyd enjoyed the view, but her thoughts were far away. For weeks she had been occupied with the children of Zambia. As a project manager for InterMark, an international consulting firm, she had been working on UNICEF's oral rehydration program for reduction of diarrheal disease in Zambia for the past six months. Her final recommendations were due in a week.

The United Nations International Children's Emergency Fund (UNICEF) contracted with InterMark to recommend how UNICEF should spend its funds over the next three years to reduce the incidence of diarrheal disease, primarily through increased use of oral rehydration salts (ORS). UNICEF spent $87,000 in 1991 to import ORS donated to the Ministry of Health for free distribution to hospitals and clinics. UNICEF was willing to spend between $87,000 and $113,000 annually for purchase of ORS or alternative programs if it could be shown that program objectives were likely to be met:

1. Substantially reduce infant and child deaths and illnesses associated with diarrheal disease, and
2. Have a high likelihood of sustainability after three years when the aid was no longer available.

The assignment had been interesting and challenging. Two month-long visits to Zambia provided a great deal of background information for her recommended program to increase the appropriate use of ORS in Zambia. Allison was expected to provide written recommendations and make a presentation to the UNICEF staff.

Zambia

The Republic of Zambia (formerly Northern Rhodesia) attained independence from Britain in 1964. Zambia was situated on an elevated plateau in south-central Africa. It had a population of 8 million in 1990 and an area of 752,614 sq. km.,

This case was prepared by Ronald Stiff, University of Baltimore. It is intended as a basis for classroom discussion rather than to illustrate effective or ineffective handling of an administrative situation. Copyright © 1994 by the *Case Research Journal* and Ronald Stiff. Used with permission from the *Case Research Journal*.

slightly larger than the state of Texas. As a land-locked country, it was dependent on either its neighbors or air transport for links with the outside world.

For many years, the mining of copper dominated the Zambian economy, although its contribution had declined significantly in recent years. The agricultural sector received the active support of the government and international donors, but it had not achieved its potential, and agricultural exports had declined. The per capita GNP, which stood at US$ 290 in 1988, placed Zambia in the low-income economies as defined by the World Bank (eighteenth poorest worldwide). Per capita GNP was expected to be as low as US$ 150 or K10,500[1] per capita in 1991. Many households earned less than K2,800 per month.

Health Expenditures and Status

In 1986 the government spent K250 per capita for health care. Estimation of morbidity (illness) and mortality (death) levels and trends were uncertain in many developing countries, including Zambia, because of problems with the quality of measurements. The national infant mortality rate fell from around 130 deaths per 1,000 in the mid-1950s to about 120 in the mid-1960s, and thence to about 115 in the early 1970s. This was considerably higher than the infant mortality rate in the twenty-five highest-income countries, which was 9 per 1,000 in 1988. Correspondingly, the proportion of children dying between birth and their fifth birthday (childhood mortality) fell from 22 percent to 20 percent, and thence to 19 percent, respectively, where it remained through 1991. In Zambia one of every five children died before reaching age five.

The national figures were within the general range of other countries in Central and Southern Africa. These statistics concealed regional differences in mortality that had implications for the effective delivery of health programs. Childhood mortality estimates for the 1960s showed a clear general pattern of highest mortality in the rural

provinces, lowest mortality in the two most urbanized provinces, and an intermediate level in the Southern province. The infant mortality rate for that period ranged from 82 (Copperbelt) to 175 (Eastern) for a national average of 121 deaths per 1,000.

Allison analyzed the most current Zambian statistical reports and grouped the Zambian provinces into three regions to evaluate geographical differences (Exhibit 5-1). She noted that the central provinces, along the main rail line, were far more urbanized than the provinces she grouped as northeastern and northwestern. The lower population densities and less developed road systems in these areas made delivery of health care services challenging. Allison wondered if UNICEF had the resources to achieve widespread distribution of ORS in both rural and urban regions.

This pattern fit well with what was known of background factors such as income levels, general economic development, nutrition, education, and fertility levels. The leading causes of mortality at Zambia's health centers in 1981 were measles (26 percent), pneumonia (14 percent), malnutrition-anemia (14 percent), malaria (10 percent), and diarrheas (10 percent). The leading causes of outpatient morbidity in children under fifteen years of age were respiratory illnesses, malaria, diarrhea, and injuries, most of which were preventable. Diarrhea cases for children under fifteen years of age at health centers are shown in Exhibit 5-2.

Most patients received free medical care through Ministry of Health, missionary, military, or mining company facilities. The number of medical facilities existing in 1988 is shown in Exhibit 5-3, and the estimated number of health care providers is shown in Exhibit 5-4.

Private Sector Health Services

There were several private medical practitioners, primarily seeing patients in Zambia's capital, Lusaka. In addition, approximately 10,000 traditional healers provided services throughout the country. It was estimated that as many as nine out

Exhibit 5-1. Population Statistics for Zambia

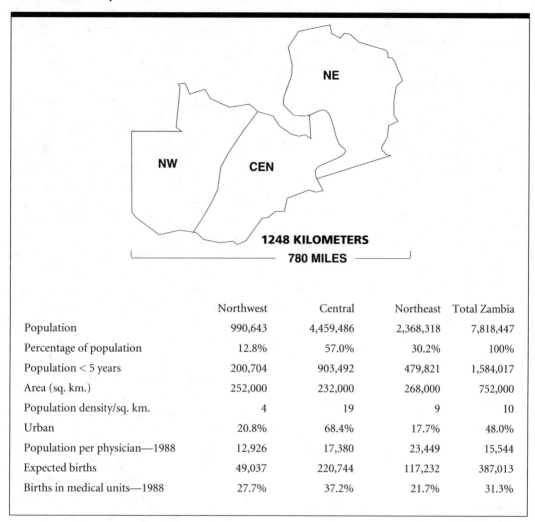

	Northwest	Central	Northeast	Total Zambia
Population	990,643	4,459,486	2,368,318	7,818,447
Percentage of population	12.8%	57.0%	30.2%	100%
Population < 5 years	200,704	903,492	479,821	1,584,017
Area (sq. km.)	252,000	232,000	268,000	752,000
Population density/sq. km.	4	19	9	10
Urban	20.8%	68.4%	17.7%	48.0%
Population per physician—1988	12,926	17,380	23,449	15,544
Expected births	49,037	220,744	117,232	387,013
Births in medical units—1988	27.7%	37.2%	21.7%	31.3%

SOURCES: *Country Profile, Republic of Zambia: 1989–1990* (Lusaka: Central Statistical Office); *Bulletin of Health Statistics: 1978–1988* (Lusaka: Ministry of Health, Health Information Unit, Republic of Zambia); *Monthly Digest of Statistics: January 1991* (Lusaka: Central Statistical Office).

NOTES: All 1990 except as noted. Analysis combines Zambian provinces as NW = North-Western and Western; CEN = Central, Copperbelt, Lusaka, and Southern; and NE = Eastern, Luapula, and Northern.

of ten patients sought help from "traditional" healers before coming for "scientific" treatment; some continued traditional medicine while hospitalized. The cost of the traditional healer's consultation fees could be greater than that paid to private medical doctors for the same symptoms.

Diarrhea Causes and Treatment

Diarrhea in Zambia results from consuming contaminated food or water. The percentage of Zambian households supplied with piped water and sewage systems declined in the latter half of the 1980s. In 1991, about 50 percent of the total popu-

Exhibit 5-2. Diarrhea Cases in Health Centers for Children Under 15 Years of Age

1986	805,880
1987	758,151
1988	842,142

SOURCE: *Bulletin of Health Statistics: 1987–1988* (Lusaka: Ministry of Health, Health Information Unit, Republic of Zambia).

Exhibit 5-3. Medical Facilities

Hospitals	
Government	42
Mission	29
Mines	11
Clinics: Rural	
Government	643
Mission	64
Clinics: Urban	
Government	142
Mines	75
Total	1,006

SOURCE: *Bulletin of Health Statistics: 1987–1988* (Lusaka: Ministry of Health, Health Information Unit, Republic of Zambia).

Exhibit 5-4. Health Care Providers

Physicians	500
Clinical officers	1,100
Nurses	5,250
Midwives	1,135
Health assistants	531
Community health workers	983

SOURCE: *Bulletin of Health Statistics: 1987–1988* (Lusaka: Ministry of Health, Health Information Unit, Republic of Zambia).

lation had access to water defined as "reasonably" safe by World Health Organization standards.

Diarrhea was one of the most critical health problems in Zambia. For children under five years of age, who constituted more than 20 percent of the total population, diarrhea was a leading cause of morbidity and mortality. In 1982, diarrhea accounted for up to 13.5 percent of total admissions, 19.2 percent of total outpatient visits, and 13.2 percent of total deaths in rural health centers. In addition, it was responsible for 7.8 percent of total admissions, 17.3 percent of total outpatient visits, and 8.6 percent of total deaths in the hospitals.

Management of diarrheal cases involved restoring and maintaining fluids by oral rehydration and, in a few cases, intravenous therapy. Often, improving or maintaining nutritional status was necessary through appropriate feeding (including breast-feeding) during and after diarrhea, as well as treating fevers and other complications with drugs. The most effective treatment was drinking oral rehydration salts, as recommended by the World Health Organization and UNICEF. ORS contained three essential salts (the formulation of ORS had some similarities to sports drinks such as Gatorade®). A typical packet is shown in Exhibit 5-5. At the onset of diarrhea, weak tea and juice were often given to children, but a correctly prepared salt-sugar solution was better. However, ORS was by far the most effective means of establishing rehydration. From a health care educator's perspective, parents had to understand that a dehydrated infant could die in less than twenty-four hours, and the parents needed to know how to provide the child with the best available rehydration solution. Parents had to be educated to recognize serious cases requiring that the child be taken to a trained health care provider.

Diarrhea produced severe dehydration especially damaging to the health of infants. The typical sequence leading to diarrheal deaths is shown in Exhibit 5-6, and factors to reduce diarrheal deaths at each stage in this sequence are given in Exhibit 5-7. In this sequence, ORS did not stop diarrhea but reduced dehydration by replacing fluids and electrolytes. Use of antidiarrheal drugs,

Exhibit 5-5.

ORAL REHYDRATION SALTS

Each sachet contains the equivalent of:

Sodium chloride:	3.5 g.
Potassium chloride:	1.5 g.
Trisodium citrate, dihydrate:	2.9 g.
Glucose anhydrous:	20.0 g.

DIRECTIONS

Dissolve in ONE LITER of drinking water.

To be taken orally:
Infants - over a 24 hour period
Children - over an 8 to 24 hour period,
according to age or as otherwise
directed under medical supervision.

CAUTION: DO NOT BOIL SOLUTION

MANUFACTURER
Jianas Bros., Packaging Co.
Kansas City, Missouri, U.S.A.

Exhibit 5-6. Typical Sequence Leading to Diarrheal Deaths

1. Low per capita income
2. Low protein diet
3. Malnourishment
4. Poor sanitation
5. Air or water infection
6. Diarrheal episode
7. Dehydration
8. Diarrheal death

such as kaolin, codeine, or activated charcoal, could cause severe life-threatening reactions in young children because these drugs did not reduce dehydration. Some pharmacists encouraged use of these drugs because either they were not educated in the use of ORS or they wanted to sell products that were higher priced than ORS.

Health care educators believed that ideal communications directed to parents should include the following informational items:

- Diarrhea, any diarrhea, was a potentially serious illness for children
- A child who had diarrhea should have received appropriate and sufficient fluids and food while diarrhea persisted and should have received extra fluids and food after an episode of diarrhea for a period equal to the duration of the illness
- The caretakers of a child with diarrhea should observe and monitor the child for danger signs, persistence of diarrhea, and the presence of blood in the stool
- Children with these danger signs must be taken for appropriate medical treatment as soon as possible

Need and Demand for ORS

Without high-quality health statistics, determining the need and demand for ORS was difficult. In 1988, 842,142 new cases of diarrhea in children under fifteen years of age were treated at hospitals or health centers. Many cases did not receive preadmission care. Additionally, the population under age five was increasing at a rapid rate. In 1991, 400,000 births were expected, with as many as 100,000 to new mothers, who were unlikely to understand the proper care of sick infants because virtually no prenatal education was provided. It was estimated that there were about five episodes of diarrhea in each of the 1.6 million children under five years of age each year; at least one-third of these required ORS. There were at least one million more cases in older children and adults each year. Effective treatment required about two liters of ORS. Treating these cases with ORS would require six million one-liter packets or the equivalent in packets of other sizes. (In Zambia, ORS was supplied as concentrated salts requiring the user to mix it with the correct quantity of water.) Only

Exhibit 5-7. Factors Reducing Diarrheal Deaths at Each Stage

STAGE ONE
Better distribution of national income
    Increase national productivity
    Additional donor aid in cash and
        materials

STAGE TWO
Add soya to mealy meal (corn meal)

STAGE THREE
Add kapenta (fish) to mealy meal

STAGE FOUR
Effective sewage system
Use of latrines
Proper disposal of the stools of young
    children
Pure water
Boiled water

STAGE FIVE
Increase persons immunized
Breast-feeding
Washing hands
Well cooked foods
Increase AIDS prevention programs

STAGE SIX
IV solutions
Manufactured oral rehydration solutions
Increased availability of health centers
Effectively trained health care professionals
    and parents
Home prepared oral rehydration solutions
Home prepared fluids

about half of this supply was available either through free distribution at health clinics or hospitals or for sale in the marketplace.

The actual demand for ORS was somewhat less than this estimate because of the difficulties in obtaining ORS and limited consumer awareness of its benefits. ORS supplied at no cost through hospitals and health centers by the Ministry of Health had limitations because of shortages, the distance and time involved in obtaining the ORS from

these sources, and frequent long waiting lines for health care services. It was estimated that 25 percent of the population lay outside a 12 km radius of a health clinic or hospital. Marketplace distribution was often ineffective because some segments of consumers were unable to pay for the ORS or unaware of its benefits. As with most products, demand varied with the price charged.

The need for education of parents was extensive. Many parents with children under fifteen years of age were not knowledgeable about oral rehydration therapy. Adult literacy in 1985 was reported to be 67 percent. Allison thought that illiteracy was likely to be higher than reported because the average amount of schooling was only 2.6 years.

Analysis of Constraints

Some constraints presented in the general economic and social environment applied specifically to a control of diarrheal disease program—constraints to the supply of ORS, or constraints to the use of ORS by mothers. Other constraints applied more broadly to delivery of all primary health care service but had a direct bearing on the success of the program.

General Environment

Although Zambia had the most highly urbanized population in sub-Saharan Africa, about 60 percent of the population lived in rural areas, where there were few points of population concentration. Household contact between mothers and the health system were common for the 75 percent of parents who lived within 12 km of clinics (average of five contacts per year for children under one year of age); however, contact was far less likely for those who lived further away. Distribution of ORS packets was expensive and delays were frequent in many rural areas where the transportation infrastructure was weak.

Cash available in households for purchases of ORS, radio batteries, public transport, and even "mealy meal" (the local term for corn meal, the major food staple) was scarce. The typical high-end expenditures for traditional medical treatment were generally between K70 and K350 for a routine course of treatment. Many households had monthly incomes of K2,800 or less. This highlighted the need for education about the most cost-effective medical treatments, such as ORS for diarrhea.

There was a large proportion of female-headed households in rural areas as result of male labor migration to urban communities in search of higher wages. The approximately 25 percent of rural households headed by females were those most likely to be at the bottom of the income scale. Because these mothers needed to produce income, they were less likely to have time to seek health services, obtain health education, or give health care at the onset of diarrhea. These households were less likely to participate in, or benefit from, a program because of financial and time constraints.

Health System Constraints

The general health system constraints in Zambia consisted of shortages of staff, shortages of supplies, inadequate support measures, and lack of appropriate supervision at all levels. Field supervision suffered from shortages of staff and inadequate provision of transportation. The large percentage of attrition found among trained community health workers and other peripheral workers was thought by Allison to be the result of infrequent or nonexistent supervisory visits. It was likely that workers at remote rural health clinics felt isolated in any case, but to never have any contact with the supervisor encouraged high employee turnover. Ideally, the supervisor's role included in-service training, checking on procedures, reinforcement, and encouragement, all vital for good performance. This support was needed for the distant workers, and transportation was very important.

Drastic cuts in the Ministry of Health budget meant that it was unlikely to be able to buy enough drugs, limiting expenditures to essential hospital supplies. It was likely that the Ministry of Health would encourage donor assistance for ORS rather than supporting an oral rehydration therapy program directly or by instituting a patient fee for drugs or services. Allison thought that UNICEF would be required to play a larger role than the Ministry of Health during the next three years.

Constraints Specific to Control of Diarrheal Disease

Allison visited hospitals and clinics with UNICEF physicians and observed inadequacies in diagnosis and treatment of diarrhea by all categories of health workers. There was a lack of awareness of the vital importance of oral rehydration therapy in clinical management and in home use for early prevention of dehydration. Health workers said that diarrheal disease was not strongly emphasized in their education, suggesting a need for refresher courses.

The doctor or clinical officer often delegated to the nurse the dispensing of ORS as well as instruction to the parent. This put the therapy in the hands of the nurse, who might not have had the same degree of therapeutic credibility as the doctor or clinical officer (physician's assistant). Similarly, pharmacists might have been the ones to instruct mothers and might have recommended less effective treatment methods than oral rehydration therapy either through lack of education or because of a desire to make profits on more expensive drugs, which were often less effective or even harmful.

ORS could be manufactured either as a premixed solution or as a powered concentrate in packets, to be mixed with water by the consumer. Although premixed ORS had the advantages of being mixed in the correct proportions and sterile, it was significantly more expensive than using packets—as much as eight times more expensive per treatment. This could discourage use; therefore, packets received considerably wider use than premixed solutions in developing countries.

ORS in packets required careful mixing. Ideally, the solution was prepared with the correct amount of boiled water. Use of unboiled water, however, was unlikely to cause serious problems because it was likely that the patient had been using the unboiled water previously and developed a resistance to most impurities. Mixtures that were too dilute were less effective than correctly prepared solutions. The most serious mixing problem was excessive concentrations of salts that could lead to severe illness and even death in infants.

Mixing instructions for ORS were complicated because there was no standardized single measuring container. For example, no standard one-liter bowl was commonly available, although there were a large number of 500 ml. cups. Once a standard packet size was selected, mothers could still be confused by having to use combinations of measuring containers.

When ORS was not readily available throughout the health system, mothers needed to know how to prepare home-mixed solutions. The occasional unavailability of either salt or sugar made home preparation problematic; this was compounded by the frequent unavailability of mixing containers or teaspoons and the lack of consumer knowledge of oral rehydration therapy. Incorrect formulations could be harmful to children, especially infants.

Information provided to the mother when oral rehydration therapy was promoted did not state that ORS was not designed to stop the diarrhea. ORS maintained hydration through the disease course. Diarrhea often ran its course if the child was kept hydrated and there was not a serious underlying cause. This needed to be described carefully to the mother or father so that rapid cessation of the diarrhea was not expected. Unfortunately, if such information was not provided, parents who believed oral rehydration therapy should stop the diarrhea might not only end the therapy when diarrhea did not cease immediately but also might be unlikely to employ oral rehydration therapy in future diarrheal episodes.

Program Alternatives

Allison considered several interrelated alternatives for increasing the use of oral rehydration therapy using ORS. These included how to ensure a reliable supply of ORS, what method of distribution would be effective in reaching consumers, what method of packaging should be encouraged, whether health care professionals needed to be trained in the use of ORS, and how to best promote ORS therapy with consumers.

Supply Alternatives

The major supply of ORS was from the Swedish International Development Agency, which supplied one-liter packets of ORS in essential drug kits, monthly, to the 707 rural health clinics. Each sealed kit included 150 one-liter packets. As a result, the supply of ORS was greater in some rural health clinics than in urban areas. There was no inventory control in place to balance supply and demand between the rural health clinics. Consequently, there could be several months' supply at some clinics while others stocked out. The Swedish International Development Agency was considering increasing the ORS in kits to 200 each next year. In addition, the agency considered supplying some stocks at the district level for reallocation to clinics on an as-needed basis, developing methods to reallocate inventories, and distribution to urban clinics. Allison was concerned that the Swedish International Development Agency's policies of free distribution were likely to have an effect on the motivation of private manufacturers and distributors of ORS.

UNICEF remained the most likely donor for additional ORS supplies; it could agree to help the Ministry of Health by continuing to donate imported one-liter packets. In the past year, 1.2 million one-liter packets had been donated at a total

Exhibit 5-8. Local Manufacturing Costs for 1-Liter Package of ORS

Materials	K3.58	
Labor	0.80	
Direct costs		4.38
Factory overhead	1.10	
Production cost		5.48
Company overhead	1.33	
Factory cost		6.81
Profit margin	1.19	
Manufacturing selling price		K8.00

SOURCE: Company interviews.

NOTES: Costs were based on an annual production volume of two million packets. Retail price was higher due to mark-ups. Costs for smaller packets were identical except that materials cost was less per packet.

imported cost of $87,000—about K5 per packet. In addition, UNICEF had the option of subsidizing the production of ORS packets by local manufacturers. UNICEF did this in two countries (Haiti and Indonesia), paying the local producers the equivalent of the imported cost of packets.

The major constraint to this type of arrangement in Zambia was the high cost of the locally produced ORS packets. The approximate cost breakdown for local manufacturing of one-liter packets of ORS is given in Exhibit 5-8.

Packets were produced for free distribution at health clinics and hospitals through the Ministry of Health by a government-owned company, General Pharmaceutical Ltd. At various times, the packets were for sale in the private sector by Cadbury Schweppes's Zambian operations and the Zambian firms Gamma Pharmaceuticals and Interchem. A UNICEF grant of K7 million (estimated at half the total cost of setting up ORS manufacturing for production of two million packets annually) helped supply the equipment necessary for General Pharmaceutical Ltd. to manufacture up to two million packets per year. General Phar-

maceutical Ltd. had produced 1.4 million one-liter packets under the brand name "Madzi-a-moyi" (Water for Life) in the past year, but General Pharmaceutical Ltd. ceased production because of the high cost of imported raw materials and packaging.

A small amount of the General Pharmaceutical Ltd. production was sold through about 100 government-owned pharmacies for K6 to K10. Although this price appeared to be less than the manufacturer's cost, it resulted from these packets being produced in 1990, when the kwacha had not devalued to its current level. The retail price was expected to be higher if they resumed production.

Gamma Pharmaceuticals and Interchem each had the capacity to manufacture two million packets of either one-liter or 250 ml. per year. Neither was producing ORS. Gamma used its machine to produce other products, and Interchem had not been able to use its Korean-made machine for two years because of failure of a part. Distribution of drug products was through deliveries either to sales agents in the Copperbelt and Livingstone areas, or to general merchandise wholesalers who came to Lusaka to purchase ORS. There was also some direct distribution to pharmacies and other outlets in Lusaka.

The manufacturer's costs and prices were expected to be approximately the same for either manufacturer. Additional production capacity was expected to cost about K14 million for each two million units produced per year for either one-liter or 250 ml. packet sizes. However, long delays were experienced in supplying equipment to General Pharmaceutical Ltd. because of shipping and building construction problems, as well as the need to install a three-phase electrical supply. Interchem's parent company was evaluating replacement of the current machine.

Cadbury Schweppes had recently received Ministry of Health approval to market orange flavored ORS in 250 ml. packets using the brand name Oresa (Oral REhydration SAlts). The company manufactured 500,000 packets; 40,000 had been distributed directly to chemists (drug stores) to test market acceptance, and the remainder were in inventory. The manufacturer's price was K12, with a suggested retail price of K15. Some chemists, however, charged K18. Flavored ORS was neither encouraged nor discouraged by the World Health Organization, although at one time they opposed flavored ORS because of its potential for unnecessary use and its increased cost relative to unflavored ORS. On the other hand, 300 ml. soft drink bottles (Coke, Fanta, Torino) were widely available in Zambia (many were distributed by Cadbury) for mixing 250 ml. ORS. Research at the University Teaching Hospital showed that children, even at very young ages, were more willing to drink flavored ORS and, as a result, consumed more total fluids than when given unflavored ORS. Cadbury Schweppes had the capacity to produce 18 million packets a year in one shift, which was also used to produce powdered Kia-Ora, a children's drink (similar to Kool-Aid®). These could be either 250 ml. flavored or one-liter unflavored. The cost of unflavored ORS was expected to be about the same as for other local manufacturers. The per packet cost of 250 ml. flavored ORS was slightly more than that of one-liter of unflavored. Cadbury could supply either flavored or unflavored ORS in bulk packages for hospitals and health clinics.

Flavored ORS was imported in limited quantities. Small quantities of Rehidrat® (manufactured by Searle) were available in lemon-lime 250 ml. packets for K30. ORS imported for resale, however, was subject to a 100 percent import duty under import substitution laws. An additional 200,000 to 400,000 packets were contributed annually by the Red Cross, churches, and other non-government organizations.

Cadbury was the only firm that had the potential to produce ORS in bottles. It was expected that the cost for 250 ml. bottles would be about the same as for soft drinks—K40 per bottle including a K20 bottle refund. Thus, a two-liter treatment would cost the consumer K320 without refund and K160 if bottles were returned, considerably more than the cost of buying packets.

Considering the low incomes of many target consumers, a need existed to price ORS at a level to maintain affordability. This approach appeared to be impossible without some type of subsidy. An ORS price subsidy to manufacturers or importers could create a financial burden that was unlikely to be sustainable over time. In the short term, UNICEF might have used the value of the raw materials as a subsidy or might have provided promotional or educational services for branded products. Another option was for industry to offer a modest price to low-income consumers and still create revenues to help pay program costs by charging a much higher price for a different, more "modern" product aimed at higher-income consumers.

Distribution

Even if there was substantial donor support for free ORS distribution through clinics and hospitals, there was a need for other modes of access to ORS as well as a need to promote home-mix solutions. The commercial sector in Zambia offered several possibilities.

As a normal business practice in Zambia, a manufacturer established the recommended consumer price for its product. Trade discounts based on the recommended consumer price were 20 percent to retailers and 20 percent to trade channel members.

Allison conducted interviews with the general manager or the marketing manager of the major organizations that expressed an interest in distributing ORS. Each reached a large number of retail outlets, as shown in Exhibit 5-9.

Gamma Pharmaceutical

Gamma Pharmaceutical, which started activities in 1984, manufactured pharmaceutical products for the Zambian market and for export. Its products were sold to private pharmacies, government and industry health facilities, and retail out-

Exhibit 5-9. Potential Distribution Outlets for ORS

	Number of Outlets
Gamma Pharmaceutical	1,000
Interchem	1,000
Cadbury Schweppes	5,000
Lyons Brooke Bond	2,200
Colgate & Palmolive	8,000

lets, including supermarkets. Gamma had a fleet of six delivery trucks and one van, along with two sales agents. Gamma was a sound, fast-growing company with a strong production and marketing team.

Interchem

Interchem manufactured a variety of pharmaceutical products. In addition to distributing ORS, its marketing manager was interested in resuming production. Interchem needed to either repair its existing packaging machine or purchase a new one. It was not certain that repair parts were available from the Korean supplier. A new machine would cost K14 million.

Cadbury Schweppes

Cadbury Schweppes was a major producer of soft drinks, drink syrups, and other consumer packaged goods. Cadbury distributed its products directly to retail outlets. Cadbury was evaluating flavored ORS and deciding if it should introduce Oresa throughout Zambia. They had about 460,000 packets in inventory and could begin production of additional packets within a month.

Lyons Brooke Bond

Lyons Brooke Bond, Zambia, formerly a Lever Brothers company, was an independent firm incorporated in Zambia. Lyons Brooke Bond manufactured and distributed processed food products. The managing director of the company had shown an interest in distributing ORS, although the organization did not handle any pharmaceutical products.

Colgate & Palmolive

Colgate, one of the largest distributors in Zambia, had five sales agents, four delivery vans, five freight trucks, and more than ten large wholesalers. Colgate & Palmolive manufactured and distributed personal care and hygiene products.

Evaluation of Distribution Alternatives

Allison's review of distribution capabilities in Zambia offered several options in terms of cost-effectiveness, marketing opportunities, sustainability, and possible future self-sufficiency. Although historically the bulk of ORS had been distributed at no cost by not-for-profit organizations, the commercial firms in Zambia could be enlisted in the implementation of an ORS program. These firms had strong experience in marketing, sound management capabilities, and financial stability; had well-developed infrastructures that allowed them access to thousands of retail outlets; and were interested in participating in a marketing program both as good corporate citizens and as a potentially profitable business. Allison believed that these firms had a good understanding of the marketing environment in Zambia and that their existing distribution channels could provide an effective method of distributing ORS. One or more firms could be encouraged to make a long-term financial commitment to supply ORS.

However, she felt that there were several problems in encouraging increased participation by local manufacturers and distributors. Would the market price to consumers be too high to encourage appropriate use? Was the market large enough to encourage sufficient participation by manufacturers and distributors? Would free distribution by the government and other organizations reduce the private sector's interest in entering the market? Finally, would an oversupply be created as a result of competition, which would lead to either reduced quality control or withdrawals from the market by manufacturers and distributors?

Packaging

The form of packaging had significant implications for correct use of ORS. ORS could be packaged as a premixed solution in bottles or cardboard containers, or as powdered salts in foil packets. Advantages and disadvantages existed for each alternative.

Premixed ORS

Pros:

ORS was sterile

Correct concentration of ORS

Less intense consumer education required for preparation

Cadbury could produce in bottles

Cons:

Only one firm had the capacity to produce bottles

As much as eight times more expensive per treatment to the consumer than packets

Required more space in delivery vehicles and on store shelves

Use of bottles required a deposit and return system due to limited supply of bottles in Zambia

No Zambian firm could produce cardboard containers suitable for ORS

Use of cardboard increased waste and litter

Packets

Simple, consistent messages were needed to effectively promote ORS packets, along with associated training and education efforts. A single packet size was likely to be most effective; risk of confusion among mothers was possible if more than one packet size was available. Two packet sizes were possible for widespread production and distribution: 250 ml. or one-liter. The following are the pros and cons.

250 ml. Packet

Pros:

Soft drink bottles of 300 ml. were widely available and could be used for 250 ml. packets; soft drinks were sold for K40 per bottle, including a K20 bottle refund

Tea cups of 250 ml. were widely available

Cons:

Half a million one-liter packets were available in the distribution system

Imported ORS was generally available in one-liter packets

Changes in syrup bottle sizes could occur

If parents mixed 250 ml. packets in one-liter containers, ORS was less effective

One-Liter Packet

Pros:

At least 500,000 existed in the supply system

UNICEF's imported cost was less than local manufacturers' price

UNICEF one-liter packets could be purchased in emergency shortages

Cups of 500 ml. were widely available

Cons:

The variety of cup sizes available at retail outlets was increasing, with many cups of nonstandard size available

If parents mixed one-liter packets in 300 ml. bottles, vomiting and serious heart and nervous problems could result, especially in younger children

Key questions were when local production could begin and whether local production would provide a substantial, reliable supply of acceptable quality. If production was delayed or unreliable, UNICEF or another supplier would have to fill the gap with one-liter packets.

Training of Health Care Professionals

Physicians, nurses, clinical officers, pharmacists, and traditional healers in their regular treatment and advice set the standards for medical care. If these professionals did not understand and have confidence in oral rehydration therapy, it was unlikely that they would establish oral rehydration as the standard treatment for diarrhea in Zambia.

Physicians needed training in appropriate clinical management of infants and children with diarrhea. Physicians needed to go beyond statements of symptoms as a basis for prescribing treatment for diarrhea. Effective treatment incorporated a patient history, an examination, and therapeutic management. Because physicians were opinion leaders, special efforts were desirable at the beginning of a program to inform them about oral rehydration therapy through seminars and refresher training courses.

Diarrheal Training Units

Diarrheal training units had been effective in training health care workers in other developing countries; however, only one existed in Zambia. The purpose of diarrheal training units was to develop the skills and confidence of physicians and nurses so they could give proper therapy to children with diarrhea. When participants attended clinical training, they developed skills in assessing and managing diarrhea. They learned to treat simple and complicated cases and how to communicate these skills to mothers and colleagues.

Experience suggested that a three- to five-day training course was needed for professionals to be effective. This approach made training expensive. Some professionals found it difficult to leave their responsibilities for the required period. Because diarrheal training units emphasized individual and practical teaching, only relatively small numbers of professionals could be trained at any time.

Exhibit 5-10. Local Costs in Kwacha

Cost per Unit per Year	
Land Cruiser truck (4WD)	K1,200,000
Annual fuel and maintenance	300,000
Driver	30,000
Trainers (if full time with program)	
Physician	72,000
Public health nurse	36,000
Public health trainer	36,000
Training Materials	
For health care persons	120
For parents	10
Jugs (one-liter)	100
Measuring spoons	30
Mugs (250 ml.)	15
"Banana" cups (500 ml.)	35
Posters—each	500

SOURCE: Interviews with health education professionals.

In effective diarrheal training units, the number of participants ranged from five to fifteen. In addition, the need to have enough diarrhea cases of various types for each trainee to handle meant that some diarrheal training units were operational only during the rainy season.

The only diarrheal training unit in Zambia was a World Health Organization–funded unit at the University Teaching Hospital in Lusaka that trained doctors and nurses. Allison felt that additional diarrheal training units could be effective, but their costs needed to be evaluated. Costs involved in training are included in Exhibit 5-10.

Promotion

There were an estimated three million radios in Zambia and two broadcasting stations; both were state owned: *Radio Mulungushi*, a very popular station, which was primarily urban, and *Radio Zambia*, primarily rural. There were as many as 250,000 television sets and one state-operated television station (operating from 5 p.m. to midnight weekdays, with longer hours on the weekend). There were seven major languages; therefore, it was considered critical to advertise in English plus several other languages to reach the population effectively. A media rate card is provided in Exhibit 5-11.

Message Content

A major challenge for ORS advertising was to persuade consumers that restoring the child's activity and preventing dehydration was a sufficient reason for using the product. Most communications/promotions efforts chose not to deliver negative messages such as "oral rehydration therapy does not stop diarrhea" or "antidiarrheals do not stop diarrhea," although both were factual. Programs chose to address these issues in other ways, such as in scientific seminars for physicians or working to change national drug policies.

A second major challenge was not only to stimulate sales of the product—the traditional goal of advertising—but also to emphasize the correct mixture and utilization of ORS. ORS product advertising needed to include brand-specific advertising from the beginning for maximum effectiveness, but generic advertising might also be appropriate within the same campaign.

The Sustainability Issue

Any donor program was considered sustainable when the flow of benefits from the program could be maintained or enhanced when donor funding ceased. Thus, sustainability did not refer to each activity undertaken as part of a control of diarrheal disease program but instead referred to the lasting impact of the program. Seen in this perspective, the global smallpox eradication program

achieved the ultimate in sustainability: the target population continued to receive the health benefits resulting from the eradication of the disease. Ultimately, the goal of any diarrheal disease program was that there be a sustained reduction in morbidity and mortality from diarrhea because of the program.

There were various levels at which diarrheal disease program activities took place, including strategies that had shorter- or longer-term impacts on diarrhea. For example, the installation of a water and sewer system would be likely to have a larger impact on diarrhea morbidity and mortality than an advertising campaign promoting oral rehydration therapy use. However, building infrastructure was a longer-term, considerably more expensive solution. Allison knew that multiple actions were possible, but it was not possible to do everything and solve all the problems. One solution would be to seek ways to ensure that mothers and health workers maintained appropriate case management practices (oral rehydration therapy use being one of them) after the initial program investment was made. More directly yet, one might concentrate on ways to sustain the resource base for program activities such as training, information systems, ORS production and distribution, or any other activities designed to reduce the incidence of diarrheal disease.

Donors wanted to invest in development efforts and then have the benefits resulting from their investment carry on without the need for continued outside support. The developing countries themselves preferred to avoid recipient country dependency on donor funding over the long term. This translated into donors trying to avoid paying recurrent costs, such as for salaries, routine supervision, and transportation. When these costs were regularly paid by donors, the program was felt to be in jeopardy of being dropped or critically underfunded when the donor project ran out and the program reverted from donor support to the routine government budget. If the government did not have sufficient funds to match the level of donor funding, the program's organization and

Exhibit 5-11. Basic Media Rates for Zambia, December, 1990

TELEVISION		RADIO	
TIME SLOT	RATE FOR 1 AD	TIME SLOT	RATE FOR 1 AD
PRIME TIME		A TIME	
60 seconds	K12,000	60 seconds	K1,800
45 seconds	9,600	45 seconds	1,500
30 seconds	6,000	30 seconds	1,200
15 seconds	3,600	15 seconds	900
7 seconds	3,000		
A TIME		B TIME	
60 seconds	K 9,600	60 seconds	K1,440
45 seconds	6,600	45 seconds	1,200
30 seconds	4,200	30 seconds	900
15 seconds	3,000	15 seconds	720
7 seconds	2,160		
B TIME		C TIME	
60 seconds	K 6,000	60 seconds	K1,080
45 seconds	6,600	45 seconds	780
30 seconds	3,600	30 seconds	720
15 seconds	1,800	15 seconds	540
7 seconds	1,200		

TV TIME DISTRIBUTIONS		RADIO TIME DISTRIBUTIONS	
PRIME TIME	18:55 to 20:00	A TIME	05:00 to 08:00
			12:00 to 14:00
A TIME	07:00 to 11:00		16:30 to 22:00
	20:00 to 23:00	Weekend	05:00 to 22:00
B TIME	06:00 to 07:00	B TIME	08:00 to 12:00
	15:00 to 18:55		14:00 to 16:30
	23:00 to Close		22:00 to 23:00
		Weekend	22:00 to 23:00
		C TIME	23:00 to Close
		Weekend	23:00 to 24:00

PRESS	ONE CENTIMETER DOWN BY ONE COLUMN WIDE
Times of Zambia	K100.80
Zambia Daily Mail	70.87

SOURCE: Zambia National Broadcasting Company Rate Card, 1991.

NOTE: Gross rates include 20 percent sales tax.

activities might break down to the point where they were no longer effective. This situation described what happened to an unsustainable program, one in which insufficient thought had been given to how the host country could support the program.

Developing UNICEF's ORS Program

Within a week, Allison had to present the program that she had developed to the UNICEF staff, both orally and in writing. Among the issues she considered were

- How to increase the supply of ORS
  —Increase imports
  —Provide subsidies for local manufacturing
  —Purchase from local manufacturers
- How to make the distribution of ORS more effective
- How to encourage private manufacturing and distribution
- How to educate effectively health care providers and parents about when ORS is necessary and the correct use of ORS

- Should packet size be standardized at 250 ml. or one-liter, or should two sizes be encouraged? Is there any role for premixed ORS?

Allison realized that she could recommend a variety of activities, but not everything could be accomplished in the UNICEF budget, which was $87,000 in 1991. UNICEF was willing to spend as much as $113,000 annually in the years 1992 through 1994 if they felt that their objectives were likely to be met. She suspected that there were some actions that would greatly improve the functioning of the system and had begun to think about the processes involved in the flow of ORS, from supply by the manufacturer to demand and use by the consumer. She was also concerned about the flow of ORS information. Where were the leverage points? How could appropriate use be achieved on a sustainable basis?

Note

1. The kwacha, the Zambian currency. In 1991, K70 equaled US$ 1.

The New York State West Nile Virus Outbreak

What Should Be Nassau County's Response?

An alert infectious disease physician from North Queens called the New York City Department of Health (NYCDOH) on August 23, 1999, to report two unusual cases of encephalitis. Dr. Farzad Mostashari from the U.S. Centers for Disease Control and Prevention (CDC) later stated, "What struck the New York physician was that he needed to rule out the possibility that these cases weren't encephalitis, but botulism. And that was because of the striking muscle weaknesses seen." The NYCDOH investigated the report and subsequently identified a cluster of six patients with encephalitis who lived in northern Queens. These initial cases were tested for antibodies to common North American arboviruses by IgM capture ELISA. On September 3, the cases were reported to be positive for antibodies to the St. Louis Encephalitis (SLE) virus. Active surveillance was initiated in New York City on August 30 and in Westchester and Nassau counties on September 3 (see Exhibit 6-1 for a map of the area). Eight of the earliest cases lived within a two-by-two-mile area in North Queens. A clinical case was defined as "a presumptive diagnosis of viral encephalitis with or without muscle weakness or acute flaccid paralysis, Guillian-Barre syndrome, aseptic meningitis, or presence of the clinical symptoms characterizing the initial cluster of cases in a patient presenting after August 1st."

New York City Responds

On September 3, the city began actions to alleviate the outbreak and educate the public. Because SLE was a mosquito-borne illness, citywide pesticide spraying and other vector control measures were taken; local firehouses served as distribution centers for Deet-based insect repellants. A hotline was established to address the public's questions about the outbreak itself or pesticide applications. Spraying schedules were published with warnings

This case was originally developed by Amy Dreibelbis, Jason Farley, William Lovett, and Stephanie Waldrop as a student project under the supervision of Susan L. Davies, Peter M. Ginter, Robert R. Jacobs, Donna J. Petersen, and Dale O. Williams at the School of Public Health, University of Alabama at Birmingham. The case was revised by Stuart A. Capper, Peter M. Ginter, and Linda E. Swayne. It is intended to be used as a basis for classroom discussion rather than to illustrate effective or ineffective handling of an administrative situation. Used with permission from Donna J. Petersen.

Exhibit 6-1. Map of Nassau County, New York

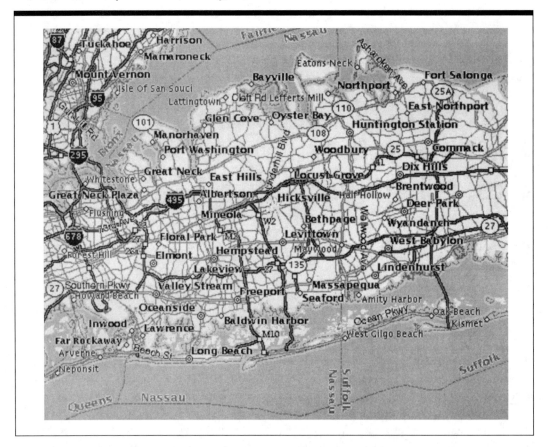

for residents to remain indoors during the pesticide applications. About 750,000 educational leaflets containing information about protection from mosquitoes were distributed throughout the city. Public service announcements encouraging people to limit outdoor activity, to wear long-sleeved shirts and long pants, and to eliminate any possible mosquito breeding grounds such as old tires were distributed to radio and television stations, newspapers, and World Wide Web sites.

Meanwhile, local health officials noticed a marked increase in deaths among birds, particularly crows, in New York City. In addition, there had been several unusual deaths among birds at the Bronx Zoo. Two captive-bred Chilean flamingos, a cormorant, and an Asian pheasant had died at the zoo, and necropsy results showed meningoencephalitis and myocarditis. On September 10,

concerned officials at the zoo sent tissue samples to the U.S. Department of Agriculture National Veterinary Services Laboratory (NVSL) in Ames, Iowa, to test for eastern equine encephalitis and other avian pathogens. None of the tests came back positive. The NVSL then sent virus samples isolated from the bird's tissues to the CDC on September 20. Polymerase chain reaction (PCR) testing and DNA sequencing begun at the CDC on September 23 indicated that the viral isolates were closely related to a virus never seen before in the Western hemisphere: the West Nile virus (WNV). Alarmingly, viral isolates from a brain sample of a human encephalitis case proved to be identical to the West Nile–like sequence isolated from the zoo birds. Officials at the New York State Department of Health concurrently sent brain tissue specimens from three encephalitis cases to the University of California at Irvine for additional testing. Testing in California confirmed what the CDC had found: the virus infecting these humans appeared to have a genomic sequence very similar to that of the West Nile virus. Health officials realized that what they had on their hands might not be an outbreak of SLE at all.

The West Nile Virus

The virus was first discovered in the West Nile District of Uganda in 1937 and was subsequently isolated in humans, birds, and mosquitoes. The virus was a member of the Japanese encephalitis antigenic complex of the genus *Flavivirus*, family *Flaviviridae*. All known members of this complex (nine to date) were transmissible by mosquito, and many caused febrile, sometimes fatal, illnesses in humans. Largely, bird-feeding mosquitoes were identified as the principal vector of West Nile virus; there was no known person-to-person transmission. The virus had been isolated from forty-three mosquito species, predominantly of the genus *Culex*.

In humans, West Nile fever was typically a febrile illness, with influenza-like symptoms, characterized by an abrupt onset of moderate to high fever (three to five days, infrequently biphasic, often with chills). The incubation period was three to six days. Other symptoms included headache (frontal), sore throat, backache, myalgia, arthralgia, fatigue, conjunctivitis, retrobulbar pain, maculopapular or roseolar rash (almost half the cases spreading from the trunk to the extremities and head), lymphadenopathy, anorexia, nausea, abdominal pain, diarrhea, and respiratory symptoms. Occasionally (in less than 15 percent of cases), acute aseptic meningitis or encephalitis (associated with neck stiffness, vomiting, confusion, somnolence, abnormal reflexes, convulsions, pareses, and coma), anterior myelitis, hepatosplenomegaly, hepatitis, pancreatitis, and myocarditis occurred. The virus could be encountered in a person's blood for ten days after recovery if they were immunocompetent and up to twenty-eight

days if immunocompromised. Peak viremia occurred four to eight days postinfection.

West Nile Virus Verified in New York

A West Nile–like virus had struck New York. *Newsday* reported that the true scale of the outbreak was "determined by scouring hospital records, the city morgue, and all lab samples of spinal fluids examined for other reasons, doctor's office records, and dozens of other sources." All serum and cerebrospinal fluid samples from the New York outbreak that initially had been reactive to SLE antigens were retested and shown to positively react to WNV antigens. The ten borderline cases and eight samples that did not react to SLE came back positive for WNV antibodies. A total of thirty-eight cases eventually were identified in New York City: twenty-six from Queens, nine from the Bronx, two from Manhattan, and one from Brooklyn. Spraying efforts begun when the outbreak was first thought to be SLE had been very effective in reducing the adult mosquito population in these areas.

The Current Situation of West Nile Virus in Nassau County

In Nassau County, concerns were increasing not only about the West Nile–like virus but also regarding the measures the county was taking and preparing to take to address the outbreak.

Nassau County, State of New York

Nassau County was one of the two counties on Long Island not associated with New York City (the other was Suffolk County). The population was at a relatively stable level of about 1.3 million people. About 15 percent of the population was over 65 years of age, and about the same percentage of the population was younger than 15, typical for an industrialized country. The county had a highly suburban population and was relatively prosperous, with a median income of approxi-

Exhibit 6-2. Nassau County Sentinel Bird Deaths (9/3/99-9/24/99)

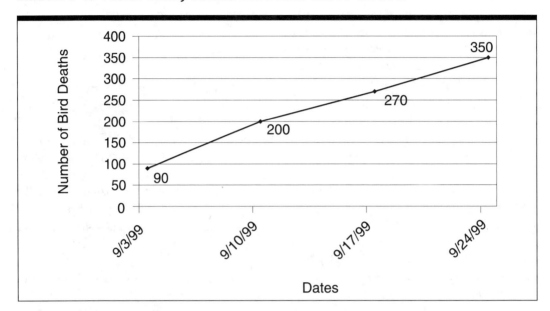

mately $58,000. Slightly more than 5 percent of the population was at the poverty level or below for Nassau County. Sixty-two farms occupied about 1 percent of the land in the county. Most of the population was involved in retail trade and services (61 percent). Unemployment in 1996 was a low 5 percent.

Nassau County Surveillance Begun

On September 3, following the lead of both Westchester County and New York City, Nassau County initiated active surveillance for both mosquitoes and dead birds carrying the virus. The public had been informed via the news media, pamphlets, radio, and World Wide Web announcements to take protective measures to avoid contracting the virus. With cooperation from the Nassau County Department of Public Works (NCDPW), the Integrated Pest Management Mosquito Surveillance and Control program had been expanded to include weekends. Five two-man teams were now inspecting and spot treating existing and potential breeding sites. All hospitals and clinics were made aware of the case definition of the disease and were informed that any sus-

pected cases should be reported to the health department immediately. Numerous hotline numbers had been set up in the department to answer the public's questions, address any concerns and complaints, and receive reports of dead birds in the area. The initial efforts, however, were not accomplishing as much as had been hoped.

The low counts of mosquitoes reported from the county public health laboratories were less reassuring than they had been a few weeks earlier. Reports of dead and sick crows around the county continued. As of September 29, the number of dead birds throughout the county was nearly 400 (Exhibit 6-2). Furthermore, live birds were now being reported as infected with the virus.

Nassau County Health Commissioner Dr. Katrina Guest was most concerned about the fact that lab results on three pigeons and four geese from two Nassau communities indicated that the birds were exposed to and contracted the virus in Nassau County, not via migration from nearby Suffolk and Westchester counties, where numerous cases and a death reportedly had occurred. All these events strengthened Dr. Guest's belief that stronger measures would need to be implemented. Laboratory analyses to make an estimate of infected mosquitoes in Nassau County were still not complete, but reports from Brooklyn and Queens indicated that the level of infected mosquitoes was greater than expected.

Nassau County presented an interesting epidemiological situation. Because there was no person-to-person transmission, reducing exposure to mosquitoes was the primary means of prevention. Nassau County, however, was known for its outdoor activities such as swimming, fishing, and boating that meant increased overall time spent outdoors. Questions arose as to how to limit contact with mosquitoes without significantly affecting the citizens' quality of life.

Ground Spraying in Nassau County

Ground spraying strategies were implemented, but two more cases were identified in Port Washington. These two cases, along with those that had been identified in Floral Park, brought the total number of cases in the county to four. No deaths had occurred yet, and that was something foremost in Dr. Guest's mind. Aerial spraying was the next line of defense and was likely to be accompanied by some resistance from community leaders, residents, and environmental advocacy groups. The news media, environmental advocacy organizations, and community agencies had criticized the health department's efforts to inform the public about the ground spraying efforts. Dr. Guest was angered by reports from one community group, the Network Neighborhood, claiming that trucks had conducted spraying while children were outside playing. She did not want to see people die from this virus and would personally support any measure possible to prevent deaths in the county from occurring.

What Next?

As Nassau County Health Commissioner, Dr. Guest knew the evidence to justify her actions needed to be concrete. She requested that each of the offices within the department provide her with recommendations. She had received the memos prepared by them. After reading all the data and opinions that her colleagues had gathered, she felt somewhat overwhelmed. Were they about to have a serious epidemic on their hands?

Input From the Department Leadership Team

Each member of the team had prepared information that would be helpful, but they also raised some very difficult questions. The county had a mosquito control program titled "Nassau County Mosquito Surveillance and Control Status Report—December 1998" (see Exhibit 6-3 for a copy of the report). Dr. Guest reviewed the memos from key staff one more time to prepare for the team's meeting later that day.

Office of Infectious Disease

The memo from Dr. Mike Stein of the office of infectious diseases indicated that at the time, no studies had been conducted about the West Nile virus within the United States. He turned to studies conducted in other countries looking for epidemiologic clues as to what persons would be at highest risk for infection and, of those persons who were infected, who would be most likely to develop serious complications. A study conducted in Romania in 1996 found 393 people infected with West Nile virus (41 percent of the population studied). The study concluded that peridomestic transmission (transmission within a residential area) was the most common mechanism for viral spread. Time spent outdoors was significantly associated with risk of transmission. Persons who spent more than six hours per day outdoors were at the greatest risk of acquiring the infection.

At the state level, information was reviewed on the incidence of various communicable diseases. Encephalitides were extremely rare, and mostly the result of a pathogen other than an arbovirus. Lyme disease, salmenollosis, campylobacteriosis, AIDS, giardiasis, and gonorrhea were the only dis-

(text continues on page 250)

Exhibit 6-3. Nassau County Mosquito Surveillance and Control Status Report—December 1998

Nassau County Department of Health (NCDH) and Public Works (DPW) receive hundreds of complaints from County residents concerning mosquitoes every year. To these complaints and to protect public health, NCDH and DPW have been working together in a joint effort to suppress mosquito population through surveillance and control. Both departments are committed to utilizing a method of pest control known as integrated pest management (IPM), which employs a number of different control strategies geared to minimizing the use of chemical pesticides.

Exhibit I indicates the number of mosquito complaints received in 1996, 1997, and 1998 by NCDH each month during the mosquito season. In 1996 there were 566; 1997, 218; and 1998, 194 complaints. This graph depicts a substantial reduction in complaints since the initiation of the present mosquito control program, which was established in 1996 as a result of more than 500 complaints in 3 months.

Exhibit I. Mosquito Complaints by Month

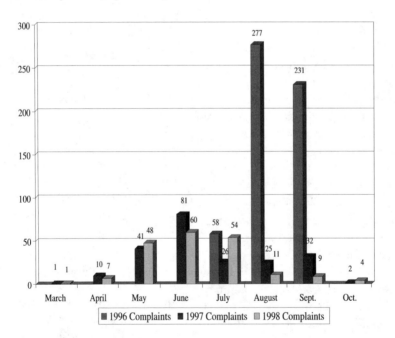

Our first line of defense against the mosquito is the elimination of stagnant water. Mosquitoes spend much of their life cycle as aquatic larvae or "wrigglers" in water in roof gutters, bird baths, street drains, storm water recharge basins, drainage ditches, old tires, artificial containers, and fresh water wetlands. In addition, there are several species that inhabit extensive saltwater wetlands on both the north and south shore of Nassau County. To reduce salt marsh mosquito populations, approximately 1,000 miles of ditches were dug in past years to improve drainage along the shoreline, on the south shore barrier islands, and the numerous hassocks and islets. Since 1997 more than 250 miles of ditches were re-established, reducing the size and number of puddles and areas of standing water suitable for mosquito egg hatching and larval development. In 1997 Nassau County Department of Public Works (NCDPW) hired additional personnel and acquired new equipment to maintain and rehabilitate the drainage ditches, and to cut access paths that facilitate inspection, maintenance, and treatment of mosquito breeding areas. Even so, it will take a number of years before all ditches are rehabilitated to their former condition. Given that natural forces such as wind, rain, tides, and major storms continu-

(Continued)

Exhibit 6-3. Continued

ally influence the marsh topography resulting in new mosquito breeding areas, ditch maintenance is an ongoing and long-term project. Well maintained drainage ditches provide a habitat for killifish that feed on mosquito larvae and also create a suitable environment for waterfowl.

Mosquito Surveillance

Surveillance of the larval and adult stages of the mosquito is an integral part of any cost effective program. During peak activities Nassau County Department of Health (NCDH) has designated staff to assist Nassau County Department of Public Works (NCDPW) in monitoring mosquito populations, responding to citizen complaints, and treating mosquito breeding habitats with larvicides by hand. The two methods of monitoring actual and potential mosquito populations are "dipping" for larvae and trapping adult mosquitoes with light traps.

Dipping for Mosquito Larvae

The most effective means of controlling mosquito populations is to identify breeding sites so that they may be modified to prevent puddling conditions conducive to mosquito breeding or treated to kill the larvae before they become adult mosquitoes. "Dipping" for larvae is the sampling technique used to estimate the number of larvae present in the standing water found in breeding areas. If the number of larvae are determined to be excessive, an appropriate larvicide can be applied. Treatment can be administered by hand to specific breeding locations or by helicopter over larger and less accessible areas. All treatments are made in compliance with the product labels and permits obtained from New York State Department of Environmental Conservation (NYSDEC). The information gained from these larvae dipping surveys allows us to determine if control measures are necessary, and if so what measures to take. Our Integrated Pest Management Program (IPM) dictates that we do not apply pest control products indiscriminately, therefore dipping plays an important role in minimizing the use of pesticides.

CDC Light Traps

CDC light traps use a combination of light and carbon dioxide to attract mosquitoes for two purposes: (1) to estimate adult populations, and (2) to trap and subsequently identify and test mosquitoes for disease, especially Eastern Equine Encephalitis (EEE), an infectious disease affecting horses and humans. If the number of adult mosquitoes are excessive, spraying with a low toxicity pesticide may be recommended, as well as a closer look at breeding areas in the vicinity, which are then prioritized for chemical or non chemical IPM strategies. If EEE were present, there would be a potential public health risk requiring extraordinary control measures.

CDC light traps were located at six sites:

- Alkers Woods in Kings Point
- Babylon Turnpike, Merrick
- Cold Spring Harbor
- High Hill at Jones Beach
- Massapequa Preserve
- Muttontown Preserve

(Continued)

Exhibit 6-3. Continued

Exhibits II and III show the number of adult mosquitoes trapped in 1998 by the six CDC light traps used to monitor adult mosquito population. A total of 4,483 mosquitoes were captured. Twelve "pools" or batches of captured specimens were submitted to the New York State Wadsworth Laboratory for EEE testing. No arboviruses were found in the twelve pools of mosquitoes submitted for testing.

Exhibit II. Number of Mosquitos by Type Captured in CDC Light Traps in 1998

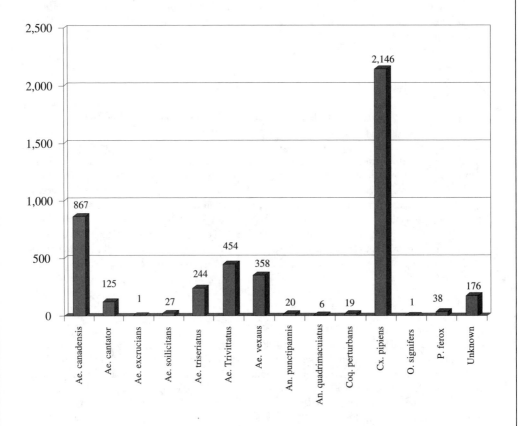

Exhibit II represents the total number of mosquitoes, by genus and species, captured between May 28 and September 16, 1998. Exhibit III shows the total number of mosquitoes captured each week from May 28 to September 16, 1998.

New Jersey Light Traps

New Jersey light traps attract mosquitoes solely by light, and are suitable for monitoring the large numbers of salt marsh mosquitoes found on the south shore of Nassau County. One limitation is the need to have an electrical outlet, since they are not battery operated like the CDC traps. The New Jersey light traps were located at the following south shore sites:

(Continued)

Exhibit 6-3. Continued

Exhibit III. Number of Mosquitos Captured by Week in CDC Light Traps in 1998

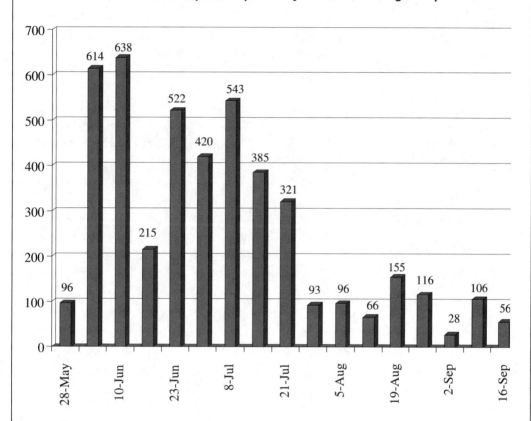

- The West End Area at Jones Beach
- The High Hill Area of Jones Beach
- The Jones Beach Sewage Treatment Plant
- The Bay Park Sewage Treatment Plant
- The Cedar Creek Sewage Treatment Plant
- The Town of Hempstead Sanitation Garage in Merrick

The New Jersey light traps operated May 20th to September 24th, 1998, generally showed light adult presence (< 50 mosquitoes per trap per night) through July 23rd, no mosquitoes from July 24th until July 30th, then moderate adult presence(> 50 and < 100 mosquitoes per trap per night) until September 24th. The highest counts were found at the three Jones Beach trap sites.

Season Duration

Mosquitoes are active from March until freezing weather. In 1997 mosquito larvae were found as late as the end of December. Mosquitoes sometimes overwinter as adults in people's homes, in street drains, and in other warm moist places, emerging on mild days. Exhibit IV indicates the mosquito species found in 1998 by dipping, those trapped in CDC light traps, and the time intervals during

(Continued)

Exhibit 6-3. Continued

Exhibit IV. Dipping and CDC Trapping Results by Type

Mosquito Species	First Larvae Dipped	Last Larvae Dipped	First Adult Trapped	Last Adult Trapped
Aedes abserratus	4/6/98	6/5/98	None	None
Aedes canadensis	None	None	5/28/98	8/12/98
Aedes cantator	3/31/98	5/7/98	6/3/98	9/16/98
Aedes excrucians	None	None	7/8/98	7/8/98
Aedes sollicitans	4/6/98	9/14/98	5/28/98	9/16/98
Aedes trisertatus	None	None	6/3/98	9/16/98
Aedes trivitatus	8/20/98	9/14/98	6/3/98	8/19/98
Aedes vexans	5/4/98	8/31/98	5/28/98	9/16/98
Anopheles punctipennis	7/14/98	9/3/98	8/17/98	9/10/98
Anopheles quadrimsculatus	None	None	7/15/98	9/10/98
Coquitlettidia perturbans	None	None	6/10/98	7/15/98
Culex pipiens/restuans	5/18/98	9/22/98	5/28/98	9/18/98
Culex salinartus	7/6/98	7/6/98	None	None
Culex territans	6/2/98	9/4/98	None	None
Orthopodomyia signifara	None	None	8/19/98	8/19/98
Psorophora ferox	None	None	7/8/98	9/2/98
Unidentified	3/24/98	12/1/98	5/28/98	9/16/98
Midgo	5/21/98	7/14/98	None	None

which they were present. It should be noted that CDC traps only operated from 5/28 to 9/16, so adult mosquitoes may have been present before and after these dates.

Complaints/Service Requests

All complaints, whether received by telephone, letter, or referral within the county system, were entered in a log, then assigned for inspection. Inspection generally involved a visit to the complainant's home, inspection of a specific situation, or more often a neighborhood survey; including but limited to streams, ponds, marshes, drainage ditches, standing water, swimming pools, artificial containers, street drains, and nearby storm recharge basins. Property owners were apprised of conditions when present, otherwise visit notices and mosquito information pamphlets were left. If appropriate, treatment was made by hand with a suitable larvicide. If a major breeding pool was identified, follow-up inspections were made in one to two weeks. Inspection results were entered in the complaint log after review by the supervisor and prior to filing.

Boat Surveys

There are more than 100 bodies of land in the south shore bays called various names (hassocks, meadows, marshes, field, island, etc.) on the maps. Most of these are hassocks and are underwater at high

(Continued)

Exhibit 6-3. Continued

tide and pose little or no mosquito problem. The few islets that do remain wholly or partially above a typical high tide and thus are capable of supporting breeding pools of *Aedes sollicitans* and other salt marsh mosquitoes were checked periodically by boat.

Upland Surveys

In addition to the salt marsh surveys, numerous surveys of streams, drains, ponds, and freshwater marshes were made to determine mosquito breeding potential, and especially to determine suitability of these sites as breeding areas for *Culiseta melanura*, a mosquito involved in the bird to bird transmission of EEE. The presence of this mosquito favors avian amplification of the EEE virus increasing the possibility of human or equine infection.

Storm Water Recharge Basin Survey

Storm water recharge basins (SWBs) are designed to return surface runoff water to the ground water table and generally perform this function well. Sometimes they retain sufficient water to become major source of mosquitoes. In 1997, mosquito larvae were found in 48 of the 332 SWBs inspected. In 1998, mosquito larvae were found in 48 of the 215 SWBs inspected.

Treatment

As stated previously, Nassau County is committed to applying the principles of IPM to all its pest control activities. What this means in practical terms is that the cornerstone of our control strategy is surveillance, so we can base control strategies on reliable information and monitor the effectiveness of that strategy. In some situations no treatment is necessary (i.e., there are mosquito eating fish present, or the puddle will dry up before larval development can be completed). In other situations, there are treatment restrictions to be observed so as to avoid harm to non-target organisms, especially in environmentally sensitive areas such as freshwater wetlands. Several of our treatment options have restrictions on the label or on our NYSDEC permits, when fish are present. NYSDEC has issued permits for each aspect of our mosquito control efforts specifying in detail what may be done, when it may be done, and by whom it may be done. All control measures must fully comply with these permits. Furthermore, all pesticides must be used in accordance with the product labels and all applicable pesticide laws.

When treatment is necessary, there are a number of options available such as:

(1) Introduction of fish

Many saltwater fishes eat mosquito larvae. Killifish are present in large numbers in the bays and in the south shore ditches. NCDPW trapped large numbers and moved them to salt water pools on the West End of Jones Beach, an area where other treatment was not possible due to the presence of a Piping Plover nesting area (access limited).

Several varieties of small top feeding fresh water fish, including Gambusia, were introduced to some storm water recharge basins (SWBs) that held water year-round.

(Continued)

Exhibit 6-3. Continued

(2) Elimination of standing water

Mosquito larvae are often found in clogged roof gutters, old tires, boat covers, swimming pools covers, and other artificial containers; although swimming pools themselves when properly maintained or periodically chlorinated, are not a problem. During complaint inspections property owners were advised of conditions conducive to larvae development of mosquitoes. The mosquito control pamphlet given out during complaint inspections emphasizes the need for eliminating these localized breeding situations.

(3) Backpack and hand treatment with a suitable larvicide

Three larvicides were used:

1. BTI (*Bacillus thuringiensis* var. israeliensis) is a naturally occurring soil bacteria that is eaten by the larvae, infecting them, and killing them. It is available in granular form or in a donut shaped briquette. It is very target specific but will not work against the pupae stage as pupae do not eat.
2. Vectolex CG (*Bacillus sphaericus*) is also naturally occurring bacteria that infect mosquito larvae. It persists well in the organic rich environments favored by the *Culex* species of mosquitoes. It also is ineffective against pupae.
3. Altosid (Methoprene) is an insect growth regulator that prevents mosquito larvae from changing into adults (it is sometimes called a juvenile hormone). It is used in a briquette form for hand treating SWBs and other sites requiring long acting control (30 days).

(4) Aerial spraying

Nassau County DPW has a contract with a private company for aerial spraying by helicopter. The helicopter is able to spray large inaccessible areas with a suitable larvicide, usually a liquid formulation of Altosid. Areas sprayed include the marshy areas of Jones Beach, Lido Beach, and a number of islets and hassocks on the south shore of Nassau County. Decisions as to when and where to treat are based upon the salt marsh survey, tidal conditions, and boat surveys. The helicopter has been a very effective control measure and will continue to be used in the future. The helicopter was used 15 times in 1998 and 15 times in 1997.

(5) Adulticiding

Adult mosquitoes are sensitive to a number of contact pesticides (Exhibit V). The adulticide of choice for mosquitoes is a product named Scourage (resmethrin 4.14% and piperonyl butoxide 2.42%), which may be sprayed by an ultra low volume generator mounted on the back of a pickup truck. Driven at a constant 5 mph rate, this method can treat large areas on either side of a roadway. Spraying must be done at time of no wind, usually early morning, to minimize drift. Adulticiding is only done when unacceptably high numbers of adult are present and other means of control are ineffective.

(Continued)

Exhibit 6-3. Continued

Exhibit V. 1998 Pesticide Usage by Nassau County Mosquito Control Program

Product Ingredient*	Target*	Quantity*	Method of Application*	Active Ingredient	Pounds of Active
Altosid liquid	Mosquitoes	14,400 ou	Helicopter	Methoprene	193.5
Altosid briquets	Mosquitoes	6,515 briq	Hand	Methoprene	6.1
Vecto Bac CG	Mosquitoes	5,440 lbs	Helicopter	BTI	10.9
Bactimos briquets	Mosquitoes	1,709 briq	Hand	BTI	4.9
Vecto Lex CG	Mosquitoes	623 lbs	Backpack blower	BS	46.7
Scourge	Mosquitoes	1,856 ou	Truck sprayer	Resmethrin	4.4
				Piperonyl butoxide	13.1
Trimec	Mosquitoes	40 gals	Spray tank	2,4-D	81.2
				Mecoprop-	43.2
				Dicamba	8.4

* Data provided by Nassau County Department of Public Works.

The Effect of Weather

Storms from April through October are a major factor leading to mosquito breeding as well as higher than normal tides. When monthly rainfall for 1996, 1997, and 1998 is compared with the 50-year monthly average, 1997 was indeed dryer than 1996, one of the wettest years in last 50 years. However, there were 43.48 inches of rain in 1997 vs. a 50-year average rainfall of 44.27 inches. The total rainfall for 1998 was 42.62 inches.

Training

NYSDEC requires that anyone applying pesticides be certified and receive continuing education in safe pesticide storage, handling, and treatment practices. In 1998, two Health Department Sanitarians completed a DEC approved thirty-hour course given by NCDPW, passed the Pesticide Applicator Certification Test and were certified in category VIII (Public Health). The course was formatted and given by Gregory Terrillion of DWP. Certification of two additional people permitted greater program flexibility and quicker response to problems found during the various complaint inspections and surveys. Both inspectors have attended three training sessions for which each received 11 CEUs, required to maintain their certification, as well as valuable information about mosquitoes and the new reporting requirements for the Pesticide Registry. NCDPW has 5 certified applicators for a total of 7 certified applicators in the program.

(Continued)

Exhibit 6-3. Continued

Conclusion

In 1998, the mosquito control efforts of NCDPW and NCDH continued to build on the successes of 1997. The ability to do regular surveys of salt marsh areas and treat by helicopter when necessary provides significant reduction of salt marsh mosquito populations. As the salt marsh ditches are rejuvenated, there should be further declines in mosquito populations in many areas of Jones Beach. In addition both departments will continue to survey and monitor upland areas to locate and prevent fresh water mosquito breeding. There were fewer mosquito complaints in 1998 than in 1997 despite a wet spring, as a result in part to the enhanced ability to hand-treat localized situations and to do effective follow-up.

NCDH and NCDPW will continue to work cooperatively to conduct an effective and environmentally safe mosquito control program with the cooperation and support of the various Nassau County departments, the office of the County Executive, the Nassau County Legislature, New York State, the towns, and the public. A mosquito control pamphlet further describes our program, and provides a phone number to which comments, complaints, or questions may be directed.

---

eases in recent records (1995–97) that had more than 10 cases per 100,000. Considerations of the impact of a new encephalitis were overshadowed by the impact of these more mundane (common) diseases. The New York State Department of Health strongly encouraged cost-benefit analysis before implementing any plans because of this discrepancy.

It appeared that mosquito eradication would be the most appropriate means of dealing with the situation. This, however, resulted in several additional epidemiologic questions that Dr. Stein listed:

1. Would the eradication programs sufficiently eliminate the target mosquito, particularly the *Culex* species?
2. Were the numbers (four cases) sufficient to make significant changes to the current mosquito control program, "Nassau County Mosquito Surveillance and Control Status Report—December 1998"?
3. What could be learned from the situation in New York City, where approximately twenty-three confirmed cases (plus twenty probable cases) and five deaths had occurred?

4. What were the seasonal implications related to the recurrence of this event if short-term control was obtained this season? What were the long-term control options?

Office of Environmental Health

"The media's sensationalism could make this thing a nightmare for us all," Terry Jones, head of the Nassau County Department of Health's (NCDH) Office of Environmental Health, told Dr. Guest as he handed her his memo. He continued, "There's even talk that it's an act of bioterrorism or a covert test by the government to assess the efficiency of the nation's health agencies and laboratories to handle a 'mysterious outbreak.'"

In his memo, Jones reported that three weeks previously, the county initiated active surveillance to monitor for mosquitoes capable of transmitting the virus as well as for dead birds that were thought to be carriers of the virus. Shortly after that, County Executive Lou Timpanini, on advice from the NCDH and the NCDPW, authorized ground spraying of a larvicide by the name of resmethrin. Nassau County had four cases, while neighboring Westchester had eight cases, and New York had reported twenty-five cases of the West Nile virus. Reports of dead crows, however, kept popping up, and numerous phone calls came from the local press and concerned citizens asking "Just what is the department doing about this?" News articles indicated that people were keeping their children indoors and described the virus as the "exotic terror."

Trapping efforts so far indicated low counts of mosquitoes throughout the county, despite surveillance reports of a concomitant increase in sentinel bird deaths, especially crows. Weather conditions for late fall and winter were not expected to differ greatly from the averages for the area. Outbreaks of West Nile virus were known to occur primarily during the late summer and early fall. It was possible that the onset of cooler temperatures and the eventual frost could reduce the mosquito populations naturally. There was a chance, however, that some mosquitoes could hibernate through part of the winter and re-emerge if the county experienced abnormally warm temperatures at any time during the season. A further concern was that eggs laid in the late fall would survive the frost and hatch in the spring. Because the virus could be transmitted vertically in mosquitoes, eggs laid late in the fall could be potential carriers of the virus, making a re-emergence of cases feasible come springtime.

Vector/Analysis

Although *Culex pipiens* was the primary vector responsible for transmitting the virus, *Aedes vexans* had also been implicated as a vector. Substantial numbers of both *Culex pipiens* and *Aedes vexans* had been recovered through surveillance efforts in previous years, but *Culex pipiens* was considered to be Nassau County's "problem mosquito." *Culex pipiens* thrived in urban environments, and it preferred polluted and organically contaminated water in which to breed. It was a persistent biter, attacking mainly after dark, usually during the dusk and dawn hours. Adults did

not migrate very far and usually stayed in close proximity to breeding sites. *Culex pipiens* had been known to exhibit aggressive biting behavior in response to spray efforts. *Aedes vexans* could also persist during September and October, when temperatures were still warm. The survival of *Aedes vexans* was partially dependent on its proper selection of a breeding site. Females usually laid their eggs in moist soil areas that were prone to flooding and that were densely covered by twigs and damp leaves. *Aedes vexans* was not at all localized to breeding sites but could travel substantial distances, even up to eight miles according to one source.

Integrated Pest Management

Because West Nile virus was transmitted by mosquitoes, the main concern held by Terry Jones and the Office of Environmental Health was controlling the vector with minimal risk to the environment, wildlife, and human populations. The NCDH and the NCDPW practiced integrated pest management (IPM), whereby a variety of strategies was used to control pest populations without resorting to the use of chemical pesticides. Initial defense tactics included increased surveillance by trapping and dipping as part of the IPM program and the identification and elimination of potential mosquito breeding sites.

Communities had been advised to drain areas of standing water that served as ideal habitats for the mosquito larvae and pupae stages. This included draining old containers, birdbaths, old tires, roof gutters, and any nearby ditches. The IPM program had been expanded to include weekend inspections of potential outbreak areas and breeding sites. Spot treatment with the larvicide resmethrin in areas with excessive numbers of virus-carrying mosquitoes had occurred every day of the week since September 10, and community residents had been informed of these activities primarily through newspapers and public service announcements broadcast via radio and television.

Aerial spraying was something Jones did not want to contemplate. He stated that "expanding and intensifying control efforts to include ground spraying using trucks has been enough of a headache." Ground spraying involved the deployment of trucks into communities. As a truck was driven down the middle of the street, the pesticide Scrounge (active ingredients: resmethrin and piperonyl butoxide) was dispersed continuously from the back of the truck at a height of about 15 feet in all directions. The spray range was about 150 feet. Only those communities with elevated numbers of dead birds were targeted for ground spraying, yet the department, in conjunction with the NCDPW, had faced challenges simply in trying to accomplish the ground spraying initiatives. For one, the weather had proven to be less than cooperative on the days that spraying had been scheduled, causing numerous delays. Temperatures had to be above 50° F, and wind velocity could not be greater than 10 mph. Other requirements for spraying included no rain and, of course, evidence of mosquito activity. In addition, the department received complaints from several environmental organizations and even the threat of a lawsuit by a coalition of environmental groups that advocated for increased surveillance and the use of more benign control measures such as the use of *Bacillus thuringiensis* var. *israelensis* (BTI), a biological pesticide.

For the most part, these advocacy groups were suggesting many of the same preventive measures that the department had already instituted as a part of its mosquito surveillance and control program two years earlier. In fact, many of these measures were being expanded to deal with the present situation. One particular not-for-profit agency, Environmental Advocates, had been urging the addition of biological pesticides such as BTI to stagnant water as a means to control larval and pupal populations and *Bacillus sphaericus* (BS) to storm sewers, as well as filling lakes and streams with mosquito-eating fish. The office had considered some of these options, but as with any pesticide, biological or chemical, there were a variety of factors to consider. Vectolex was usually recommended for control of *Culex* mosquito larvae, but it had limited effects on other mosquito genera.

The use of BTI and BS could leave residual products that could have effects on non-target populations. The hazards of Scrounge used for ground spraying and Anvil (active ingredients: sumithrin and piperonyl butoxide) considered for aerial spraying were minimal to none compared to the choices that other counties had made. New York and Suffolk County had decided to conduct aerial spraying using malathion, which had been implicated as the cause of pesticide-related illnesses in California and Florida. Anvil was not nontoxic, but it was less toxic than malathion (Exhibit 6-4).

Both resmethrin and sumithrin were pyrethroids, which were considered to be the safest class of chemical insecticides available (Exhibits 6-5 and 6-6). Pyrethroids were synthetic analogues of pyrethrins, a naturally occurring group of compounds found in chrysanthemum flowers. Pyrethroids alone exhibited low toxicity in humans and other mammals, largely because they were rapidly detoxified via the metabolic processes. Toxicity varied depending on the route of exposure, however. Oral and dermal absorption usually produced moderate to unmeasurably low toxicity. Pyrethroid insecticides were rarely used alone. Most often they were combined with synergistic agents that increased their potency and extended the length of their effects. Piperonyl butoxide was the most common synergist used in conjunction with pyrethroids, and it was known to inhibit mammalian enzyme systems responsible for metabolism and detoxification.

The ability of the body to metabolize pyrethroids was the primary determinant of toxicity. When the normal metabolic mechanisms of detoxification were inhibited by synergists such as piperonyl butoxide, the potency of pyrethroids increased. In addition, organophosphate pesticides had an inhibitory effect on detoxification enzymes, and their use in conjunction with pyrethroids was known to increase the potency of the insecticides.

Terry Jones's memo speculated about the thousands of interactions possible among these chemicals. With so many counties electing to spray and

(text continues on page 263)

Exhibit 6-4. Pesticide Information Profile for Malathion

EXTOXNET
Extension Toxicology Network
Pesticide Information Profiles

A Pesticide Information Project of Cooperative Extension Offices of Cornell University, Oregon State University, the University of Idaho, and the University of California at Davis and the Institute for Environmental Toxicology, Michigan State University. Major support and funding was provided by the USDA/Extension Service/National Agricultural Pesticide Impact Assessment Program.
EXTOXNET primary files maintained and archived at Oregon State University
Revised June 1996

Malathion

Trade and Other Names: Malathion is also known as carbophos, maldison and mercaptothion. Trade names for products containing malathion include Celthion, Cython, Dielathion, El 4049, Emmaton, Exathios, Fyfanon and Hilthion, Karbofos and Maltox.
Regulatory Status: Malathion is a slightly toxic compound in EPA toxicity class III. Labels for products containing it must carry the Signal Word CAUTION. Malathion is a General Use Pesticide (GUP). It is available in emulsifiable concentrate, wettable powder, dustable powder, and ultra low volume liquid formulations.
Chemical Class: organophosphate
Introduction: Malathion is a nonsystemic, wide-spectrum organophosphate insecticide. It was one of the earliest organophosphate insecticides developed (introduced in 1950). Malathion is suited for the control of sucking and chewing insects on fruits and vegetables, and is also used to control mosquitoes, flies, household insects, animal parasites (ectoparasites), and head and body lice. Malathion may also be found in formulations with many other pesticides.
Formulation: It is available in emulsifiable concentrate, wettable powder, dustable powder, and ULV liquid formulations. Malathion may also be found in formulations with many other pesticides.
Toxicological Effects:
- Acute toxicity: Malathion is slightly toxic via the oral route, with reported oral LD50 values of 1000 mg/kg to greater than 10,000 mg/kg in the rat, and 400 mg/kg to greater than 4000 mg/kg in the mouse [2,13]. It is also slightly toxic via the dermal route, with reported dermal LD50 values of greater than 4000 mg/kg in rats [2,13]. Effects of malathion are similar to those observed with other organophosphates, except that larger doses are required to produce them [2,8]. It has been reported that single doses of malathion may affect immune system response [2]. Symptoms of acute exposure to organophosphate or cholinesterase-inhibiting compounds may include the following: numbness, tingling sensations, incoordination, headache, dizziness, tremor, nausea, abdominal cramps, sweating, blurred vision, difficulty breathing or respiratory depression, and slow heartbeat. Very high doses may result in unconsciousness, incontinence, and convulsions or fatality. The acute effects of malathion depend on product purity and the route of exposure [33]. Other factors which may influence the observed toxicity of malathion include the amount of protein in the diet and gender. As protein intake decreased, malathion was increasingly toxic to the rats [78]. Malathion has been shown to have different toxicities in male and female rats and humans due to metabolism, storage, and excretion differences between the sexes, with females being much more susceptible than males [79]. Numerous malathion poisoning incidents have occurred among pesticide workers and small children through accidental exposure. In one reported case of malathion poisoning, an infant exhibited severe signs of cholinesterase inhibition after exposure to an aerosol bomb containing 0.5% malathion [44].

(Continued)

Exhibit 6-4. Continued

- **Chronic toxicity:** Human volunteers fed very low doses of malathion for $1\frac{1}{2}$ months showed no significant effects on blood cholinesterase activity. Rats fed dietary doses of 5 mg/kg/day to 25 mg/kg/day over 2 years showed no symptoms apart from depressed cholinesterase activity. When small amounts of the compound were administered for 8 weeks, rats showed no adverse effects on whole-blood cholinesterase activity [2]. Weanling male rats were twice as susceptible to malathion as adults.
- **Reproductive effects:** Several studies have documented developmental and reproductive effects due to high doses of malathion in test animals [2]. Rats fed high doses of 240 mg/kg/day during pregnancy showed an increased rate of newborn mortality. However, malathion fed to rats at low dosages caused no reproductive effects [8]. It is not likely that malathion will cause reproductive effects in humans under normal circumstances.
- **Teratogenic effects:** Rats fed high doses (240 mg/kg/day) showed no teratogenic effects. Malathion and its metabolites can cross the placenta of the goat and depress cholinesterase activity of the fetus [8]. Chickens fed diets at low doses for 2 years showed no adverse effects on egg hatching [8]. Current evidence indicates that malathion is not teratogenic.
- **Mutagenic effects:** Malathion produced detectable mutations in three different types of cultured human cells, including white blood cells and lymph cells [2,8]. It is not clear what the implications of these results are for humans.
- **Carcinogenic effects:** Female rats on dietary doses of approximately 500 mg/kg/day of malathion for 2 years did not develop tumors [2]. Adrenal tumors developed in the males at low doses, but not at the high doses [80], suggesting that malathion was not the cause. Three of five studies that have investigated the carcinogenicity of malathion have found that the compound does not produce tumors in the test animals. The two other studies have been determined to be unacceptable studies and the results discounted [2,8,80]. Available evidence suggests that malathion is not carcinogenic but the data are not conclusive.
- **Organ toxicity:** The pesticide has been shown in animal testing and from use experience to affect the central nervous system, immune system, adrenal glands, liver, and blood.
- **Fate in humans and animals:** Malathion is rapidly and effectively absorbed by practically all routes including the gastrointestinal tract, skin, mucous membranes, and lungs. Malathion undergoes similar detoxification mechanisms to other organophosphates, but it can also be rendered nontoxic via another simple mechanism, splitting of either of the carboxy ester linkages. Animal studies indicate it is very rapidly eliminated though urine, feces and expired air with a reported half-life of approximately 8 hours in rats and approximately 2 days in cows [2]. Autopsy samples from one individual who had ingested large amounts of malathion showed a substantial portion in the stomach and intestines, a small amount in fat tissue, and no detectable levels in the liver. Malathion requires conversion to malaoxon to become an active anticholinesterase agent. Most of the occupational evidence indicates a low chronic toxicity for malathion. One important exception to this was traced to impurities in the formulation of the pesticide [2].

Ecological Effects:
- **Effects on birds:** Malathion is moderately toxic to birds. The reported acute oral LD50 values are: in mallards, 1485 mg/kg; in pheasants, 167 mg/kg; in blackbirds and starlings, over 100 mg/kg; and in chickens, 525 mg/kg [2,6]. The reported 5- to 8-day dietary LC50 is over 3000 ppm in Japanese quail, mallard, and northern bobwhite, and is 2639 ppm in ring-neck pheasants [6]. Furthermore, 90% of the dose to birds was metabolized and excreted in 24 hours via urine [79].
- **Effects on aquatic organisms:** Malathion has a wide range of toxicities in fish, extending from very highly toxic in the walleye (96-hour LC50 of 0.06 mg/L) to highly toxic in brown trout (0.1 mg/L) and the cutthroat trout (0.28 mg/L), moderately toxic in fathead minnows (8.6 mg/L) and slightly toxic in goldfish (10.7 mg/L) [13,8,16]. Various aquatic invertebrates are extremely sensitive, with EC50 values from 1 ug/L to 1 mg/L [28]. Malathion is highly toxic to aquatic invertebrates and to the aquatic stages of amphibians. Because of its very short half-life, malathion is not expected to bioconcentrate in aquatic organisms. However, brown shrimp

(Continued)

Exhibit 6-4. Continued

showed an average concentration of 869 and 959 times the ambient water concentration in two separate samples [12].
- **Effects on other organisms:** The compound is highly toxic to honeybees [13].

Environmental Fate:
- **Breakdown in soil and groundwater:** Malathion is of low persistence in soil with reported field half-lives of 1 to 25 days [19]. Degradation in soil is rapid and related to the degree of soil binding [12]. Breakdown occurs by a combination of biological degradation and nonbiological reaction with water [12]. If released to the atmosphere, malathion will break down rapidly in sunlight, with a reported half-life in air of about 1.5 days [12]. It is moderately bound to soils, and is soluble in water, so it may pose a risk of groundwater or surface water contamination in situations which may be less conducive to breakdown. The compound was detected in 12 of 3252 different groundwater sources in two different states, and in small concentrations in several wells in California, with a highest concentration of 6.17 ug/L [33].
- **Breakdown in water:** In raw river water, the half-life is less than 1 week, whereas malathion remained stable in distilled water for 3 weeks [12]. Applied at 1 to 6 lb/acre in log ponds for mosquito control, it was effective for 2.5 to 6 weeks [12]. In sterile seawater, the degradation increases with increased salinity. The breakdown products in water are mono- and dicarboxylic acids [12].
- **Breakdown in vegetation:** Residues were found mainly associated with areas of high lipid content in the plant. Increased moisture content increased degradation [33].

Physical Properties:
- **Appearance:** Technical malathion is a clear, amber liquid at room temperature [13].
- **Chemical Name:** diethyl (dimethoxy thiophosphorylthio) succinate [13]
- **CAS Number:** 121-75-5
- **Molecular Weight:** 330.36
- **Water Solubility:** 130 mg/L [13]
- **Solubility in Other Solvents:** v.s. in most organic solvents [13]
- **Melting Point:** 2.85 C [13]
- **Vapor Pressure:** 5.3 mPa @ 30 C [13]
- **Partition Coefficient:** 2.7482 [13]
- **Adsorption Coefficient:** 1800 [19]

Exposure Guidelines:
- **ADI:** 0.02 mg/kg/day [38]
- **MCL:** Not Available
- **RfD:** 0.02 mg/kg/day [53]
- **PEL:** 15 mg/m3 (8-hour) (dust) [39]
- **HA:** 0.2 mg/L (lifetime) [53]
- **TLV:** Not Available

Basic Manufacturer:
Drexel Chemical Company
1700 Channel Avenue
Memphis, TN 38113
- **Phone:** 901-774-4370
- **Emergency:** Not Available

References:
References for the information in this PIP can be found in Reference List <u>Number 5</u>

DISCLAIMER: The information in this profile does not in any way replace or supersede the information on the pesticide product labeling or other regulatory requirements. Please refer to the pesticide product labeling.

Exhibit 6-5. Pesticide Information Profile for Resmethrin

EXTOXNET
Extension Toxicology Network
Pesticide Information Profiles

A Pesticide Information Project of Cooperative Extension Offices of Cornell University, Oregon State University, the University of Idaho, and the University of California at Davis and the Institute for Environmental Toxicology, Michigan State University. Major support and funding was provided by the USDA/Extension Service/National Agricultural Pesticide Impact Assessment Program.
EXTOXNET primary files maintained and archived at Oregon State University
Revised June 1996

Resmethrin

Trade and Other Names: Trade names include Chryson, Crossfire, Derringer, FMC 17370, Isathrine, NRDC 104, Pynosect, Raid Flying Insect Killer, Respond, Scourge, Sun-Bugger #4, SPB-1382, Synthrin, Syntox, Vectrin, and Whitmire PT-110.

Regulatory Status: Resmethrin is a slightly toxic to practically non-toxic compound in EPA toxicity class III. Products containing resmethrin must bear the Signal Word CAUTION on the label. All products containing resmethrin for pest control at or near aquatic sites are classified as Restricted Use Pesticides (RUP) by the EPA because of potential fish toxicity. RUPs may be purchased and used only by certified applicators.

Chemical Class: pyrethroid

Introduction: Resmethrin is a synthetic pyrethroid used for control of flying and crawling insects in homes, greenhouses, indoor landscapes, mushroom houses, industrial sites, stored product insects and for mosquito control. It is also used for fabric protection, pet sprays and shampoos, and it is applied to horses or in horse stables. Technical resmethrin is a mixture of its two main isomers (molecules with the same chemical formula but slightly different configurations); a typical blend is 20 to 30% of the (1RS)-cis-isomer and 70 to 80% of the (1RS)-trans-isomer.

Formulation: Technical resmethrin is a mixture of its two main isomers (molecules with the same chemical formula but slightly different configurations); a typical blend is 20 to 30% of the (1RS)-cis-isomer and 70 to 80% of the (1RS)-trans-isomer.

Toxicological Effects:
- **Acute toxicity:** Resmethrin is slightly to practically non-toxic by ingestion. The oral LD50 for technical resmethrin in rats is variously reported as greater than 2500 mg/kg or 1244 mg/kg [3,12]. Resmethrin is only slightly toxic through the dermal route as well. The reported dermal LD50s for technical resmethrin are: greater than 3000 mg/kg in rats, greater than 2500 mg/kg in rabbits, and greater than 5000 mg/kg in mice [3,12]. It is slightly toxic via inhalation, with a 4-hour inhalation LC50 for resmethrin of greater than 9.49 mg/L [3]. Symptoms of exposure by any route may include incoordination, twitching, loss of bladder control, and seizures [12]. Dermal exposure may lead to local numbness, itching, burning, and tingling sensations near the site of exposure. Resmethrin is reported to be nonirritating to the skin and eyes of test animals and not to cause skin sensitization in guinea pigs [3].
- **Chronic toxicity:** In a chronic feeding study with rats, 25 mg/kg/day (the lowest dose tested) caused liver enlargement. At 125 mg/kg/day, there were pathological liver changes in addition to increased liver weights. Doses of 250 mg/kg/day caused increased thyroid weight and thyroid cysts [3]. In another study over 90 days, doses of 150 mg/kg/day did not produce any adverse effects in exposed rats [12]. Increased liver weights occurred in dogs fed 30 mg/kg/day for 180

(Continued)

Exhibit 6-5. Continued

days. No effects were observed in dogs in this study at dose rates of 10 mg/kg/day [3]. In a 90-day inhalation study with rats, 0.1 mg/L, the lowest dose tested, produced behavioral changes, decreased blood glucose levels in males, and decreased body weights and increased serum urea levels in females [3]. Resmethrin was not neurotoxic to rats at doses of 62.5 mg/kg/day for 32 weeks, 250 mg/kg/day for 30 days, or 632 mg/kg/day for 7 days [4]. It is unlikely that chronic effects will be seen in humans under normal circumstances.

- **Reproductive effects:** A three-generation study with rats showed a slight increase in premature stillbirths and a decrease in pup weight at 25 mg/kg, the lowest dose tested [4]. Since these doses are much higher than expected human exposures, it is unlikely such effects will occur in humans.
- **Teratogenic effects:** No birth defects were observed in the offspring of rabbits given doses as high as 100 mg/kg/day [4]. Skeletal aberrations were seen in the offspring of rats given doses higher than 40 mg/kg/day [3]. No teratogenic effects were observed in mice at dose levels of 50 mg/kg/day over an unspecified period [12]. It is unlikely that teratogenic effects will be seen in humans under normal circumstances.
- **Mutagenic effects:** Resmethrin was not mutagenic in a test performed with the bacterium, Salmonella typhimurium [6].
- **Carcinogenic effects:** No evidence of tumor formation was observed in a 2-year rat feeding study with doses as high as 250 mg/kg/day, nor in an 85-week study with mice given doses as high as 50 mg/kg/day [3,4].
- **Organ toxicity:** Pyrethroids may cause adverse effects on the central nervous system. Long-term feeding studies have shown increased liver and kidney weights and adverse changes in liver tissues in test animals [12].
- **Fate in humans and animals:** Resmethrin is quickly eliminated by chickens. When oral doses of 10 mg/kg resmethrin were given to laying hens, 90% of the dose was eliminated in urine and feces within 24 hours [46]. In another study with hens given the same treatment, residues were low in hens sacrificed 12 hours after the treatment, with the highest levels found in the liver and kidneys. Low levels were found in the hens' eggs, with levels peaking 1 day after treatment in the whites and 4 to 5 days after treatment in the yolks [47].

Ecological Effects:

- **Effects on birds:** Resmethrin is practically nontoxic to birds. Its LD50 in California quail is greater than 2000 mg/kg [3]. In Japanese quail, the five-day dietary LC50 is greater than 5000 ppm [48].
- **Effects on aquatic organisms:** Resmethrin is very highly toxic to fish with 96-hour LC50 values generally at or below 1 ug/L (0.001 mg/L) for most species tested. The LC50 for resmethrin in mosquito fish is 7 ug/L [49]. The LC50 for resmethrin synergized with piperonyl butoxide in red swamp crawfish, *Procambarus clarkii*, is 0.00082 ug/L [48]. The LC50 in bluegill sunfish is 0.75 to 2.6 ug/L, and 0.28 to 2.4 ug/L in rainbow trout [3]. Other reported 96-hour LC50s are 1.8 ug/L in coho salmon, 1.7 ug/L in lake trout, 3.0 ug/L in fathead minnow, 16.6 ug/L in channel catfish and 1.7 ug/L in bluegill sunfish [50]. Fish sensitivity to the pyrethroids may be explained by their relatively slow metabolism and elimination of these compounds. The half-lives for elimination of several pyrethroids by trout are all greater than 48 hours, while elimination half-lives for birds and mammals range from 6 to 12 hours [20].
- **Effects on other organisms:** Resmethrin is highly toxic to bees, with an LD50 of 0.063 ug per bee [3].

Environmental Fate:

- **Breakdown in soil and groundwater:** Resmethrin is of low to moderate persistence in the soil environment. Its half-life has been estimated at 30 days [51]. Observed half-lives will depend on many site-specific variables. In aerobic Kentucky loamy sand, the compound showed a half-life of nearly 200 days. Degradation end-products reported for resmethrin are chrysanthemic acid,

(Continued)

Exhibit 6-5. Continued

benzaldehyde, benzyl alcohol, benzoic acid, phenylacetic acid, and various esters [52]. Resmethrin is tightly bound to soil and would not be expected to be mobile or to contaminate groundwater, especially in light of its extremely low solubility in water [51].

- **Breakdown in water:** Resmethrin may enter surface waters through particulate run-off or misapplication. In pond waters and in laboratory degradation studies, pyrethroid concentrations decrease rapidly due to sorption to sediment, suspended particles and plants. Microbial and photodegradation also occur [22]. The half-life in water is 36.5 days.
- **Breakdown in vegetation:** No information was found.

<u>Physical Properties:</u>
- **Appearance:** Resmethrin is a waxy, off-white to tan solid with an odor characteristic of chrysanthemums [12].
- **Chemical Name:** 5-benzyl-3-furylmethyl (1RS)-cis,trans-2,2-dimethyl-3-(2-methylprop-1-enyl)cyclopropanecarboxylate [12]
- **CAS Number:** 10453-86-8
- **Molecular Weight:** 338.45
- **Water Solubility:** mg/L at 30 C [12], insoluble in water
- **Solubility in Other Solvents:** s. in hexane, kerosene, xylene, methylene chloride, isopropyl alcohol, and aromatic petroleum hydrocarbons; m.s. in methanol [12]
- **Melting Point:** 43-48 C [12]
- **Vapor Pressure:** 0.0015 mPa @ 30 C [12]
- **Partition Coefficient:** Not Available
- **Adsorption Coefficient:** 100,000 [51]

<u>Exposure Guidelines:</u>
- **ADI:** Not Available
- **MCL:** Not Available
- **RfD:** 0.03 mg/kg/day [30]
- **PEL:** Not Available
- **HA:** Not Available
- **TLV:** Not Available

<u>Basic Manufacturer:</u>
Roussel Uclaf Corp.
95 Chestnut Ridge Road
Montvale, NJ 07645
- **Phone:** 201-307-9700
- **Emergency:** Not Available

<u>References:</u>
References for the information in this PIP can be found in Reference List <u>Number 2</u>

DISCLAIMER: The information in this profile does not in any way replace or supersede the information on the pesticide product labeling or other regulatory requirements. Please refer to the pesticide product labeling.

Exhibit 6-6. Fact Sheet for Pyrethrins and Pyrethroids

NPTN fact sheets are designed to answer questions that are commonly asked by the general public about pesticides that are regulated by the U.S. Environmental Protection Agency (U.S. EPA). This document is intended to be educational in nature and helpful to consumers for making decisions about pesticide use.

National
Pesticide
Telecommunications
Network

Pyrethrins and Pyrethroids

The Pesticide Label: Labels provide directions for the proper use of a pesticide product. *Be sure to read the entire label before using any product.* A signal word on each product label indicates the product's toxicity after a single dose.

CAUTION—low toxicity WARNING—moderate toxicity DANGER—high toxicity

What are pyrethrins?
- Pyrethrins are insecticides that are derived from the extract of chrysanthemum flowers (pyrethrum) (1).
- The plant extract, called pyrethrum contains pyrethrin I and pyrethrin II collectively, called pyrethrins.
- Pyrethrins are widely used for control of various insect pests.

What are pyrethroids?
- Pyrethroids are synthetic (human-made) forms of pyrethrins. There are two types that differ in chemical structure and symptoms of exposure.
- Type I pyrethroids include allethrin, tetramethrin, resmethrin, d-phenothrin, bioresmethrin, and permethrin (1, 2).
- Some examples of type II pyrethroids are cypermethrin, cyfluthrin, deltamethrin, cyphenothrin, fenvalerate, and fluvalinate (1, 2).
- Both type I and II pyrethroids inhibit the nervous system of insects. This occurs at the sodium ion channels in the nerve cell membrane. Some type II pyrethroids also affect the action of a neurotransmitter called GABA (3).

How do pyrethrins (and pyrethroids) work?
- Nerve cell membranes have a specific electrical charge. Altering the amount of ions (charged atoms) passing through ion channels causes the membrane to depolarize which, in turn, causes a neurotransmitter to be released. Neurotransmitters help nerve cells communicate. Electrical messages sent between nerve cells allow them to generate a response, like a movement in an animal or insect.
- Pyrethrins affect the nervous system of insects by causing multiple action potentials in the nerve cells by delaying the closing of an ion channel (3).
- Pyrethrins and pyrethroids act as contact poisons, affecting the insect's nervous system (1, 4).
- Even though pyrethrins and pyrethroids are nerve poisons, they are not cholinesterase inhibitors like organophosphate or carbamate insecticides.
- Pesticide products containing pyrethrins usually contain a synergist (such as piperonyl butoxide). Synergists work by restricting an enzyme that insects use to detoxify the pyrethrins. A synergist allows the insecticide to be more effective (4).

(Continued)

Exhibit 6-6. Continued

There are many different types of pyrethroids, but the remainder of this fact sheet will deal with pyrethrins. Information on specific pyrethroids is available in other fact sheets.

What are some types of products that contain pyrethrins?
- indoor bugbombs or foggers
- human head-lice treatments
- pet flea sprays
- Dragon
- Drione
- Pyrenone
- Pyrocide

How toxic are pyrethrins?
Animals
- Pyrethrins are one of the least poisonous insecticides to mammals (2).
- Rats fed high doses (1,000 milligrams per kilogram of body weight or mg/kg) of pyrethrins showed liver damage (5).
- Rats exposed to pyrethrins exhibited difficulty or rapid breathing, incoordination, sprawling of limbs, tremors, aggression, sensitivity to external stimuli, twitching, and exhaustion (6). See box on **laboratory testing**.

> Laboratory Testing: Before pesticides are registered by the U.S. EPA, they must undergo laboratory testing for short-term and long-term health effects. In these tests, laboratory animals are purposely fed a pesticide at high doses to cause toxic effects. These tests help scientists judge how these chemicals might affect humans, domestic animals, and wildlife in cases of overexposure. When pesticide products are used according to label directions, toxic effects are not likely to occur because the amount of pesticide that people and animals may be exposed to is low compared to the doses fed to laboratory animals.

Humans
- Inhaling pyrethrins can cause coughing, wheezing, shortness of breath, runny or stuffy nose, chest pain, or difficulty breathing (7).
- Skin contact can cause a rash, itching, or blisters (7).

> Effects of pyrethrins on human health and the environment depend on how much pyrethrin is present and the length and frequency of exposure. Effects also depend on the health of a person and/or certain environmental factors.

Do pyrethrins cause sensitization?
Animals
- The crude pyrethrum (initial plant extract) contains about 30 to 35 percent pyrethrins and about 50 percent impurities (2, 5).
- Various extracts from pyrethrum flowers have caused allergic contact dermatitis in sensitized and unsensitized guinea pigs (8).
- The commercially refined extract, which is present in insecticides today, did not produce any allergic reactions in guinea pigs (8, 9).
- Sensitization sometimes occurs in some individuals after a single exposure which causes either an asthmatic condition or a skin rash or inflammation. After the initial exposure to the sensitizing agent, the sensitized individual responds to a dose smaller than the initial dose.

Humans
- In one study, a person with a history of allergic contact dermatitis experimentally exposed to crude pyrethrum developed contact dermatitis, although this may have been caused by impurities in the extract (10).

(Continued)

Exhibit 6-6. Continued

Do pyrethrins break down and leave the body?
Animals
- Pyrethrins are low in toxicity to mammals because they are quickly broken down into inactive forms and pass from the body in the urine and feces (2, 5).

Humans
- Pyrethrum (the plant extract) may be absorbed by the digestive tract and the lungs. However, it is poorly absorbed through the skin (5).
- Based on animal studies, any amount of pyrethrins absorbed by humans would be expected to be rapidly excreted. Therefore, it is unlikely that pyrethrins would accumulate in humans.

Are pyrethrins likely to cause cancer?
Animals
- In one study, rats were fed moderate to very high doses (100, 1000, or 3000 mg/kg) of pyrethrum (the plant extract) for 104 weeks. There was an increase in the non-cancerous (benign) thyroid tumors in females exposed to all doses and in males exposed to high to very high doses (11).
- In the same study, some females fed high doses (3000 mg/kg) of pyrethrum developed ovarian and benign liver tumors and males exposed to high doses (3000 mg/kg) developed benign parathyroid tumors and benign skin lesions.
- In another study, rats were fed low doses (up to 10 mg/kg) of pyrethrins, flavoring agents, and other pesticides showed no increase in tumors (6).

See **Cancer** box

Humans
- Scientists have no data from work-related, accidental poisonings, or epidemiological studies that indicate whether or not pyrethrins are likely to cause cancer in humans. Initially, the Health Effects Division Carcinogenicity Peer Review Committee (CPRC) at the U.S. EPA recently reviewed the carcinogenicity data of pyrethrins in animals and decided that they showed carcinogenicity.
- However, the CPRC could not classify pyrethrins into a carcinogenicity group until some of the tissue specimens from rats and mice were re-read. Subsequently, the CPRC will perform a second review of the carcinogenicity of pyrethrins (11).

> **Cancer:** The U.S. EPA has strict guidelines that require testing of pesticides for their potential to cause cancer. These studies involve feeding laboratory animals large daily doses of the pesticide for up to 2 years. These animals are compared with a group of animals that did not receive the chemical. Animal studies help show whether a chemical is a potential human carcinogen. If a pesticide does not cause cancer in animal tests, then the EPA considers it unlikely the pesticide will cause cancer in humans.

Do pyrethrins cause reproductive problems or birth defects?
Animals
- Rabbits fed moderate doses (up to 90 mg/kg) of pyrethrins during a sensitive period of pregnancy had normal litters (5).
- Rats fed very high doses (5000 mg/kg) of pyrethrins for three weeks before their first mating produced low birth weight pups (5).
- There were no birth defects in pups of rabbits exposed to pyrethrins (12).

Humans
- There are no epidemiological, work-related or accidental exposure data on the potential of pyrethrins to cause reproductive problems or birth defects.

(Continued)

Exhibit 6-6. Continued

What happens to pyrethrins in the environment?

Soil

- Pyrethrins have a soil half-life of 12 days (13). They have an extremely low pesticide movement rating because they bind tightly to the soil (13). See box on **half-life.**

Photodegradation

- Pyrethrins are unstable in light or air (2). Pyrethrins are rapidly degraded in sunlight at the soil surface and in water.

> **Half-life** is the time required for half of the compound to degrade.
>
> **1 half-life** = 50% degraded
> **2 half-lives** = 75% degraded
> **3 half-lives** = 87% degraded
> **4 half-lives** = 94% degraded
> **5 half-lives** = 97% degraded
>
> Remember that the amount of chemical remaining after a half-life will always depend on the amount of the chemical originally applied.

What effect does pyrethrins have on wildlife?

- Pyrethrins are highly toxic to fish and tadpoles. They affect their skin touch receptors and balance organs (4).
- Pyrethrins are toxic to beneficial insect (such as honeybees) and many aquatic invertebrates (4).
- Pyrethrins are low in toxicity to humans, other mammals, and birds (4).

Selected References:

1. Klaassen, C. D., Amdur, M. O., & Doull, J. (Eds.). (1996). *Casarett & Doull's Toxicology. The Basic Science of Poisons* (5th ed.). Toronto: McGraw-Hill Companies, Inc.
2. Ray, D. E. (1991). Pesticides derived from plants and other organisms. In W. J. Hayes, Jr. & E. R. Laws (Eds.), *Handbook of Pesticide Toxicology. Vol. 2.* (pp. 585-593). Toronto: Academic Press.
3. Costa, L. G. (1997). Basic Toxicology of Pesticides. In M. C. Keifer, M. D., M. P. H. (Ed.), *Human Health Effects of Pesticides. Occupational Medicine. State of the Art Reviews.* (Vol. 12, No. 2). (pp. 251-268). Philadelphia: Hanley & Belfus, Inc.
4. Tomlin, C. (Ed.). (1994). *A World Compendium. The Pesticide Manual. Incorporating the agrochemicals handbook.* (10th ed.). Bungay, Suffolk, U.K.: Crop Protection Publications.
5. Hayes, W. J. (1982). *Pesticides Studied in Man.* Baltimore: Williams & Wilkins.
6. Leahey, J. P. (Ed.). (1985). The pyrethroid insecticides. Philadelphia: Taylor & Francis Ltd.
7. Sittig, M. (1991). *Handbook of Toxic and Hazardous Chemicals and Carcinogens.* (3rd ed.). (Vol. 2). New Jersey: Noyes Publications.
8. Rickett, F. E., Tyszkiewicz, K., and Brown, N. C. (1972). *Pyrethrum dermatitis. I. The allergenic properties of various extracts of pyrethrum flowers.* Pestic. Sci. 3:57-66.
9. Rickett, F. E. and Tyszkiewicz, K. (1973). *Pyrethrum dermatitis. II. The allergenicity of pyrethrum oleoresin and its cross-reactions with saline extract of pyrethrum flowers.* Pestic. Sci. 4:801-810.
10. Mitchell, J. C., Dupuis, G. H. N. (1972). *Allergenic dermatitis from pyrethrum (Chrysanthemum spp.). The roles of pyrethrosin, a sesquiterpene lactone, and of pyrethrin II.* Br. J. Derm. 86:568-573.
11. United States Environmental Protection Agency (U.S. EPA). Office of Prevention, Pesticides and Toxic Substances. *Carcinogenicity Peer Review of Pyrethrins.* February 22, 1995. Washington, DC.
12. Vettorazzi, G. (1979). *International Regulatory Aspects for Pesticide Chemicals. Toxicity Profiles.* (Vol. 1). Boca Raton, Florida: CRC Press, Inc.
13. Wauchope, R. D., T. M. Butler, A. G. Hornsby, P. M. Augustijn-Beckers, & J. P. Burt. (1992). The SCS/ARS/CES pesticide properties database for environmental decision making. *[Online].* ftp://ftp.nrcs.usda.gov/centers/itc/applications/wqmodels/gleams/

(Continued)

Exhibit 6-6. Continued

For more information, call or write:

NPTN
Oregon State University
333 Weniger Hall
Corvallis, Oregon 97331-6502
Phone: 1-800-858-7378
Fax: 1-541-737-0761
E-mail: nptn@ace.orst.edu
Internet: NPTN at http://ace.orst.edu/info/nptn/
or see EXTOXNET at
http://ace.orst.edu/info/extoxnet

Date reviewed: December 1998

> NPTN is sponsored cooperatively by Oregon State University and the U.S. Environmental Protection Agency. Data presented through NPTN documents are based on selected authoritative and peer-reviewed literature. The information in this profile does not in any way replace or supersede the restrictions, precautions, directions or other information on the pesticide label/ing or other regulatory requirements.

using different chemicals, there were likely to be many opportunities for potentially harmful chemical interactions and the development of mosquito resistance without adding another pesticide. His questions included the following:

1. How would the decision to begin aerial spraying affect control efforts in the immediate and distant future, and how would it affect the health of the public?
2. To what extent would these pesticides affect wildlife, fish, soil, and water?
3. Should the Nassau County Department of Health recommend aerial spraying?

Office of Health Education

Stacey Ciero, DrPH and head of the Office of Health Education, considered using social marketing approaches to convince the public that the proposed decision made—and the actions taken by the NCDH—were sound and necessary. The other main focus of the office was to continue to make the public aware of how it could prevent contracting the virus. She knew that the strategy of aerial spraying was now the key topic in the health department, the NCDPW, and the New York State Department of Environmental Conservation (NYSDEC). The role of her office was critical in that the public's acceptance of more intense spraying efforts would depend on an understanding of the problem at hand as well as the level of pesticide exposure hazard. It was her job to explain the issues. Steps needed to be taken to mitigate the public's fears about pesticides and the risk of cancer, as well as to accurately inform the public of the likelihood of respiratory side effects and skin and mucous membrane irritation. She had certain specific questions in her mind that needed to be answered.

1. What did the public already know?
2. What risks were there for each step in the action process? How should the NCDH communicate that risk?
3. Did the public perceive that there was a risk?
4. What role had the media played in the New York epidemic as well as in the Nassau County outbreak?
5. What preparations (materials, training) should be made to head off future epidemics that might occur during the next mosquito season?
6. To what extent were the news articles and television and radio reports accurately reporting information regarding control efforts and informing people concerning methods to protect themselves from the mosquitoes and pesticide exposure?
7. How were people processing the information they had received so far? Did different communication media have different effects on people's perception of the severity of the disease or pesticide exposure? Were some communication media more effective at getting the word out than others?

These were all questions that needed to be thought through prior to the implementation of a risk communication campaign. After these decisions were made, the media could be chosen. Because the summer season was coming to a close, it was likely that transmission would cease simply because of a change in behavior (less time spent outdoors). Dr. Ciero knew that campaigns had to begin providing information about current transmission while providing lasting knowledge for the next summer season. Beginning a risk reduction campaign during the fall might provide sufficient time to change behavior in groups typically slow to make change.

Policy Issues

Dr. Quentin Burns wrote that consideration had to be given to both present and future policy issues when dealing with this outbreak. He questioned whether aerial spraying of an adulticide was really the answer in this case. The current policy on mosquito control, "Nassau County Mosquito Surveillance and Control Status Report—December 1998" (included as Exhibit 6-3), provided for aerial spraying of larvicides over inaccessible, marshy areas. The spraying was done by helicopter and normally performed around fifteen times a year. The decision to spray was based on surveillance data collected from salt marsh and boat surveys. Adulticiding was normally done via ground spraying and was reserved for instances when extremely high numbers of adult mosquitoes were present or when other efforts at control failed. If aerial spraying of an adulticide was used in this instance, it might be necessary to alter the current policy to include provisions and recommendations for spraying during outbreaks of West Nile fever. Future surveillance for West Nile virus in both birds and mosquitoes could easily be added to the current surveillance programs.

Dr. Burns asked in his memo:

1. At what point would aerial spraying or other control methods be initiated, and would these additional control methods be cost effective?
2. Should we always do aerial spraying when a certain number of cases have been detected?
3. Was spraying the best way to spend money on this outbreak?
4. Was this outbreak of great enough public health importance to draw funds away from other efforts?

Decision Time

The meeting was scheduled for five o'clock—minutes from now—to review the options before the department, discuss strategies for implementing those options, address the pros and cons of each alternative, and determine the proper way to communicate the control strategies and the rationale for such strategies to the public. Tomorrow morning Dr. Katrina Guest would present the health department's recommendation on the question of aerial spraying to County Executive Lou Timpanini. The lives and livelihoods of the community that she served could be greatly affected by the decisions she was about to make.

CASE 7

Indian Health Service

Creating a Climate for Change

"As an enrolled member of the Laguna Pueblo in New Mexico, I am a member of the Sun Clan and have the name of my great grandfather, Osara, meaning 'the sun,'"[1] Dr. Michael Trujillo told the United States Senate Committee on Indian Affairs in 1994 during his confirmation hearing as Director of the Indian Health Service (see Exhibit 7-1). He told the committee that he had known the remoteness of Neah Bay at the northwest tip of Washington on the Makah reservation, lived in the Dakotas, and experienced the winters and geographic barriers to health care in Eagle Butte, Rosebud, and Twin Buttes. He had come before them, he also told them, "as the President's nominee for the Director of a national health care program that is essential to the well-being of 1.3 million American Indians and Alaska Natives belonging to more than 500 federally recognized tribes."

Three years later, Dr. Trujillo was in front of the same committee discussing the fiscal year 1998 budget request for the Indian Health Service (IHS). For the fourth consecutive year, IHS would get no after-inflation increase in its budget alloca-

tion. But what Dr. Trujillo said in 1994 was still true: "We, who are involved in Indian health care, are facing a changing external environment with new demands, new needs, and a shifting political picture. The changing internal environment demands increased efficiency, effectiveness, and accountability."

Dr. Trujillo knew that in order to accomplish the agency's mission, IHS must honor past treaties as well as respect the beliefs and spiritual convictions of the various tribes. The need to respect local traditions and beliefs was formally recognized in Indian self-determination.

The Indian peoples had always managed with very scarce resources; however, Dr. Trujillo was concerned. IHS had not developed an adequate third-party payor billing system, it faced difficulty recruiting professional staff, and it served a population whose health status was below that of the rest of the United States.

IHS was considered a discretionary agency in the congressional budget process. Dr. Trujillo recognized the need to increase the health status of IHS's population in order to gain continued con-

This case was prepared by Robert Tusatto; Terrie C. Reeves, Texas Woman's University; and W. Jack Duncan and Peter M. Ginter, University of Alabama at Birmingham. It is intended as a basis for classroom discussion rather than to illustrate effective or ineffective handling of an administrative situation. Copyright © 1998 by the *Case Research Journal*. Used with permission from the *Case Research Journal*.

Exhibit 7-1. Dr. Michael Trujillo: Chief Advocate for Indian Health

Dr. Michael H. Trujillo was named Director of the Indian Health Service on April 9, 1994. His appointment was noteworthy for two reasons: (1) he was the first IHS Director appointed by the President of the United States and confirmed by the Senate, and (2) he was the first full-blooded American Indian to be appointed Director of IHS. Dr. Trujillo was a member of the Sun Clan in the Laguna Pueblo in New Mexico. His parents were elementary school teachers for the Bureau of Indian Affairs and were active in the political life of the pueblo. His grandfather was a governor of the pueblo and was instrumental in drafting the first Laguna Pueblo constitution. From an early age, Dr. Trujillo had been taught and shown by example to feel an obligation to the Indian people.

The first American Indian to graduate from the University of New Mexico School of Medicine, Dr. Trujillo received both his undergraduate and medical degrees from that institution. Family practice and internal medicine were his specialties, but he was also chosen for a clinical fellowship in preventive medicine at the Mayo Clinic. In addition, he received a MPH in Public Health Administration and Policy from the University of Minnesota School of Public Health.

Dr. Trujillo had numerous assignments within IHS prior to becoming Director. As an IHS physician, he worked with many tribes in diverse locations. As an IHS administrator, he was Deputy Area Director and Chief Medical Officer for the Phoenix, Aberdeen, and Portland Areas, as well as a Clinical Specialty Consultant to the Bemidji Area. He initiated nationwide quality assurance programs and a medical provider recruitment program for urban Indian health centers.

Shortly after being sworn in as Director, Dr. Trujillo released his vision for the Indian Health Service. He envisioned a new IHS: one that adapted to the challenges it faced, yet continued to be the best primary care, rural health system in the world; one that recognized the contributions and dedication of employees, as well as the active participation of tribal members; one that was redesigned to be more effective, efficient, and accountable. Dr. Trujillo cautioned that any change must be accomplished in such a way that the Indian people noticed only improved quality of care.

Dr. Trujillo's position as IHS Director allowed him to be a strong advocate for Indians in all matters regarding health. Not only did he want to improve IHS, but he also wanted improvement for the entire Indian health care system. IHS leadership and direction would provide the course the agency would take in making these improvements.

gressional funding and support. He needed to answer some difficult and complex questions. How could Indian self-determination be implemented? What should be IHS's role in the future? How should IHS change to best serve the self-determination of the Indian peoples?

Dr. Trujillo knew that his most difficult task was to provide additional, much needed health services to a growing and needy population when there was little prospect of increasing resources. Simultaneously, he had to ensure that local health needs were recognized and addressed.

Indian Self-Determination

In January, 1994, Dr. Trujillo told the same committee that the local tribes and communities needed to be more involved in decision making to facilitate Indian self-determination, the process by which the Indian people may choose to assume some degree of the administration and operation of their health services. The Indian Self-Determination and Educational Assistance Act was passed by Congress in 1975 and gave federally recognized tribes the option of staffing, managing, and operating IHS programs in their communities. Dr. Trujillo was on record as fully supporting greater self-determination of all tribes as a means of enabling Indian people to operate their own health care systems. He emphatically stated that "During my tenure, there is going to be continued emphasis throughout the agency and in our interactions with other health partners for complete recognition of the Indian self-determination process."

Dr. Trujillo knew that self-determination was far from complete. Although IHS still had many important functions to fulfill, putting health care back into the hands of the tribes was proving to be difficult. Each tribe had different concepts of health, and it was difficult to accommodate such variety in a government agency. Moreover, in the face of scarce resources there was always an inclination to centralize rather than decentralize decision making, and Dr. Trujillo knew that if IHS created the impression that it could fulfill all the needs of local communities, it would contribute to false expectations and disappointment.

Historical Perspective

IHS had a clear mandate: to provide high-quality health services to American Indians and Alaska Natives (AI/ANs). The basis for this responsibility was established and confirmed by numerous treaties, statutes, and executive orders. The first treaty between the U.S. government and an American Indian tribe was signed in 1784 and promised that the federal government would provide physician services to members of the Delaware Nation as partial payment for rights and property ceded to the United States. Treaties were signed with many individual tribes, and periodic appropriations were made by Congress to control specific diseases such as smallpox and tuberculosis and to educate the tribes about disease. Recurring appropriations were not made until the Snyder Act of 1921, which authorized health care services for AI/ANs by an act of Congress.

Health care for Native Americans was originally the responsibility of the Bureau of Indian Affairs; however, the services provided were, in general, very poor. Despite the employment of field nurses, the building of hospitals for Native Americans, and the addition of dental services, the health status of AI/ANs remained far behind that of the general population. For example, Indian infant mortality was more than double that of the general population and life expectancy for Indians was ten years less than that of the rest of the United States.

The major health problems found in the Native American population became evident during World War II, when thousands of Indians volunteered for service in the U.S. armed forces. The poor health of many Indian volunteers was noted during induction physical examinations. Citing the AI/AN health statistics, various state, medical, and professional groups began a push to put the U.S. Public Health Service (USPHS) in charge of health care for Native Americans. They argued that the Bureau of Indian Affairs could not run a quality health care system because health was only one its many concerns. Years of debate and political maneuvering followed. Finally, IHS officially became a division of the USPHS on July 1, 1955. The Transfer Act stated "that all functions, responsibilities, authorities, and duties relating to the maintenance and operation of hospital and health facilities for Indians, and the conservation of Indian health shall be administered by the Surgeon General of the United States Public Health Service."

Although the overall health status of AI/ANs did not improve immediately, much progress appeared over the longer term. Since 1973, infant mortality among AI/ANs decreased 60 percent and death due to tuberculosis dropped 80 percent. During the same period, life expectancy for AI/ANs increased by more than 12 years; life expectancy for AI/ANs was just 2.6 years below that of the general population in the early 1990s.

Over the years after the transfer, IHS developed a model for the provision of high-quality, comprehensive health services. A major component of

Exhibit 7-2. Timeline of Key Events in IHS History

1784	**First treaty between the U.S. government and an American Indian tribe signed.**
1849	Bureau of Indian Affairs transferred from War Department to Department of the Interior. Physician services extended to Indians.
1880s	First federal hospital built for Indians.
1908	Professional medical supervision of Indian health activities established with position of chief medical supervisor.
1921	The Snyder Act authorized Indian health services by the federal government (under control of the Bureau of Indian Affairs).
1955	The Indian Health Service officially became a division of the United States Public Health Service (USPHS).
1975	Congress passed the Indian Self-Determination and Education Assistance Act.
1976	Congress passed the Indian Health Care Improvement Act.
1988	IHS was elevated to agency status within the USPHS. IHS allowed to bill third-party payors where applicable.
1994	Dr. Michael Trujillo appointed as Director of the Indian Health Service.
1995	Preliminary recommendations of the Indian Health Design Team (a task force composed of tribal leaders and IHS employees) published.
1997	Final recommendations of the Indian Health Design Team published.

Exhibit 7-3. IHS Mission

The mission of the Indian Health Service, in partnership with American Indian and Alaska Native people, is to raise their physical, mental, social, and spiritual health to the highest level.

this model was the involvement of the tribes in the provision of health services to their people. This provision had a "snowballing" effect. As the health status of their tribes improved, more tribal members began to get involved in the provision of health care, which, in turn, allowed the tribes to provide even more services.

Congress followed up the Indian Self-Determination and Educational Assistance Act with the Indian Health Care Improvement Act in 1976 and attempted to elevate the health status of AI/ANs to a level equal to that of the general population. This act gave IHS a larger budget, allowed expanded health services, and provided for new and renovated medical facilities and construction of safe drinking water and sanitary disposal facilities. In addition, it established scholarship and loan payback programs to increase the number of Indian health professionals. IHS was elevated to agency status within the USPHS in 1988. This reflected the improving reputation of IHS as an institution as well as the growth of support for Indian self-determination and the IHS mission. See Exhibits 7-2 and 7-3.

Exhibit 7-4. Service Population

Area	1990 (Census) Population	1997 (Estimated) Population
Aberdeen	74,789	94,313
Alaska	86,251	103,713
Albuquerque	67,504	78,851
Bemidji	61,349	79,930
Billings	47,008	55,630
California	104,828	119,976
Nashville	48,943	73,042
Navajo	180,959	215,232
Oklahoma	262,517	297,888
Phoenix	120,707	140,969
Portland	127,774	148,791
Tucson	24,607	27,612
All Areas	1,207,236	1,435,947

The Service Population: American Indians and Alaska Natives

Traditional AI/AN beliefs concerning wellness, sickness, and treatment were different from the modern public health approach or the medical model. American Indians' and Alaskan Natives' beliefs included close integration within family, clan, and tribe; harmony with the environment; and a continuing circle of life—birth, adolescence, adulthood, elder years, the passing-on, and then rebirth. Individual wellness was conceived of as the harmony and balance among mind, body, spirit, and the environment. Effective health services for AI/ANs had to integrate the philosophies of the tribes with those of the medical community.

Of the more than 2.4 million AI/ANs in the United States, approximately 1.4 million belonged to the 545 federally recognized Indian tribes. All American Indian tribes were sovereign nations. Therefore, AI/ANs were citizens both of their tribes and of the United States. This meant that AI/ANs had a unique relationship with the federal government. Based on the "treaty rights" established between most tribes and the United States,

the federal government had a "trust responsibility" to these tribes that entitled the Indian people to services such as education and health care. However, because not all tribes signed treaties with the United States, less than two-thirds of all people with an Indian heritage were eligible to participate in the federal programs. Since October, 1978, the Bureau of Indian Affairs had received 215 letters of intent and petitions for federal recognition. Forty-one of these petitions had been resolved, with twenty-one "new" tribes being recognized.

The total number of AI/ANs eligible for IHS services in 1997 was approximately 1.43 million, and the number increased about 2.2 percent each year. Selected demographics and health factors of the service population are shown in Exhibits 7-4 through 7-10. Tribal members lived mainly on reservations and in rural communities in thirty-four states.

Similar to the nation's health care system, IHS operated in an environment of increasing health care costs, growing numbers of beneficiaries, and excess demand for services. The shift in disease patterns (from acute to chronic diseases) and the increasing elderly population played an impor-

(text continues on page 272)

Exhibit 7-5. Age Distribution (by percentage of total population)

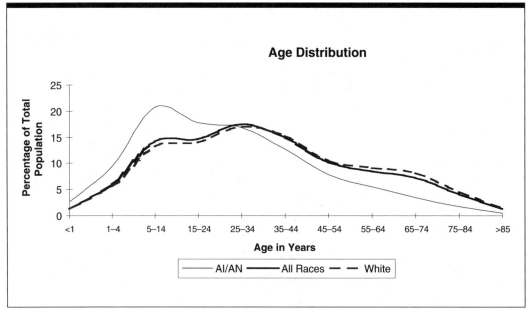

SOURCE: Adapted from *Trends in Indian Health 1996*.

Exhibit 7-6. Median Household Income (1990 Census)

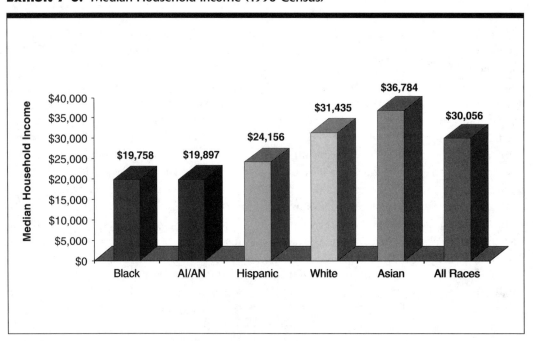

SOURCE: Adapted from *Trends in Indian Health 1996*.

Exhibit 7-7. Percentage of Total Population Below Poverty Level

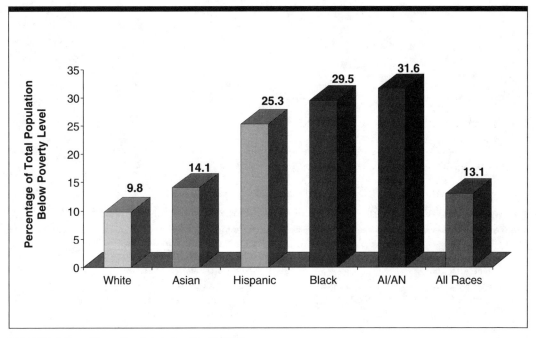

SOURCE: Adapted from *Trends in Indian Health 1996*.

Exhibit 7-8. Infant Mortality Rates

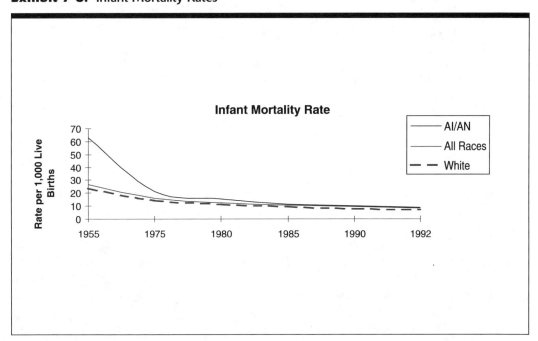

SOURCE: Adapted from *Trends in Indian Health 1996*.

Exhibit 7-9. Overall Measures of Health

	AI/AN	All Races	White
Life expectancy at birth (years)	73.5	75.5	76.3
Years of productive life lost (rate per 1,000 population)	83.0	55.6	49.9
Age-adjusted mortality rate (per 100,000 population)	598.1	513.7	486.8

SOURCE: Adapted from *Trends in Indian Health 1996*.

Exhibit 7-10. AI/AN Leading Causes of Death, Hospitalization, and Outpatient Visits

Leading causes of death
Heart diseases
Accidents (motor vehicle and other)
Chronic liver disease and cirrhosis
Pneumonia and influenza
Chronic obstructive pulmonary diseases
Cancer
Diabetes mellitus
Cerebrovascular disease
Suicide
Homicide

Leading causes of hospitalization
Obstetric deliveries and complications
of pregnancy
Injury and poisoning
Genitourinary system diseases
Endocrine, nutritional, and metabolic
disorders

Respiratory system diseases
Digestive system diseases
Circulatory system diseases
Mental disorders
Skin diseases

Leading causes of outpatient visits
Respiratory diseases
Endocrine, nutritional, and metabolic
disorders
Musculoskeletal system diseases
Complications of pregnancy and childbirth
Nervous system diseases
Injury and poisoning
Skin diseases
Circulatory system diseases

SOURCE: Adapted from *Trends in Indian Health 1996*.

tant role in health planning for IHS as well. As with the Veterans Administration (VA), IHS was a health care provider within the U.S. governmental system—though unlike the VA, IHS was not a Cabinet department and had no voice in policy making at the White House. Unlike *any* other health care system in the country, IHS was subject to both the mandates of Congress and the approval of more than 540 sovereign Indian Nations.

IHS Today: A Key Component of the Indian Health Care System

Health care for AI/ANs was delivered through a system of interlocking programs. The system was composed of IHS, the tribal programs, and the urban programs. IHS programs, called service units, were those projects and facilities that were directly staffed, operated, and administered by IHS per-

Exhibit 7-11. Elements of the Indian Health Care System

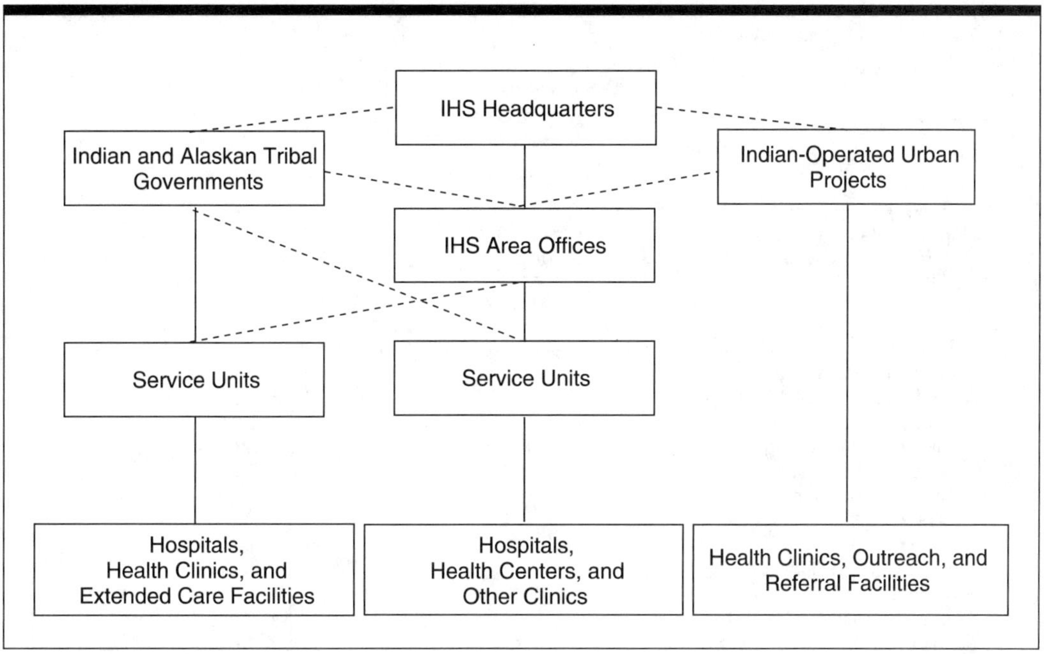

SOURCE: Adapted from *Trends in Indian Health 1996.*

NOTE: Solid lines reflect formal relationships; dashed lines (––––) reflect important but less formal relationships.

sonnel. As of October, 1995, there were sixty-eight IHS-operated service units that administered 38 hospitals and 112 health centers, school health centers, and health stations. Tribal programs were those developed through the process of Indian self-determination. Administered through seventy-six tribal-operated service units were 11 tribal program hospitals and 372 health centers, school health centers, health stations, and Alaska village clinics. Urban programs were relatively new but were expected to face a future of brisk demand because of the relocation of significant Indian populations from reservations to urban settings. The urban programs ranged from information referral and community health services to comprehensive primary health care services. As of October, 1995, there were thirty-four Indian-operated urban programs.

IHS headquarters and IHS area offices had ties to the tribal governments as well as to the Indian-operated Urban Projects. The Indian and Alaskan tribal governments had input into the decisions of IHS-operated service units. This interrelation between the federal government, tribal governments, and urban Indian groups was a key component of Indian health care management. Exhibit 7-11 shows various features of the Indian health care system.

To further complicate the organizational structure, IHS was an Operating Division within the Department of Health and Human Services (DHHS). Exhibit 7-12 shows the position of IHS on the organizational chart of the executive branch of the federal government.

Within IHS, the organizational structure consisted of three levels: headquarters, area offices, and service units. IHS Headquarters, located in Rockville, Maryland, was ultimately responsible for all policy, operations, and management decisions. The twelve area offices (see Exhibit 7-13) represented geographical regions and were responsible for performing various roles in admin-

Exhibit 7-12. Executive Branch Organizational Chart

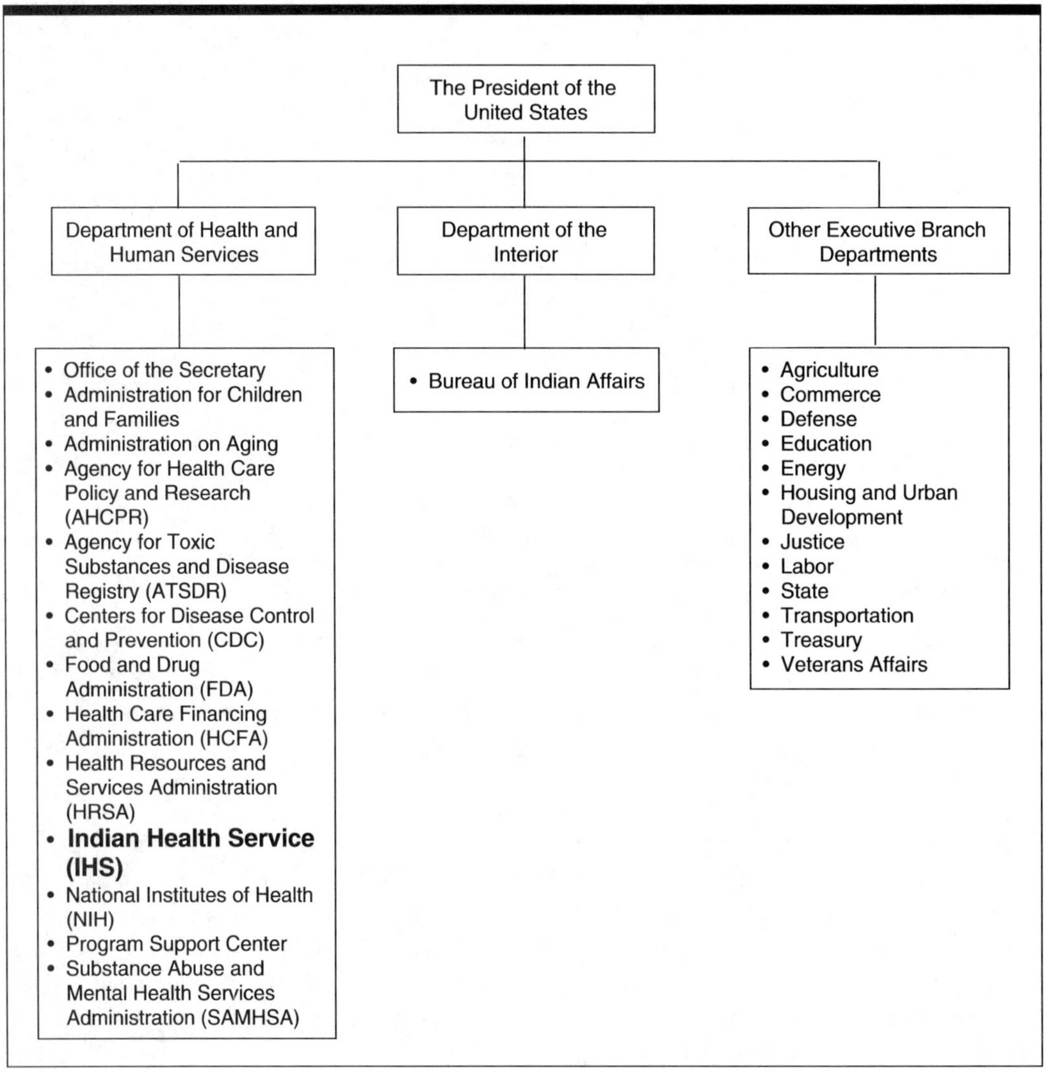

```
                    ┌─────────────────────┐
                    │ The President of the │
                    │    United States     │
                    └─────────────────────┘
        ┌────────────────────┼────────────────────┐
┌──────────────────┐ ┌──────────────────┐ ┌──────────────────┐
│ Department of     │ │ Department of the│ │ Other Executive  │
│ Health and Human  │ │    Interior      │ │ Branch           │
│ Services          │ │                  │ │ Departments      │
└──────────────────┘ └──────────────────┘ └──────────────────┘
```

- Office of the Secretary
- Administration for Children and Families
- Administration on Aging
- Agency for Health Care Policy and Research (AHCPR)
- Agency for Toxic Substances and Disease Registry (ATSDR)
- Centers for Disease Control and Prevention (CDC)
- Food and Drug Administration (FDA)
- Health Care Financing Administration (HCFA)
- Health Resources and Services Administration (HRSA)
- **Indian Health Service (IHS)**
- National Institutes of Health (NIH)
- Program Support Center
- Substance Abuse and Mental Health Services Administration (SAMHSA)

- Bureau of Indian Affairs

- Agriculture
- Commerce
- Defense
- Education
- Energy
- Housing and Urban Development
- Justice
- Labor
- State
- Transportation
- Treasury
- Veterans Affairs

istrative and program support for the local service units.

Service units were composed of several types of facilities, including hospitals, health centers, health stations, and clinics. Depending on local preferences and circumstances, these service units could exist as single entities or as combinations of facilities. For example, the Fort Hall Service Unit in Idaho included only a single health center, while the Pine Ridge Service Unit in South Dakota consisted of a hospital in Pine Ridge, health centers in Kyle and Wanblee, and small health stations in Allen and Manderson.

IHS Programs and Initiatives

In many (but not in all) cases, IHS provided comprehensive health care services to eligible AI/ANs. To be eligible for services, AI/ANs had to be members of federally recognized tribes with whom the United States had treaty agreements. Services were provided through various programs

Exhibit 7-13. IHS Area Offices

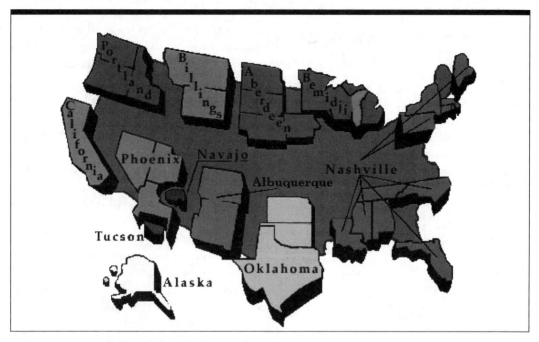

SOURCE: IHS home page (www.ihs.gov).

and initiatives administered by IHS, covering a full range of preventive health, behavioral health, medical care, environmental health, and engineering services. The initiatives focused on timely issues such as care of the elderly, women's health, AIDS, traditional medicine practices, and injury prevention, as shown in Exhibit 7-14. However, in some locations, IHS did not have the necessary equipment or facilities to provide comprehensive services. In these instances, services which were not readily accessible to AI/ANs could be provided under contracted health services with local hospitals, state and local health agencies, tribal health institutions, and individual health care providers.

In its relatively short history, IHS had contributed to tremendous improvements in the health status of its service population. Some of the many reasons for these status improvements included increased primary medical care services, sanitation facility construction, and community health education programs. IHS was often instrumental in the infrastructure changes. Exhibit 7-15 shows

some of the more impressive accomplishments of IHS.

IHS Personnel

IHS employed a workforce of approximately 15,000 people. Of these, more than 62 percent were of American Indian or Alaska Native heritage. IHS personnel consisted of nearly every discipline involved in the provision of health, social, behavioral, and environmental health services. The IHS clinical staff was composed of primary care professionals and other providers, as well as clinical technicians and assistants. Primary care providers included physicians, physician assistants, dentists, nurse practitioners, and nurse midwives. Other providers included pharmacists, optometrists, public health nurses, clinic nurses, physical therapists, and dietitians (see Exhibit 7-16). Over the past few years, because of the "Reinventing Government" initiative of the Clinton Administration resulting from a national preference for

Exhibit 7-14. IHS Programs and Initiatives

IHS Services and Programs

Preventive health
    Prenatal and postnatal care
    Well baby care
    Immunizations
    Family planning services
    Women's health program
    Nutrition program
    Health education program
    Community health representative program
    Accident and injury reduction program
Medical
    Inpatient hospitalization
    Outpatient services
    Emergency services
    Pharmacy program
    Laboratory program
    Nursing program
    Contract health services
Behavioral health
    Mental health program
    Social services
    Alcohol and substance abuse program
    Diabetes program
Environmental health and engineering
    Water and waste treatment
    Food protection
    Environmental safety and planning
    Pollution control
    Insect control
    Occupational safety and health
    Facility construction and maintenance

IHS initiatives

AIDS initiative
Traditional medicine initiative
Indian youth initiative
Maternal and child health initiative
Sanitation facilities initiative
Indian women's health initiative
Injury prevention initiative
Elder care initiative
Otitis media initiative
State initiative

getting government decision making closer to "the people," as well as the IHS redesign process initiated by Dr. Trujillo, the trend in IHS staffing was toward an increase in personnel at the service unit level and decreases at the area and headquarters levels (Exhibit 7-17).

An ongoing personnel problem concerned the recruitment and retention of dedicated, qualified professionals. Most IHS sites were remote, and many lacked adequate schools, stores, and amenities. To compensate for some of these quality-of-life imbalances, IHS offered financial incentives in the form of scholarships, loan payback agreements, and summer employment to selected health care professionals. For most professionals, however, the pay scales continued to lag behind those in the private sector.

Further exacerbating the personnel recruitment and retention problems, many employees were concerned about the changes that were occurring within IHS. Federal employees at the service unit level wondered how long they could remain in their positions once the local tribes assumed responsibility for health services. Area and headquarters employees were concerned about the future of their careers because there were so many cuts being made in these programs. All such issues concerning the organizational changes were addressed often by IHS leaders in memorandums, reports, and speeches. Information technology resources, particularly the Internet and electronic mail, were used to disseminate information. Upper management felt that it was imperative to keep the lines of communication open and to involve IHS personnel at all levels in the change process, but the uncertainty could not be eliminated.

The Indian Self-Determination and Educational Assistance Act gave federally recognized tribes various options for their involvement in the staffing. The original act allowed tribes to contract with the federal government. These contracting tribes could redesign and assume responsibility

Exhibit 7-15. Program Accomplishments

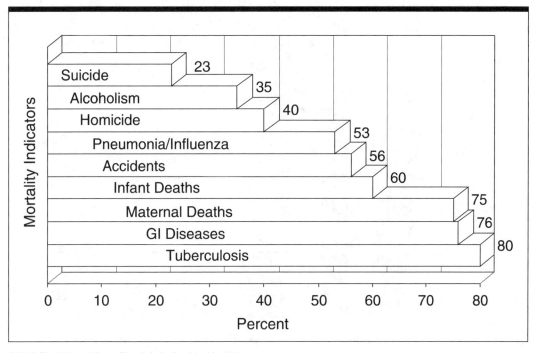

SOURCE: Adapted from *Trends in Indian Health 1996.*

Exhibit 7-16. Percentage of Outpatient Visits by Type of Provider

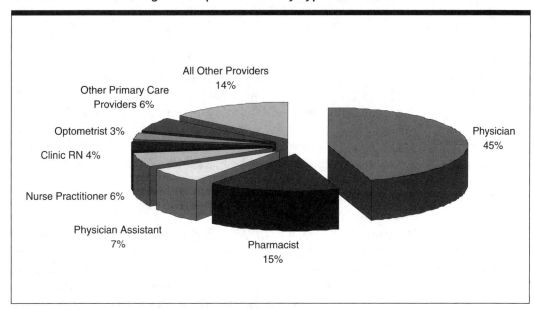

SOURCE: Adapted from *Trends in Indian Health 1996.*

Exhibit 7-17. IHS Staffing Trends

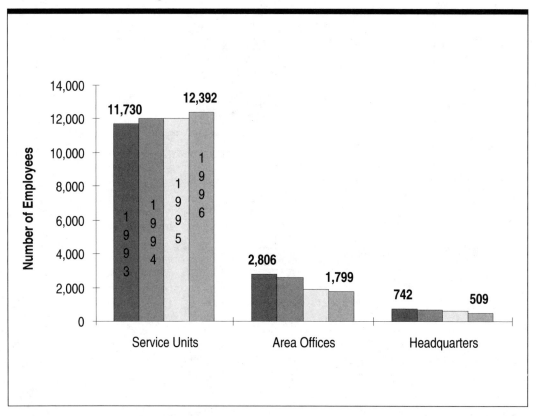

SOURCE: Adapted from *Trends in Indian Health 1996.*

for any aspect of their health care services. Some tribes made the choice to contract all of their health care services. A limitation of the contracting process was that the IHS had to approve and allow all redesign proposals.

Amendments to the act removed this limitation by creating the Tribal Self-Governance Demonstration Project. This project allowed selected tribes to compact their health care services; that is, they took over complete responsibility without the need for IHS approval or oversight. The project originally called for thirty tribes to be selected for inclusion, but by 1997 there were already thirty-four participating tribes, with several more anticipating their inclusion. The number of tribes choosing to deliver at least some portion of their own health care had increased steadily. Although

contracts and compacts accounted for only an estimated 22 percent of the total IHS budget in 1987, these obligations grew to more than 32 percent by 1995 and were expected to reach 50 percent by the turn of the century. Exhibit 7-18 shows the trend in funding for tribal contracts and compacts.

IHS Funding

Sources of funding for IHS included appropriations from the federal budget and collections from third-party billing. Congress passed the Indian Health Care Amendments of 1988, which authorized IHS to bill third parties for both inpatient and outpatient services. Medicaid, Medicare, and other insurance payors were all defined as third-party payors, and these were considered the

Exhibit 7-18. Tribal Contract and Compact Funding (in millions of dollars)

Fiscal Year	Contracts	Compacts	Total
1987	200.9	9.8	210.7
1988	217.2	13.1	230.3
1989	306.6	23.5	330.1
1990	320.7	27.4	348.1
1991	410.1	40.1	450.2
1992	511.6	50.9	562.5
1993	491.5	59.9	551.4
1994	648.1	114.5	762.6
1995	297.5	335.0	632.5

SOURCE: Adapted from *Trends in Indian Health 1996.*

only new revenue source for IHS programs. IHS did not collect the copayments or deductibles that were required with some policies, and those eligible individuals who did not have insurance coverage were not charged for the services they received. Although collections from third-party payors were increasing, there were still many concerns over the inability of IHS to bill and collect adequately for all the services that it provided. In fact, a 1995 review published by the Office of the Inspector General of the Department of Health and Human Services estimated that IHS underbilled by about $8.5 million each quarter because of untrained staff, shortage of staff, or lack of controls.

Because IHS was considered a discretionary program within the confines of the federal budget and because any attempts to balance the federal budget would involve cuts in discretionary programs, stakeholders of IHS were very concerned about the level of funding that the organization received from the federal government. The term "discretionary" referred to funds controlled by the annual appropriations process. This included most of the regular operating funds for the federal agencies, as well as funds for the thousands of large and small programs that had no binding

legal obligations to their beneficiaries. Estimates were made that many IHS programs were underfunded by 30 to 40 percent, although some went as low as 70 percent below their level of need. Exhibits 7-19 and 7-20 show the trends for these funding sources. The 1998 budget request allowed no fund increases to account for inflation, population growth, or newly recognized tribes. Exhibits 7-21 and 7-22 show the financial position of IHS for fiscal year 1996 and fiscal year 1997.

The shift from direct federal funding to state block grant funding of health care programs (such as a Medicaid managed care program) was another great concern of IHS and tribal leaders. It was a common occurrence for states to overlook or ignore Indian concerns when developing programs. Many state governments had the misconception that Indian tribes had relationships only with the federal government and were not eligible for state resources, when in fact AI/ANs were entitled to the same privileges and resources as any other state citizens. In response to these concerns, a state initiative workgroup was created by IHS to focus on the social, economic, legal, and policy issues pertaining to state health reform initiatives and Indian health programs.

(text continues on p. 283)

Exhibit 7-19. Trends in IHS Budget Appropriations (in millions of dollars)

Category	FY87	FY88	FY89	FY90	FY91	FY92	FY93	FY94	FY95	FY96	FY97	FY98
Services												
Clinical	748	817	883	1,031	1,235	1,276	1,252	1,325	1,370	1,418	1,452	1,468
Preventive Health	66	70	73	78	90	65	70	75	77	78	81	82
Other[1]	56	60	63	70	85	90	204	246	260	264	274	285
Total Services	870	947	1,019	1,179	1,410	1,431	1,526	1,646	1,707	1,760	1,807	1,835
Facilities	71	62	62	72	166	274	334	297	253	239	248	287
Total Appropriations	941	1,009	1,081	1,251	1,576	1,705	1,860	1,943	1,960	1,999	2,055	2,122

SOURCE: Adapted from *Trends in Indian Health 1996.*

1. Other services include urban health, Indian health professions, tribal health management, direct operations, self-governance, and contract support costs.

Exhibit 7-20. Trends in Third-Party Collections (in millions of dollars)

Category	FY88	FY89	FY90	FY91	FY92	FY93	FY94	FY95	FY96
Medicare/Medicaid	66	75	88	94	122	141	160	162	177
Private Insurance	—	—	3.5	8	12	18	23	31	34
Total Collections	66	75	91.5	102	134	159	183	193	211

SOURCE: Adapted from *Trends in Indian Health 1996.*

Exhibit 7-21. Statement of Financial Position (in millions)

	1996	1997
Assets		
Entity Assets:		
Fund Balances with Treasury	$1,172	$1,108
Investments	—	—
Accounts Receivable, Net:		
From Federal Agencies	19	6
From the Public	4	16
Interest Receivable	—	—
Advances:		
To Federal Agencies	13	—
To the Public	10	40
Inventories	13	15
Property and Equipment, Net	497	647
Non-Entity Assets:		
Accounts Receivable, Net:	—	—
Total Assets	$1,728	$1,832
Liabilities		
Funded Liabilities:		
Payables:		
Due Federal Agencies	$ 24	$ 26
Due the Public	42	48
Advances:		
From Federal Agencies	47	64
From the Public	—	—
Accrued Payroll and Benefits	29	30
Unfunded Liabilities:		
Annual Leave	60	60
Workers' Compensation Benefits	44	45
Other Liabilities	1	2
Pensions	—	—
Total Liabilities	$ 247	$ 275
Net Position		
Unexpended Appropriations	991	954
Invested Capital	511	662
Cumulative Results of Operations	84	48
Future Funding Requirements	(105)	(107)
Total Net Position	1,481	1,557
Total Liabilities and Net Position	$1,728	$1,832

SOURCE: DHHS Web site (http://www.hhs.gov).

Exhibit 7-22. Statement of Operations and Changes in Net Position (in millions)

	1996	1997
Revenues and Financial Sources		
Appropriated Capital Used:		
General Appropriations	$1,991	$2,135
Matching Contributions	—	—
Employment Taxes	—	—
SMI Premium Collected	—	—
Interest Revenue	—	—
Sales of Goods and Services	310	415
Imputed Financing	—	71
Other Revenue and Financing	—	—
Total Revenue and Financing Sources	$2,301	$2,621
Expenses		
Operating:		
Personnel Costs	$ 745	$ 755
Travel and Transportation	46	48
Rent, Communications and Utilities	43	40
Printing and Reproduction	2	1
Contractual Services	738	851
Supplies and Materials	80	180
Grants	516	605
Insurance Claims and Indemnities	—	1
Other Operating Expenses	81	—
Depreciation and Amortization	24	24
Imputed Personnel Costs	—	71
Other Non-Operating Expenses	—	1
Total Expenses	$2,275	$2,577
Excess of Revenues and Financing Sources	$ 26	$ 44
Net Position, Beginning Balance	$1,464	$1,481
Adjustments	—	178
Net Position, Restated Beginning Balance	1,464	1,659
Excess of Revenues and Financing Sources	26	44
Non-Operating Changes	(9)	(146)
Net Position, Ending Balance	$1,481	$1,557

SOURCE: DHHS Web site (http://www.hhs.gov).

Also, a strategic business plan was being developed by a working group composed of tribal leaders, IHS personnel, and private sector consultants. This plan would focus on revenue generation, cost control, internal business improvements, and allocation of tribal shares. Although the business plan was still in the development stage, this committee represented the IHS commitment to a new style of leadership, one that focused not only on the efficient and effective use of resources but also on the partnership with the Indian people.

The Future of IHS

Dr. Trujillo knew that IHS was a very dynamic organization, that it was staffed by professional personnel, that the AI/AN populations were unique, and that tribal cultures, values, religions, and traditions must always be considered and respected when delivering health services to this population. In addition, he knew that IHS was at a crucial juncture in its existence. Stakeholders in Indian health were calling for major changes in the organization. Various economic changes were signaling the need for new and innovative ways to fund programs. Tribes were asking for more control over health care for their members. At the same time that IHS was constrained by treaties, it was also considered a discretionary agency of the United States.

Dr. Trujillo was committed to Indian self-determination and knew that the spirit of self-determination required local assessment and definition of health service requirements. At the same time, he was responsible for improving the health status of the American Indians and Alaska Natives to the highest level possible. Although there was no inherent conflict between self-determination and improvements in health status of all the Indian peoples, in the face of scarce resources, Dr. Trujillo knew there were limits to the services that could be provided to any single community. He needed to carefully manage the expectations created by self-determination while not discouraging local communities from becoming involved in their own health affairs. The creation of false expectations could be as damaging as not involving tribes in local health affairs. Balancing expectations with local support required some serious thinking about the future mission and role of his.

Note

1. All quotations are taken from statements made before committees of Congress and/or the houses of Congress by the person quoted. Sources are shown in the references.

References

Kendrick, T. (1997). *A Future of Possibilities for Health, Indian Health, and Indian Health Leaders.* Available: http:\\www.ihs.gov.

Trujillo, M. H. (January 27, 1994). *Confirmation Hearing Statement Before the United States Senate Committee on Indian Affairs.* Available: http:\\www.ihs.gov.

Trujillo, M. H. (May 11, 1995). *Opening Statement Before the Interior Subcommittee of the Senate Appropriations Committee.* Available: http:\\www.ihs.gov.

Trujillo, M. H. (November 28, 1995). *Time of Change . . . Time for Change: The State of the Indian Health Service.* Paper presented at the National Indian Health Board 13th Annual Consumer Conference. Available: http:\\www. ihs.gov.

Trujillo, M. H. (February 20, 1996). *Challenges and Change: The State of the Indian Health Service.* Available: http:\\www.ihs.gov.

Trujillo, M. H. (December, 1996). Message From the Director: Looking to the Future of the Indian Health Service. *IHS Primary Care Provider, 21,* no. 12, pp. 157–160.

Trujillo, M. H. (March, 1997). *The Future Indian Health Care System.* Available: http:\\www.ihs.gov.

Three Vexing Cases in Health Care Ethics

Prologue

Mr. Blackwell decided to consult the Institutional Ethics Committee (IEC) of Regional Memorial Hospital. Blackwell was the CEO of this large public health facility, which had more than 900 beds and served a countywide population of more than one million. His concerns centered on two clinical cases that had plagued his medical and administrative staff for months and one ethical dilemma in which he felt the hospital might have harmed babies by giving away infant formula. These questions just did not go away.

The first two cases, Baby Boy-X and Annie O., were not typical, but they raised ethical issues that were troublesome, fairly common, and not easily managed. The major issue was cost. Even with a combined expenditure of more than $0.5 million, questions remained about the nature, duration, and efficacy of care provided. Blackwell sought the advice of the hospital's IEC regarding the appropriateness of the care given and special help on what would constitute a fair level of care in cases such as those of Baby Boy-X and Annie O. In addition, the third case was an important policy issue that had ethical implications: Should the hospital provide free baby formula? This issue was more complex than it first appeared.

Background

Cranford and Doudera's description of hospital ethics committees was useful: "Institutional Ethics Committees are interdisciplinary groups within health care institutions that advise about pressing ethical problems that arise in clinical care."[1] A primary assumption on which IECs are founded was that cooperative, reasoned reflection was likely to assist decision makers in reaching better conclusions. These committees provided information and education to staff and surrounding communities about ethical questions, proposed policies related to ethically difficult issues, and reviewed patient care situations (prospectively and retrospectively) in which ethical questions were at stake. Contributions provided by IECs included the following: (1) they served as a locus for discussion, clarification, dialogue, and advice (not decision); (2) they supplied protection and support for health care providers making difficult decisions; and (3) they increased aware-

These cases were prepared by John M. Lincourt, the University of North Carolina at Charlotte. The first two situations come from *Ethics Without a Net, a Case Workbook in Bioethics* by John M. Lincourt (Dubuque, IA: Kendall/Hunt Publishing Company, 1991). Reproduction of the cases is by permission of the publisher. The prologue, background sections, and third situation were written especially for *Public Health Leadership and Management: Cases and Context*. Used with permission from John M. Lincourt.

ness of and sensitivity to ethical dimensions of clinical cases.

IECs were not without their critics. Some claimed that such advisory groups threatened to undermine the traditional doctor/patient relationship and impose new and untested regulatory burdens on patients, families, physicians, and hospitals. Labeling an issue as *ethical* removed it from the category of those issues that were strictly medical and declared that relevant considerations were not solely technical in nature. Many health care providers were unaccustomed to working in this area of ethical values, and some insisted that their training and experience provided scant preparation for it. Conversely, other health care providers claimed that ethics was woven into the very fabric of medicine, thereby rendering them eminently capable, if not the most capable, to make such decisions. These individuals tended to view IECs as "God Squads," that is, generally lacking moral authority and ill-equipped to handle the ethical challenges of life and death decisions. Such attitudes still persisted in some quarters.[2]

The operation of IECs was similar to that of other hospital committees, but there were some important differences. These included the interdisciplinary composition, sliding orientation period, and varied utilization patterns. IECs tended to be large committees with between ten and twenty members. Membership included nurses and physicians (frequently from Oncology and Pediatrics), administrators including an outside attorney, members of the clergy and social services, a citizen or two, plus an ethicist (if available). Orientation for a new committee or new members ranged from a week or two up to a full year. Typically, this period was devoted to a careful review of institutional and community standards of care, an introduction to the bioethical literature (which was becoming vast), and, most important, practice sessions involving ethics cases. Such reviews usually were retrospective in nature and came from that institution, one of similar status, or the literature.

Committee utilization patterns varied. The IEC might be convened for a case requiring immediate action, the careful review of past cases that were known to include ethical misjudgments, or cases that on review were not ethical at all but centered on some other problem or issue, such as a legal or procedural one. Finally, The Patient Self-Determination Act (PSDA), passed by Congress as part of The Omnibus Reconciliation Act of 1990, became effective on December 1, 1991, and helped to legitimize IECs and socialize them more completely into hospital medical practice.

Case 1—Baby Boy-X

Baby Boy-X was born to a thirty-seven-year-old woman at thirty-six weeks gestation. The birth was a spontaneous vaginal delivery, and the patient's medical history gave no clue to the future difficulties associated with the birth of this child. The first indications of fetal risk were revealed when the Apgar scores were computed. This child had scores of 2 at one minute and 1 at five minutes. These scores were used to assess the general condition of the neonate by rating the child's status using the following criteria: color, pulse, respiration, reflex response, and muscle tone. A total score of 10 denoted a newborn in the best condition. Neonatal mortality rose rapidly as the total Apgar score approached 0. For example, scores of 1 and 2 predict a 12 to 15 percent survival rate. Baby Boy-X's score was cause for serious concern for the medical staff at Regional Memorial.

The patient's clinical, physical, and social histories supported the Apgar assessment. These included

- Deformed right leg
- Hydrocephalus
- Nonfunctioning G.I. tract
- Irregular cessation of breathing that required a ventilator
- Chronic anemia that required transfusions and nutritional supplements
- Repeated grand mal seizures during the first two months
- Probable blindness
- Lowered and malformed ears

- Severe contractions of the limbs, including fingers and toes
- Cerebral shrinkage and degeneration due to lack of oxygen to the brain
- Little brain activity except during seizures
- Gastrostomy, colostomy, and ileostomy tubes inserted surgically for proper nutrition and excretion

Baby Boy-X was kept in the neonatal intensive care unit (NICU) for four months. He was on a ventilator and given drugs for his seizure disorder. The consensus among the NICU personnel was that the prognosis was poor, and they expected the patient to die from massive infection or following violent seizure activity. The cost at four months was $182,265. The mother and father were separated, and the family was on welfare. The father had not visited the child.

On numerous occasions, members of the medical and administrative staffs initiated discussions with the mother about her son's grim prognosis and poor quality of life. These conversations were started in the hopes she would realize the futility of all the heroic measures being employed and allow her son to die naturally and soon. Staff members stated privately that scarce and costly medical resources were being wasted. This patient would never leave the hospital alive, and his life in the hospital was severely compromised and painful. Some administrators asked pointed questions about rethinking the "medical full-court press" for this patient. Resources expended on Baby Boy-X could be redirected to clients whose chances for survival and normal lifestyles were markedly better.

In the face of all these remarks, the mother remained adamant. The following text was taken from the NICU nursing notes and reflected poignantly the mother's attitude at the time.

She [mother] does not identify her child as a person with serious health problems. She does not understand the nature and extent of his high-risk problems plus his levels of pain and discomfort. She feels the baby is alright and she seems quite unrealistic about treatment outcomes. Because of car problems, she visits only once each week and usually for about one hour. She holds the baby briefly and combs his hair. The child's father has yet to visit the patient. She continually insists that everything medically possible should be done for her child.

Case 2—Annie O.

This case ranged over three years, cost the taxpayers in excess of $310,000, and could be considered a "classic worst-case scenario" in allocation. The initial encounter with the patient occurred in the Emergency Room of Regional Memorial Hospital. A description of some of the medical and nonmedical facts that shaped the case and led to the ethical dilemma for Annie O. follows.

The patient was a forty-one-year-old white female who was hospitalized forty-one times over a period of three years. The hospitalizations ranged from four to twenty-one days, and on several occasions, the patient signed herself out of the hospital against medical advice. She was a wheelchair-bound paraplegic subsequent to a gunshot wound to the spine. Her former husband was tried and convicted of the assault and was in prison. The patient's only child was placed in a foster home because the court deemed the patient "an unfit mother."

The patient presented to the Emergency Room with the following problems and history:

Fever > 103° F
Insulin dependent diabetic
Chronic urinary tract infection
Recurrent depression
Allergies to most antibiotics
Recurrent vaginal infection and pelvic rash
Intermittent alcohol and substance abuse
Multiple fractures due to osteoporosis
Poor nutrition and overweight—5'4" and 197 pounds
Deep and pitting ulcers on both buttocks due to poor hygiene/sanitation

The social history was relevant. The patient lived in an abandoned garage owned by a local farmer. There was no electricity and no running water, and the garage had a dirt floor. Water and electricity were supplied by way of a garden hose and extension cord from the farmer's house. There were no toilet facilities. The patient was well known to the local medical community for her consistent noncompliance. Over the years, many adjectives had been used by health care providers and others to describe her behavior. These included "rude," "hostile," "obstinate," "uncooperative," "cunning," "mean," and "blatantly self-destructive." One physician described Annie as "a bitch on wheels." Even though Annie had many serious medical problems, her uncooperative attitude and risky lifestyle made her case extremely difficult to manage. On her most recent admission, she spiked a fever of > 103° F, she had a raging urinary tract infection, and one of her ulcers was infected. This combination of medical problems, though serious, was fairly typical for this patient. However, a new problem surfaced on this visit to the hospital. Annie O. was also pregnant.

Case 3—Free Baby Formula

At question was a curious phenomenon. Health professionals were virtually unanimous in the belief that breast milk was best for infants. Evidence was overwhelming that breast milk reduced a baby's susceptibility to illnesses such as ear infections and stomach flu and played a positive role in many other ways such as mental and hormonal development. Why, then, did so many mothers who gave birth in hospitals choose synthetic baby formula? The reasons were many and varied, including opposition to breast-feeding from family and friends, lack of good information, unsympathetic work settings, and reasons of custom and fashion.

Many health professionals believed hospitals undermined breast-feeding by the widespread practice of giving new mothers free formula supplied by formula manufacturers. Research indicated the practice did make a difference. One study at Boston City Hospital, cited in *The Wall Street Journal*, found that 343 low-income women, who received free formula from the hospital, breast-fed their infants for a median duration of forty-two days, compared with sixty days for those who received no free formula—a difference of 30 percent. The article concluded with the observation that breast-feeding rates were not much higher than they were ten years ago.

At a joint meeting of the IECs of the three local hospitals, this issue of conflict of interest between formula manufacturers that supplied the free formula and the three hospitals was raised. All three hospitals accepted free baby formula. One breast-feeding proponent candidly described her suspicion of the close ties between hospitals and formula companies hoping to promote their product. Discussion of the issue by IEC members at this joint meeting resulted in four main options for dealing with the issue: (1) accept no free formula at all despite its availability; (2) give no free formula to those who breast-feed; (3) charge patients a nominal fee for the free formula, so families considered the cost of formula when making the breast-feeding decision; and (4) continue to issue free formula but also distribute information about the benefits of breast-feeding. The four options were not prioritized.

The Meeting

At Mr. Blackwell's request, the IEC of Regional Memorial Hospital was to meet to advise him on a morally justifiable course of action relative to the hospital's free baby formula practice and to offer advice on what to do about Baby Boy-X and Annie O.

Notes

1. R. E. Cranford and A. E. Doudera, "The Emergence of Institutional Ethics Committees," *Proceedings of the American Society of Law and Medicine* (April, 1983), p. 13.

2. M. Siegler, "Ethics Committees: Decision by Bureaucracy," *Hastings Center Report* 16 (June/July, 1986), pp. 3, 22.

DeKalb County Board of Health (A)

Selecting a New Director

It was 10 a.m. on a bright spring day as Cynthia Pallozi pulled into the DeKalb County Board of Health (DCBOH) parking lot. Pallozi was an hour early for her first meeting with the selection committee. Three weeks ago, she had accepted one of three community representatives' positions on the committee for the selection of the new director of DCBOH. Pallozi was still trying to understand why she had been nominated and why she had accepted. The only thing she knew about public health in general and the DeKalb County Board of Health in particular was that it gave immunization shots and reviewed the sanitation of restaurants. When she had visited Egypt, she had used DCBOH for her shots.

Pallozi had read in the *Atlanta-Journal* about the director, Dr. Bohn, dying in an automobile accident. That was in October of last year, and she had forgotten about it. Then, about four weeks ago, Dr. Derril Gay, DCBOH Interim Director, had called. At that time, Dr. Gay told Pallozi she was nominated because of her community work and professional experience as a realtor—activities that he believed would help her understand the needs of the community.

In a follow-up call, Dr. Gay provided a brief overview of Dr. Bohn's leadership. He recalled,

> Dr. Bohn assumed the director's position in 1976. She believed in the traditional medical model. That means she believed in generating services based on a professional assessment of the needs of the community. She was a committed professional. She recruited a noted physician to head the physical health unit in 1984–85. In addition, she replaced the Director of Environmental Health with an experienced professional in that area. Dr. Bohn actively sought grants to develop new programs. For example, she started the first AIDS task force in the state of Georgia. She was an outstanding leader and is greatly missed.

As required by Georgia statute, the selection of a public health agency director was a two-step process. First, a screening committee (consisting of state and local officials) reviewed all applicants and prepared a pool of candidates. Second,

---

These cases were prepared by Jane C. Nelson, Emory University, and Thomas C. Neil, Clark Atlanta University. They are intended as a basis for classroom discussion rather than to illustrate effective or ineffective handling of an administrative situation. Used with permission from Tom Neil.

a selection committee composed of individuals from the area served by the agency chose the next director from among the pool of candidates. The selection committee for DeKalb County was composed of the interim director, Dr. Derril Gay, two members from the DCBOH advisory board, Pallozi, and two other prominent members from the community.

In preparation for the selection committee's first meeting, Dr. Gay had asked all members to identify the characteristics and competencies suitable for the new director and to think about the leadership role the new director should play in carrying the agency into the new century. In addition, he had asked that each member prepare questions for the candidates that the group would review. Dr. Gay set two goals for the first meeting: establish the criteria to be used to review the résumés of the candidates and determine the questions that committee members wanted each candidate to answer. He sent a brief analysis of the status of DCBOH as well as a synopsis of continuing health programs and those initiated during the previous administrative year (Exhibit 9-1). Also in the packet was an overview of DeKalb County in terms of population, employment, human services, and number of patients served (Exhibit 9-2). Dr. Gay recognized that the community members had limited understanding of public health—especially in terms of the future of public health. Therefore, he provided a copy of *The Future of Public Health* (1988), prepared by the Institute of Medicine (see Exhibit 9-3).

To further prepare for this important task, Pallozi talked on the phone with the senior managers who had worked with Dr. Bohn. (See Exhibit 9-4 for her notes.) After speaking with the managers, she realized that leading an organization of 1,400 professionals—with myriad diverse service programs in a dynamic environment—was a monumental task. Further, she visited the local library and discovered that under Dr. Bohn's guidance, the DeKalb County Board of Health had become the leader in providing public health services within the state of Georgia. Numerous articles indicated that DCBOH was viewed as highly professional and that its management under the leadership of Dr. Bohn had initiated many programs that were adopted by other public health boards within the state.

Although she had been diligent in her preparation, Pallozi still had to write down the desirable characteristics, competencies, and the role to be played by the new director—as well as her questions. She decided to review—one more time—the notes she had made during the interviews with the senior managers and her notes from *The Future of Public Health*. She realized that the role played by the DeKalb County Board of Health in the twenty-first century would be vital to the county's continued growth and the diversity of issues it faced. Was that why she was having difficulty determining the characteristics for the next leader of DCBOH? Pallozi was committed to selecting the most qualified candidate and fervently hoped that her judgment would be beneficial. She looked at her watch. "Goodness, only forty-five minutes left. Better get cracking," she thought.

Exhibit 9-1. DeKalb County Board of Health Programs: Continuing and Initiated During 1987–88

Teenage Pregnancy Task Force: Developed because of continuing concern with the increased number of teen pregnancies. Benchmarking was done on successful programs across the United States, and San Francisco's was selected as a model.

Chlamydia Testing and Treatment of Prenatal Patients: Initiated because chlamydial infections were the most prevalent sexually transmitted infections affecting both women and children. These infections increased the risk of premature birth, ectopic pregnancies, stillbirths, and neonatal deaths.

Services to Homeless Persons: Based on a $22,025 grant from the Georgia General Assembly, provided nursing services between fifteen and twenty hours a week to three shelters.

Tuberculosis at DeKalb County Jail: Consisted of screening, contact investigations, and education.

Women, Infants, and Children (WIC): Increased 26 percent since 1986 for a total of 7,363 participants. An outreach program was established along with a priority system because of limited funding.

Early and Periodic Screening, Diagnosis, and Treatment (EPSDT): Provided valuable services to children on Medicaid.

Nutrition Project: Funded from a $19,407 grant from the U.S. Department of Agriculture, provided a nutritionist to conduct follow-up for high-risk infants.

Refugee Health: Screened 330 African, Southeast Asian, and Eastern European refugees.

School Health: Screened 24,443 children for hearing, 18,511 for vision, and 12,965 for scoliosis.

Mother and Infant Outreach: Provided intensive services to 688 infants. The Maternal Team contacted 4,155 pregnant women for education and follow-up services and received national recognition from the "Healthy Mothers and Children" organization.

Dental Health: Provided educational services to 42,438 school-age children, screened 32,685, and treated 9,956.

DUI Pilot Project: Assessed 118 individuals during the first six months. Those identified as high risk were required to attend a twenty-hour program.

The Food Protection Newsletter: Distributed quarterly to food service establishments. The newsletter focused on products, equipment, training, regulations, and policies.

Exhibit 9-2. DeKalb County: The Essence of the New South

The following summary was developed from information taken from the publication *Atlanta Region Outlook* (Atlanta, GA: Atlanta Regional Commission, 1989).

DeKalb County was recognized as one of Georgia's leaders. With the city of Atlanta on its western border and Stone Mountain rising on its eastern perimeter, DeKalb was at the hub of the region's growth. Traversed by Interstate Highways I-85, I-285, and I-20, it offered access for commercial and industrial traffic. DeKalb County, in cooperation with Fulton County, funded MARTA, a comprehensive public transportation system consisting of both buses and heavy rail.

Education was an important element in the county, which developed a public-supported community college with three campuses. Other institutions of higher learning in the county were Oglethorpe University, Agnes Scott College, and Emory University—offering undergraduate, graduate, and professional degree programs including a Master's of Public Health.

Population

In 1988, the population in DeKalb County was 539,770—an increase of 0.8 percent over 1987. Growth in the county was uneven, with the southeastern section growing the fastest because of lower land prices, large tracts of undeveloped land, and good infrastructure. Minority population growth continued to be slightly ahead of nonminority growth, with minorities accounting for 31.9 percent of the population. The Atlanta Regional Commission's projections for 2010 included a population of 701,318 (27 percent increase) and a rank of fourth in the Atlanta metro area.

Trends

1. Population growth would continue primarily in the southern half of the county. In the central section, a shift would occur as older couples retired out of DeKalb and younger families with children moved into the county.
2. The area south of I-285 would experience growth because of large tracts of undeveloped land with good infrastructure.
3. The growth in population would be largely from relocation of individuals from outside the Atlanta area seeking proximity to established schools and shorter drive times.
4. The percentage of children ages 0-19 was projected to remain constant through the year 2000.
5. All minority groups, especially Asians and Hispanics, would increase in percentages and actual numbers.
6. The elderly—those 55 or older—accounted for 9.8 percent (50,267) of the population in 1986. Their proportion was projected to grow to 18.9 percent by 2000. The percentage of elderly Asians and Hispanics was expected to grow significantly as the younger adults established themselves and provided for their parents.

Employment

An average of 313,518 residents was employed from a total labor force of 329,661. An additional 13,293 were added to the labor force in 1988. During the period from 1980 to 1988, DeKalb increased its working population more than any other Georgia county (81,629). DeKalb County accounted for

(Continued)

Exhibit 9-2. Continued

approximately 27 percent of the jobs in the seven-county Atlanta regional area. For the past five years, DeKalb averaged less than 5 percent unemployment. This low unemployment rate was attributed to the diversified economic base.

Human Services Activities

In addition to the DeKalb County Board of Health, the following human services were available:

DeKalb-Atlanta Human Services Center—a 54,000-square-foot structure—served the southwest DeKalb population. During 1988, 112,000 clients received services through one of the eight agencies: DeKalb-Grady Hospital Clinic, Dental Services, Community Health Assessment and Promotion Project, DeKalb County Department of Family and Children Services, Food Stamp Office, Kirkwood Mental Health/Mental Retardation Center, Economic Opportunity Neighborhood Services Center, and Georgia Power's Community Services Program.

DeKalb-Atlanta Senior Center—a 9,000-square-foot structure—opened in 1981 adjacent to the Human Services Center. Congregate meals, arts and crafts classes, fellowship, and other social activities were provided.

South DeKalb Senior Center—a 7,000-square-foot facility opened in 1979—provided services related to health (mental and physical), education, and recreation as well as home-delivered meals, transportation services, and shopping assistance.

Hamilton Community Center—a 45,000-square-foot facility that formerly was a high school—housed a 258-child Head Start Program; the Board of Education's Alternative High School; a gymnasium; and office space for departments of recreation, parks, and cultural affairs as well as for Georgia Power's Community Services Program.

Bruce Street/East DeKalb Center—housed within an old elementary school—provided services similar to those found at the South DeKalb Center.

The following table describes patients served in the DeKalb Health District in 1987.

Race/Sex	Number	Percentage
Black females	61,210	34.9
Black males	50,482	28.8
White females	33,888	19.3
White males	29,881	17.0
Total	175,461	

The budget for the DeKalb Health District for 1988 was $20,217,117; for 1989, it was $22,932,987.

Exhibit 9-3. Cynthia Pallozi's Notes on *The Future of Public Health*

The mission of public health seemed to emphasize generating organized community effort to address the interest the public had in health. The public health agency should provide scientific and technical knowledge to prevent disease and promote health among all citizens. The involvement of private organizations and individuals in a community's health was strongly recommended.

The core functions of public health agencies were identified as assessment, policy development, and assurance:

- Assessment for a public health agency entailed collecting and analyzing information on the health of the community and providing this information to the community.
- Lead in developing public health policy through strategic initiatives, in conjunction with the political process at the state and local levels.
- Assurance placed public health agencies in the position of actively ensuring community health through encouraging action by the private or public sectors, through development of regulations, or through direct services. Key policy makers and the general public were involved in prioritizing community-wide health services.

Exhibit 9-4. Cynthia Pallozi's Notes on Senior Managers' Perceptions of the DeKalb County Board of Health

Alan Siefert, MD, Director of Physical Health—started as a clinician in sexually transmitted diseases (STD) in 1986 and took over as head of physical health after seventeen or eighteen months. He stated that Dr. Bohn ran a tight ship. DCBOH was very organized, services were good, and DeKalb consistently received the highest rating for public health agencies in the state. The department developed service protocols, sent these to the state where they were approved, and then they were frequently adopted throughout the state. Focus was on clinical services delivered in an efficient manner.

Bill Fields, Director of Administration—image of DCBOH was positive and enjoyed a high level of public support. The general public saw DCBOH as a place for services for the poor and a place to get shots. Professionals throughout the state viewed us as the most effective health department because of the depth and professionalism of the staff, a health director who was a driving perfectionist, and a commitment to quality. DCBOH's mission was to protect the community from infectious disease. DCBOH saw its responsibility as providing preventive care to those who couldn't afford it. Through Medicaid, DCBOH began getting into more direct patient services. The vision for new regional centers began. Patient flow analysis and computerized records increased efficiency. Although DCBOH operated from a traditional medical service model, there was some innovation within the constraints set by Dr. Bohn.

Josephine Gordon, Lead Nurse—mission was to provide preventive health care in the county. Each community within the county seemed to view the Health Department in terms of its own needs. Management tried to integrate services with other agencies to benefit clients.

Mike Smith, Director, Environmental Health—when he arrived, DCBOH was doing a good job in traditional areas. With a few exceptions, DCBOH was ahead of other public health agencies in responding to the environmental needs of the county.

DeKalb County
Board of Health (B)

Redefining the Paradigm of Success

Among the candidates who made it through the screening committee and were presented to the selection committee for consideration as the new director of DeKalb County Board of Health was Paul Wiesner, MD. Dr. Wiesner had been a last-minute applicant who, even as he applied, was unsure about whether he really wanted to be the director of a local public health agency.

I was in my seventeenth or eighteenth year at the Centers for Disease Control—CDC is a federal agency located in Atlanta, Georgia. I had administrated the sexually transmitted disease (STD) program and been involved with the research program on smoking in Washington, D.C., under the Secretary of Health. Although I was only two or three years away from retirement at CDC, I wasn't happy with the direction the agency seemed to be taking. So, I was looking for a new challenge. I thought directing a local public health agency might be it. I have always enjoyed working directly with service delivery. It's fun to see a program work—to try and institute change and improve the quality of service. At the national level, I had been involved in the development of APEX-PH. That stands for assessment protocol for excellence in public health. It's a tool for assessing the status of a public health department, so I was aware of what public health could be doing.

Dr. Wiesner continued.

I decided to apply for the DeKalb County Board of Health Director position, and that's when I discovered how the process of selecting a director of a local public health agency works. The state of Georgia has a significant role. The Commissioner of the State Department of Human Resources designates the new director with approval by the local public health board. In part, this decision process is required because public health is delivered on a district basis, which typically includes two or more counties. That's why the official title is "District Director of Public Health." DeKalb County is one of the few single-county agencies in Georgia. I discovered that the director was responsible for physical health as well as mental health/mental retardation/ substance abuse. I had no background in mental health, mental retardation, or substance abuse, but I believed my background in working with the sexually transmitted disease program at the federal level could help. In physical health, I was strong. . . . But dealing with the chronically mentally ill was not my area.

I do believe my values are in line with the philosophy underlying MH/MR/SA's treatment mission. I recognized that I'd have to articulate this very clearly to those on the screening and selection committees. I looked for common connections based on my experience in physical health and the direc-

295

tion I saw public health heading. I identified three commonalties: caring, competence, and connections with the community.

In preparation for the selection process, I talked with people at the state and local level. I discovered that a major concern of the decision makers charged with oversight for public health within the Georgia Department of Human Resources was the categorical focus of the federal government. Basically, categorical focus means the federal decision makers select certain health issues and establish funding for the designated issues. The state and district departments thought they had to respond to these funding initiatives even if they believed another need was more pressing for their state or community. Because I was an employee of the Centers for Disease Control, I believed this would be a sensitive area.

Dr. Wiesner recalled the questions asked by the selection committee members as indicating they wanted a manager with good technical skills and someone who would get along well with others. He said, "I was prepared to discuss my enthusiasm for public health's broad mission as articulated in the Institute of Medicine's report on the future of public health: 'Public Health is what we all do individually and collectively to create the conditions in which people can be healthy.' We never discussed it."

Much to his surprise, Dr. Wiesner was selected as the new director of the DeKalb County Board of Health.

Assuming Leadership

Since his appointment, Dr. Wiesner had assessed the agency's strengths and needs for improvement by visiting more than 100 DeKalb County residents. He wanted to know what the community thought of the Board of Health and what could be done to improve the agency's performance. He discovered that although the agency had an excellent reputation within the profession, its visibility within the community was low. He concluded that the agency needed to shift its focus

from "the most needy" to "the most to benefit" and to broaden the base of resources and support. He wanted the provision of public health services in DeKalb County to be a true community venture.

Dr. Wiesner engaged the community by accepting every opportunity to speak to groups in a variety of forums as well as at breakfast clubs. At these meetings, he presented the linchpins for his vision:

1. Establish a democratic procedure that encompassed all stakeholders in making decisions about community health.
2. Rediscover ways to maintain prevention and provide primary care through community involvement.
3. Acknowledge and come to grips with the limits of the collective resources.

He envisioned a continuous connection between the DeKalb County Board of Health and the people it served. His vision would require community participation in strategic decisions to focus on the community becoming healthier. The goal of health orientation would require the technical expertise and information of the professional public health practitioners as well as the community's wisdom, insight, and energy. Dr. Wiesner recognized that DCBOH had an excellent reputation for analyzing health data and using it to direct clinical services. Service delivery focused on professional, medically related activities rather than on the community and its lay leaders. The mental health section of the agency under the specific statutory mandate to serve the "neediest" people suffering from mental illness, mental retardation, and substance addictions significantly influenced DCBOH's concept of care. MH/MR/SA accounted for approximately 1,000 of the 1,400 employees. Promotion of wellness and health, policy development, surveillance, epidemiology, and broad community collaboration were all secondary considerations to providing for the "neediest" people. Dr. Wiesner had come to believe that the future of public health in general—and DeKalb County Board of Health in particular—rested on a fundamental transformation of its historical vision and mission. Yet, DeKalb County Board of Health's track record of professionalism and service under the traditional paradigm was exemplary.

Dr. Wiesner recalled a conversation he had with a friend, with whom he often discussed his ideas and concerns. He confided,

> When I arrived at DCBOH, I soon realized its mission was very different from what I envisioned we would need for the next century. Population-based services were not central to the cultural lore or to the practice of decision making. If our agency continues with the paradigm that has worked so well in the past, we will die a slow death, and the potential of public health to provide a broad spectrum of care will be lost. Unfortunately, the transformation of public health in DeKalb County is not about responding to an external threat or meeting a specific crisis. Our problem—perhaps our opportunity—is how do I convince individuals that our existing success is insufficient and may be contradictory for our future success?

Dr. Wiesner could still hear his friend's reply. "Paul, your quandary is twofold: One, where do you initiate strategic transformation of this agency in the face of its historical as well as its relatively near-term success? And two, How do you initiate this transformation so the amount and intensity of resistance is minimal?"

As the light from the setting sun faded and the colorful autumn leaves became shades of gray, Paul Wiesner knew he had to answer the "where" and "how" if he was to be successful in leading DCBOH into the twenty-first century.

Red Tide and Red Ink in Escambia County, Florida

8 a.m., June 30, 2000

"Hello, Escambia County Health Department, Peter Lanza speaking," Dr. Lanza, medical director for Escambia County, said into the telephone.

"Hi Peter. This is John Smith from Okaloosa Health Department. I've just faxed you the latest report from the Department of Environmental Protection. I think you need to take a close look at it. Red tide is going to be an unwelcome visitor this summer by the looks of things," he concluded.

Lanza replaced the receiver. The day had just begun, and he could already feel a migraine coming on. He reached for the fax and began reading (Exhibit 10-1). Scattered fish kills were reported in Okaloosa County on June 30. Many dead fish, including twelve to eighteen dolphins, had been washed up. Sampling of the water supply one mile offshore indicated the presence of *G. breve* red tide bloom. The bloom was moving inland toward Pensacola.

Scanning farther down the page, Lanza's eyes fell on the cell count concentrations. He felt a sinking feeling in his stomach. The *G. breve* cell count reading was high. There were greater than a million cells per liter. This kind of level would result in a high number of fish kills, not to mention major respiratory irritation to humans. The resulting fish kills would pose severe problems regarding cleanup initiatives. Lanza's brow became furrowed as he pondered the consequences of an influx of respiratory irritants that could affect many of the area's population, residents and visitors alike. He thought, "I'd better review our last red tide data and also what happened in North Carolina."

2 p.m., June 30, 2000

The phone rang again. "Hello, this is Peter Lanza."

This case was originally developed by Tina Cummings, Willie Lipato, Mustafa Mohd, and Alan Rowan as a student project under the supervision of Susan L. Davies, Peter M. Ginter, Robert Jacobs, Donna J. Petersen, and Dale O. Williams at the School of Public Health, University of Alabama at Birmingham. The case was revised by Stuart A. Capper, Peter M. Ginter, and Linda E. Swayne. It is intended to be used as a basis for classroom discussion rather than to illustrate effective or ineffective handling of an administrative situation. Used with permission from Donna J. Petersen.

Exhibit 10-1. Department of Environmental Health Fax Received June 30/2000/8:00 a.m.

R E D   T I D E   S T A T U S   * * * * NW Coast * * * * 06/28/00 * * * * *

Summary On June 29, samples were collected in Choctawhatchee Bay because scattered fish kills had been reported. With regard to *G. breve* red tide, conditions remained above normal. As of June 29, reports of many dead fish and 12-18 dolphins and of 'spinning' fish continued regularly. On June 28, the bayous on either side of Niceville were particularly mentioned, so Panhandle state employees arranged samples. On 06/29, a bloom was present in samples 1 mi off Pensacola moving inland. Choctawhatchee Bay samples contain very high counts of red tide organism.

ALONGSHORE & NEARSHORE results & observations   [WEST to EAST]

Escambia / Santa Rosa

	Bloom appears to be moving inshore will arrive on beach approx. 06/29/00.	high*	

Okaloosa/Walton

	[all samples below included surface and bottom collections]		P	
06/29	Choctawhatchee Bay: Cinco & Garnier bayous	high*		DOACS (SEAS), Panama City
06/29	Destin Buoy	high*		DOACS (SEAS), Panama City
06/27	Choctawhatchee Bay: Boggy Bayou	high*		DOACS (SEAS), Panama City
06/27	Choctawhatchee Bay: 10 sites associated with shellfish harvesting areas	high*		DOACS (SEAS), Panama City

* a bloom of *Prorocentrum belizeanum* (also a dinoflagellate) was present. There is no indication that this species will cause any effects. However, discoloration of the water is possible, and, depending on how concentrated the bloom becomes, it could reduce oxygen levels in the water during night-time hours, which can cause marine mortalities in the early morning hours.

OFFSHORE results and observations

6/29	Transect off Pensacola ■ 1 and 5 miles = HIGH ■ 10 miles = HIGH ■ 20 miles = HIGH ■		FMRI volunteer

Shellfish (=bivalves [clams, oysters, but not scallops]) Harvesting Bans:
For current open/closed status of shellfish areas for harvesting, please call the DOACS Division of Aquaculture Automated Shellfish Information Line (tollfree) 1-877-304-4024 (& listen carefully though the CLOSED list); otherwise, contact one of the following field offices of the FL Dept. of Agriculture and Consumer Services: **Panama City at 850/747-5252, Apalachicola at 850/853-8317, Cedar Key at 352/543-5181, Murdock at 941/255-7406, or Palm Bay at 407/984-4890.**

NOTE: As of the 6/25 Information Line message, ALL approved or conditionally approved harvesting areas in the Panhandle are closed due to red tide.

Comments: none

Anticipated Actions: FMRI staff are obtaining water (surface and bottom) specifically from the sites of the most recently observed mortalities and odd behaviors so that the water itself can be tested for brevetoxins. This chemical method is still experimental and the analysis indicates only positive or negative for detectable toxin. When the samples are collected and analyzed, results will have to be interpreted with reservations.

Key for Results:	Gymnodinium breve cells/liter	Possible Effects
VERY LOW	< 10,000	Continued shellfish harvesting ban and possible respiratory irritation
LOW	< 100,000	Respiratory irritation and maybe fish kills
MEDIUM	100,000 to < 1,000,000	Respiratory irritation and probable fish kills
HIGH	> 1,000,000	As above plus discoloration

P = preserved samples   PRESENT = normal levels of 1000 cells or less

Prepared by Beverly Roberts, FWC FL Marine Research Institute, St. Petersburg 727-896-3625, status web site = www.fmri.usf.edu/redtide.com

"Hi. I'm Tom Zelose from the *Pensacola News Journal*. We're hoping to run an article on red tide in tomorrow's edition. Can you spare a few minutes to give me some information on red tide?"

Journalists made Lanza's skin crawl. He thought, "The press is notorious for sensationalizing environmental problems. They were responsible for the majority of misinformation about red tide the last time we had an occurrence, and as a result property values fell and resorts and hotels suffered cancellations, even when the beaches were not affected!" This irked Lanza; however, he thought, "Maybe this time I can somehow use the press to assist us." He realized he was going to have to be extremely cautious about what he told the reporter. He mused to himself, "I do not want any information about the high cell counts of red tide being revealed to the press at this stage—at least until we have time to weigh all the possible options. The last thing we need is the media causing panic among residents and visitors with a misinformed article."

To the reporter, Lanza said, "I'll give you some information on red tide, but I'd like you to run the article past me before you go to print tonight."

Zelose replied, "No problem. We can do that."

"Okay, what do you want to know?" Lanza asked.

"Well, first of all, what is red tide, and is it a new phenomenon?" the reporter responded.

"Red tide is caused by a phytoplankton, specifically, a microscopic alga called *Gymnodinium breve*, usually referred to as *G. breve*. This harmful algal bloom produces a toxin that in normal conditions is of no great concern to the surrounding environment. However, when there is a large concentration of the organism such as during a bloom, the toxin can overwhelm environmental resources of the organisms in the vicinity. Red tide isn't a new phenomenon. In fact, red tide has been reported along Florida's coast since the 1500s," Lanza reminded the reporter.

"So what are the effects to humans and wildlife of a large concentration of red tide?" the reporter continued. Lanza had anticipated that the reporter would ask this question. He had to be careful about how he communicated the risk. He answered, "Organisms are exposed to toxins through ingestion of the cells, by consumption of toxic prey, such as birds and fish, and also by aerosol transport. Fish receive the highest exposure to the toxin and therefore have the highest mortality rate. As a consequence, fish kill is the main effect."

"But what about affects on humans? Aren't shellfish affected, also?" the reporter queried.

"Yes, they can be. If *G. breve* concentrations of greater than five times ten to the third [5×10^3] cells per liter are recorded, it results in the immediate closure of shellfish beds because of the potential for neurotoxic shellfish poisoning. Although the majority of the red tide blooms are usually associated with mortality of invertebrates, fish, and birds, there have been numerous accounts of other marine animal mortality, especially dolphins and sea turtles. In 1996, 149 manatees died in southwest Florida during the winter and spring period," Dr. Lanza explained.

"Neurotoxic shellfish poisoning? That sounds pretty serious!" exclaimed the reporter.

"Well, that's the worst-case scenario. There is constant monitoring of the water, so shellfish beds are closed if the concentrations are above safe limits. Then the public will be advised not to consume any shellfish. If infected shellfish were to be consumed, the most likely effects would be gastrointestinal diseases," Dr. Lanza stated carefully.

"So besides consumption of shellfish, aren't there direct affects from just being on the beach if red tide is present—breathing problems and that sort of thing?" the reporter pressed.

"Well, the main public health concern is infection from stepping on the dead fish and also the smell. However, aerosols from the red tide can produce respiratory ailments. People may experience shortness of breath, but these symptoms cease if the affected person simply moves about 100 feet from the beach. Those most at risk are asthmatic sufferers, young children, and the elderly. If you like, I can fax a document that describes the health concerns about red tide," Dr. Lanza offered. (See Exhibit 10-2.)

Exhibit 10-2 The Health Impact of Red Tide

Mechanism of action:

- *G. breve* produces two types of lipid soluble toxins: hemolytic and neurotoxic. The neurotoxic toxins are known as brevetoxins.
- The major brevetoxin produced is PbTx-2; lesser amounts of PbTx-1, PbTx-3, and hemolytic components are produced.
- These toxins are depolarizing substances that open the voltage-gated sodium (Na+) ion channel in cell walls, leading to uncontrolled Na+ influx into the cell. This alters the membrane properties of excitable cell types in ways that enhance the inward flow of Na+ ions into the cell; this current can be blocked by external application of tetrodotoxin. It is believed that the respiratory problem associated with the inhalation of aerosolized Florida Red Tide toxins are due in part to the opening of sodium channels by the brevetoxin.

Clinical Presentation:

- The two forms of red tide toxin–associated clinical entities first characterized in Florida are an acute gastroenteritis with neurologic symptoms following ingestion of contaminated shellfish (NSP).
- Aerosolized red tide toxins respiratory irritation consists of conjunctival irritation, copious catarrhal exudates, rhinorrhea, nonproductive cough, and bronchoconstriction with the inhalation of the aerosol of Florida Red Tides, the toxins of *G. breve*.
- Some people also report other symptoms such as dizziness, tunnel vision, and skin rashes.
- In the normal population, the irritation and bronchoconstriction are usually rapidly reversible by leaving the beach area or entering an air-conditioned area.
- Asthmatics are apparently particularly susceptible, a finding confirmed in recent investigations with an asthmatic sheep aerosolized red tide toxins respiratory irritation model.
- Furthermore, there are anecdotal reports of prolonged lung disease, especially in susceptible populations such as the elderly or those with chronic lung disease.

Diagnosis:

- The diagnosis of Florida Red Tide toxin–associated clinical entities has been based on the clinical scenario of persons becoming ill with gastrointestinal and neurologic symptoms after eating shellfish or with acute respiratory symptoms similar to asthma after inhaling aerosols associated with exposure to Florida Red Tide toxins.
- Recent promising research includes: an FPLC methodology for the identification of the *G. breve* toxins, as well as antibodies to brevetoxin and a possible cell-based assay.

Treatment and Prevention:

- In 1999, the Florida Department of Health added NSP to their list of reportable diseases; however, aerosolized red tide toxins respiratory irritation is not a reportable illness.
- In the case of aerosolized red tide toxins respiratory irritation, the use of particle filter masks or retreat to air-conditioned environment will anecdotally provide relief from the airborne irritation.
- In sheep exposed to aerosolized red tide toxins, the use of cromolyn or chlorpheniramine may treat, and if used prophylactically, even prevent the bronchoconstrictive response; this may have implications for asthmatics and other susceptible persons exposed to aerosolized red tide toxins.
- The Florida Department of Environmental Protection (DEP) since the mid-1970s has conducted a control program with the closure of shellfish beds when *G. breve* concentrations are greater than 5000 cells/liter, until 2 weeks by testing for toxin with mouse bioassay testing. This should prevent cases of ingestion NSP related to contaminated shellfish consumption in most of the Florida human population, but not the respiratory irritation associated with exposure to aerosolized red tide toxins.

"Please do. It should help with my article. What are you guys doing over there to try and prevent this problem? I mean this sounds like a pretty dangerous situation," Zelose commented.

Dr. Lanza knew that Zelose was trying to get him riled. Calmly, he replied, "The state's role mainly focuses on prevention of red tide blooms by preventing nutrient loading of the water that flows into the marine environment. Scientists are not sure about the interaction of red tide blooms, but there does appear to be an association because the incidence of red tides has increased proportionately to the population growth in Florida."

"What exactly causes these *nutrient* increases, anyway?" the reporter pressed.

Dr. Lanza could hear the derision in Zelose's voice, and he would not allow himself to rise to the bait. Dr. Lanza knew that the Escambia Health Department was carefully monitoring the situation daily. At this stage, there were limited solutions to dealing with red tide. Perhaps in another five years there would be more solutions available to them. He carefully explained, "Nutrients flowing into the river, bays, and marine environments have many and varied sources. Some sources include septic tanks, crop and animal farming, storm water runoff, fertilizer from yards, and many others. Some studies have examined the application of clay to reduce toxic load. The clay is lightly spread across the water and it binds with the toxin. However, you can imagine the efficacy of this in the field is much lower than in the lab. It is also an expensive operation, and you can understand that we here at the Health Department have to weigh the possible benefits against the likely costs."

"Yeah, yeah, that's very interesting," the reporter replied, clearly finding the information to be less than titillating.

Dr. Lanza was beginning to lose his patience. He had important information he needed the public to understand, and this journalist was getting on his nerves.

The reporter had another question. "Do you think this red tide is going to be a problem this summer, then? It's Fourth of July weekend soon. What will happen if you have to close the beaches? That could have some serious consequences."

Dr. Lanza broke in, "Look, all I can tell you is that we're monitoring the situation closely. We cannot tell far in advance what the concentration in the water will be and which way the bloom will travel, or even how long it will last. The Escambia Health Department is on alert, though, and we will take the necessary precautions if the situation arises." Dr. Lanza felt he had suitably dodged the question, but he needed to get off the phone. "I am afraid I'm going to have to finish now, as I have some other issues pressing today. Remember that you said I could see the article before it goes to print."

"Yeah, sure. No problem," the reporter responded.

Hanging up the phone once more, Dr. Lanza was thankful that he did not have to prolong his conversation with the journalist. Zelose had raised a very important point, though. The Fourth of July weekend was in a few days. The weekend was one of the busiest of the year, with more than 100,000 visitors during the holiday last year. During the 1997 tourist season, well over a million visitors came to Pensacola. The area had always been popular with residents of the nearby states of Louisiana, Alabama, Georgia, Mississippi, and Texas, but visitors also came from as far north as Missouri and Michigan. Florida's beaches were nationally acclaimed. Perdido Key was among the top twenty beaches in the nation.

Reaching for his copy of *The Insiders' Guide to Florida's Great Northwest*,[1] Lanza reread the descriptive passage on Pensacola. The book stated:

> Come to our beaches. Wiggle your toes in the powdery white sand. Gaze out over the waves crashing at sea, then breaking gently on the shore. You'll come to understand why we've worked so hard to preserve this natural splendor.

Dr. Lanza had lived his entire life in and around Pensacola, and he could understand why visitors would flock to the region. Gazing out the window, he caught a glimpse of a bronzed young man skimming across the water on a jet ski. He loved water sports himself and understood the reasons why tourists were willing to part with their hard-earned dollars to go fishing, rent jet skis, charter boats, or go diving in the area around Pensacola, especially Perdido Beach. The water was beautiful. The whole area was beautiful.

Escambia County was home to 301,613 residents. More than half of the residents were between eighteen and fifty-four years of age, and most were white (76.6 percent). More than half of the residents were employed full-time within the county. Fifty-one percent of the working population in Pensacola was employed in either a service industry or retail trade. There were 558 restaurants in the area, with seating capacity for 47,709. There were thirteen hotels with a total of 1,304 rooms and sixty-six motels with 4,899 rooms. All these businesses and their employees (as well as many others) could suffer huge economic consequences if the beaches had to be closed this summer. Dr. Lanza remembered reading that in 1987, closure of shellfish harvesting areas alone caused a loss of $25 million in North Carolina. He thought, "The red tide concentration levels in the report I just read are far higher than levels in North Carolina in 1987."

The per capita income in Escambia County was $19,852 in 1999. Local residents worked hard for a living, and although people grumbled about the tourists, there was no doubt that without them, life would be very difficult. Dr. Lanza recalled, "Red tide occurred last year and the beaches remained open. However, the cell count per liter was less than 10,000. This had resulted in some fish kill and an increase in the number of asthma cases in the ER during the summer period." He continued to ponder the situation. "Will I really have to order the close of the beaches? We could just put the ER on red alert and warn the public. Those who are most susceptible are asthma sufferers—young children and elderly. However, the G. breve cell count was very likely to cause respiratory irritation in non-asthmatics too, and just about anyone who was exposed."

Examining data from the federal Centers for Disease Control and Prevention, Dr. Lanza quickly calculated the predicted number of asthmatic visitors to the region. He calculated that 6 to 8 percent of the population had asthma. This meant that there could be more than 8,000 persons with severe respiratory problems during the holiday weekend in Escambia County. Last year, visitors had reported symptoms of dizziness, tunnel vision, and skin rashes. Although there was a lack of sound scientific data that red tide caused bronchoconstriction, Lanza knew himself that G. breve in the reported concentration could result in breathing difficulties for any people on the beach.

"Warning the public of the health risk is essential," he thought, "but how can a public health education campaign reach out-of-state visitors?" The Pensacola News Journal and the local television and radio stations (WCOA and WEAR) could be involved in informing residents. "But how can we reach those people traveling from Missouri, Michigan, and Texas? And what did the public already know about red tide? Was the information accurate? How can I communicate the risk but at the same time not cause panic? Can I just inform those who were most vulnerable, or do I need to warn everyone who planned to go to the beaches? Closing beaches would require mobilizing more police units to ensure that people did not try to go onto the beaches. . . ." These questions and many others would need to be addressed, and rather quickly. Dr. Lanza was not confident that the current surveillance system was able to quickly detect an increase in respiratory problems. He glanced at the clock. It was already after 5:30 p.m. He decided that there wasn't much more he could do today.

8 a.m., July 1, 2000

The following morning, as Lanza picked up the newspaper and opened his office door, the phone was already ringing. He rushed to answer it.

"Dr. Lanza? This is the Mayor." The urgency of the Mayor's tone was apparent. Lanza was worried. "Have you seen the paper this morning?" queried the Mayor.

"No sir," responded Dr. Lanza.

"Well, I want to have a decision by noon today about what the hell we're going to do. We may have to close the beaches," he speculated.

The Mayor hung up, and Lanza replaced his receiver. Pulling the morning paper out of its plastic wrapping, he saw, to his horror, the front page headline:

CHILD DIES ON DESTIN BEACH, RED TIDE SUSPECTED

Shaking his head in disbelief, Dr. Lanza reached for his coffee. "I don't have much time to decide what to do about the beaches. Can they possibly remain open over the Fourth of July weekend after this sort of publicity?" he wondered.

Note

1. Robin H. Rowan and Clark Perry, *Insiders' Guide to Florida's Great Northwest*, 2d ed. (Monteo, N.C.: Insiders' Publishing, 1995), p. 357.

The New Mexico Meningococcal Outbreak

Prologue

The vastness of the landscape that was the northwestern region of New Mexico could not be overstated. It was "where a single glance can take in several hundred square miles of land and several hundred million years of history."[1] Within this circumscribed area of nearly 75,000 square miles was Chaco Canyon, the heart of the ancient Anasazi culture; Los Alamos, where the nuclear age began; a large portion of the Navajo Nation and all of the Jicarilla Apache Homelands; the fabled San Juan trout waters and the Bisti Badlands; great expanses of the Santa Fe, Carson, and Cibola National Forests; and the sacred mountains of Shiprock, Taylor, and Cabazon. The area was vast, sparsely populated, and ethnically and racially diverse.

It was in this part of northwestern New Mexico in the late spring of 1993 that a mysterious outbreak of unexplained respiratory failure and death occurred in otherwise healthy young persons. During a nineteen-day period, twenty-four cases (with twelve deaths) were identified with what would later be called the *Hantavirus* pulmonary syndrome—the first illness attributable to the exotic class of viral hemorrhagic fever viruses to be described in North America. The worldwide public and media attention focused on the area was unprecedented. The fear and pain that directly affected virtually every person, family, clan, and community in the region was compounded by the discrimination, ostracism, and stigmatization of being associated with the deadly disease. It was against this backdrop that the following events occurred.

From Measles to Meningitis

"Mary, you're not going to believe this!" Those seven words were to make it a day that Dr. Mary Cooperman would not soon forget. Dr. Cooperman was the health officer for District I of the New Mexico State Public Health Division of the New Mexico Department of Public Health (NMDOH). (The glossary on page 316 provides a list of acronyms.) Sitting in her Albuquerque office with other members of the staff, she was about to participate in a scheduled 4:00 p.m. conference call with the NMDOH's State Epidemiology Division regarding the ongoing measles outbreak in Albuquerque. (See Exhibit 11-1 for a description of the New Mexico Department of Health.)

This case was prepared by Gary Simpson, Maria Goldstein, Patricia Barnett, Paul Ettestad, Judith Candelaria, and Stuart Capper, University of Alabama at Birmingham. It is intended as a basis for classroom discussion rather than to illustrate effective or ineffective handling of an administrative situation. Used with permission from Gary Simpson.

Exhibit 11-1. New Mexico Department of Health

The New Mexico Department of Health (NMDOH) was a large, multifaceted, centralized organization with more than 4,000 employees and an annual budget of $300 million. The department provided direct services for the developmentally disabled as well as services for citizens in need of mental health care, substance abuse treatment, and long-term care. Additionally, the department provided statewide public health services, public health laboratory services, and epidemiologic investigation for communicable disease outbreak control. The Public Health Division; the Division of Epidemiology, Evaluation, and Planning; and the Scientific Laboratory Division were three of eight divisions within the Department of Health that routinely worked together on outbreak control.

A classic, yet decentralized, bureaucracy, the Public Health Division was organized into seven program-specific bureaus and four geographic districts. A staff of more than 1,000 included 15 physicians, 25 nurse practitioners/physician assistants, 125 registered nurses, and more than 200 other public health professionals. Fifty-five public health offices were scattered throughout the state. Several of these offices were mobile units. Staff in the offices were state rather than county employees.

The organization stated its mission as

> The mission of the Public Health Division of the Department of Health is to work with individuals, families, and communities in New Mexico to achieve optimal health. We provide public health leadership by developing health policy, sharing expertise with the community, assuring access to coordinated systems of care, and delivering services to promote health and to prevent disease, injury, disability and premature death.

District 1 of the New Mexico Public Health Division consisted of seven counties covering the central and northwest area of the state (see map). The district contained the most populous and only truly urban area of

Map of Cuba, New Mexico, Area

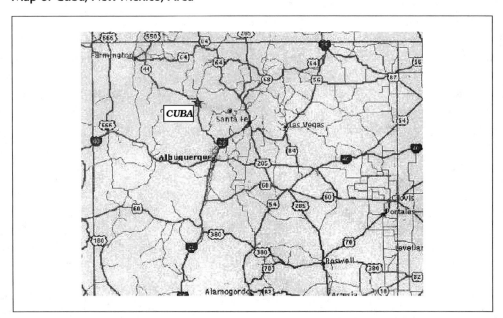

(Continued)

Exhibit 11-1. Continued

the state—Albuquerque. It contained six other counties that were very rural, some with population densities of fewer than four persons per square mile. The district served an ethnic population that was representative of the state. In the northwestern portion of the district, especially in McKinley and northern Sandoval counties, a large proportion of the population was Native American, either Navajo or Jicarillo Apache. Because the boundaries of these reservations and state, federal, and private lands followed a serpentine course, this area was known as the "checkerboard" area.

Fifteen public health offices in District I covered the seven counties. Each public health office was managed by a team of public health workers that varied from office to office but usually consisted of a public health nurse, a clerk, a WIC nutritionist, health promotion staff, and a social worker. The programs offered varied somewhat, but the core public health programs of immunizations, family planning, WIC, infectious disease investigation and control, wellness education, and community organizing were present in differing degrees in most health offices. Communicable disease investigation and control was usually carried out by public health nurses following orders and protocols from the District Health Officer and the Division of Epidemiology, Evaluation, and Planning (a division of NMDOH).

The Division of Epidemiology, Evaluation, and Planning conducted surveillance for communicable diseases and provided epidemiologic investigation and evaluation services for the state. The division had four physician epidemiologists, seven PhDs, two veterinary epidemiologists, three RNs (one with an MPH), and five master's level epidemiologists. The division's information system was supported by a systems analyst manager and two systems analysts. Surveillance data were stored, plotted, and analyzed using a complement of hardware and software.

The Scientific Laboratory Division (another division of NMDOH) was a public health and environmental laboratory centrally located in Albuquerque on the campus of the University of New Mexico School of Medicine. Its mission was to provide laboratory support services for tax-supported agencies and groups administering programs for New Mexico citizens. It provided routine and specialized laboratory testing in the areas of microbiology, cytopathology, chemistry, and toxicology. Its services were routinely provided to the Division of Epidemiology, Evaluation, and Planning as well as the Division of Public Health. In addition, the laboratory provided reference services for clinical facilities throughout the state for tests not available on-site. The scientific laboratory division played a crucial role in the national infectious disease surveillance activities of the Centers for Disease Control and Prevention (CDC) by serving as a link between clinicians in New Mexico and CDC. A twenty-four-hour overnight courier service in support of specimen delivery to the laboratory was provided to all local public health offices.

Other organizations involved in this outbreak included the University of New Mexico Hospital, the Office of the Medical Investigator, Emergency Medical Services, Indian Health Service, and the San Juan Regional Medical Center.

University Hospital was a 300-bed acute care hospital in Albuquerque affiliated with the University of New Mexico School of Medicine. It was located on the School of Medicine campus just adjacent to the Scientific Laboratory Division (SLD). The largest concentration of infectious disease specialists in the state was affiliated with the University Hospital and the School of Medicine.

The Office of the Medical Investigator (OMI) at the University of New Mexico School of Medicine was the centralized statewide medical examiner agency for New Mexico. The OMI investigated all deaths in New Mexico that were sudden, suspicious, violent, unnatural, unexpected, or unexplained. In addition, the agency contracted with the Navajo Nation to provide autopsies. An OMI death investigation included a review of the scene and circumstances of death. A final classification of the cause and manner of death was produced after full investigation, which could include autopsy and multiple laboratory tests.

(Continued)

Exhibit 11-1. Continued

Emergency Medical Services (EMS) was a system in New Mexico that provided timely emergency medical care to the entire population. In some of the smallest and most rural communities, the EMS system was the only locally available source of medical care for residents and visitors. It was a vital public safety service and an integral component of the health care system. EMS had a dedicated communications system that allowed field-to-hospital interaction for medical direction. The field component across the state involved thousands of paid and nonpaid (volunteer) certified first responders and licensed emergency medical technicians.

The Indian Health Service (IHS) provided comprehensive health care and public health services to Native Americans throughout New Mexico. Epidemiology and disease control programs were central to these activities. The Epidemiology Branch of IHS acted directly and through technical consultation to (1) coordinate, facilitate, and lead public health responses to disease outbreaks on Indian lands; (2) develop, maintain, and monitor surveillance systems; and (3) provide direction to disease control programs.

The Navajo Area Office (one of the two IHS area offices with jurisdiction in New Mexico) was located in Window Rock, Arizona. It provided services to more than 200,000 members of the Navajo Nation in Arizona, Utah, and New Mexico. The Navajo Nation was a sovereign nation within the United States. Any outbreak response needed the cooperation of the president of the Navajo Nation as well as the Navajo Nation Department of Health (NNDOH). Care was provided through a system of 6 hospitals, 7 health centers, and 132 health stations. In addition, IHS stationed public health nurses throughout communities in the Navajo area.

The other IHS area office was located in Albuquerque. All IHS hospitals and some of its health centers had medical laboratories, but frequently specimens were sent to SLD for testing. The Navajo Nation had a group of grass-roots community health workers called community health representatives (CHRs) stationed in each community that were counted on for their interpreting skills.

One of the IHS hospitals was located in Crownpoint. The Director of Community and Preventive Health for the hospital was responsible for communicating any outbreak response efforts to the hospital CEO and other executives as well as the medical staff. IHS had public health nurses, drivers/interpreters, and secretarial support to contribute to outbreak control efforts. Staff were experienced in interviewing community and case contacts. The IHS and the NMDOH functioned under two different chains of command, rules and regulations, and budgets.

The San Juan Regional Medical Center (SJRMC) was located in the Four Corners area. The center included an emergency room, an immediate care center, diagnostic laboratory and X-ray services, and a full range of medical specialties. The hospital had 145 medical/surgical beds and 15 licensed skilled-nursing beds.

District I encompassed the northwestern quadrant of New Mexico as well as Albuquerque, New Mexico's largest city, and its surrounding counties. During the first week of March, the district experienced a serious measles outbreak in and near the Albuquerque area. Dr. Cooperman and her staff had been putting in long hours setting up clinics, screening, doing contact investigation, and maintaining follow-up. Staff time was stretched almost to its limit. A final effort to contain the outbreak was the main focus of the conference call.

Dr. Cooperman thought that Alice Navarro, a state epidemiology nurse, was joking when, after her attention-getting first statement, she went on to say, "There are three more meningitis cases in the Cuba area!" It became apparent that Navarro was dead serious. She continued, "There are two siblings, ages seventeen and eighteen, who attend Cuba High school and another eight-year-old child who attends Torreon Grade School. They are being admitted to University Hospital with diagnoses of meningococcal infection." (See Exhibit 11-2 for a description of the communities in the Cuba, New Mexico, area.)

Dr. Cooperman did a quick mental inventory of the events of the past week. On Sunday, March 5, Dr. Michael Session, the State Epidemiologist, was on weekend call. Dr. Session's job was routine surveillance and communication to monitor outbreak investigations and determine when control efforts might be indicated. A call came in from Dr. Garland Underwood, Pediatric Infectious Disease Specialist at the University of New Mexico Hospital (UNMH) in Albuquerque, to report that a three-year-old female had been admitted with signs and symptoms compatible with infectious meningitis. Cerebral spinal fluid (CSF) and blood cultures were pending, but Dr. Underwood was fairly certain of his diagnosis.

Dr. Session contacted Dr. Cooperman at home. Dr. Cooperman called the public health nurse epidemiologist in Albuquerque and asked her to call the family of the sick child to identify contacts. The nurse called back that evening after talking to the parents and reported that no one else in the family had been sick. She learned that the child attended a day care center. The household contacts had been given Rifampin prophylaxis. A plan was developed to go to the day care center first thing the next morning to check on the health status of the other children and staff and to deliver a letter informing parents and staff of the exposure, symptoms to watch for, and recommendations for prophylaxis.

On Monday, March 6, Dr. Session gave the information to the surveillance nurse in the NMDOH Division of Epidemiology who was on call for the day and would follow up on the investigation. She contacted the state SED lab in Albuquerque, which had the blood and CSF specimens. The Gram stain of the CSF contained Gram-

negative diplococci and reinforced the concern that the organism was indeed *Neisseria meningitidis*. Culture results were still pending.

More Meningitis

That evening, Dr. Session received a call from the UNMH about a thirteen-year-old boy in the intensive care unit (ICU) with signs and symptoms of meningococcal meningitis. The boy was from the small Navajo community of Ojo Encino, ninety miles northwest of Albuquerque. He had been seen on Friday, March 3, at a clinic in Cuba but was initially diagnosed with sinusitis. He was seen again in the clinic on Monday with cough, fever, headache, and a rash on the anterior trunk and arms—all consistent with meningococcal infection. The boy was sent to UNMH by ambulance that evening. Blood cultures were pending, and Indian Health Service (IHS) in Crownpoint was notified. A public health nurse was sent out from that facility to interview contacts and give Rifampin prophylaxis. Parents and employees of the day care center in Albuquerque were in need of reassurance. Dr. Session knew that the NMDOH Division of Epidemiology probably would be dealing with the press very soon.

On Tuesday, March 7, as efforts were continuing, the infection control nurse from UNMH called Alice Navarro to update her on the condition of the two known cases. The thirteen-year-old had *Streptococcus pneumoniae* growing from a sputum culture, was responding to painful stimuli, and was being given clindamycin and ceftriaxone. This diagnosis confused the issue on whether this was meningococcal disease, but signs and symptoms were compatible with the original diagnosis.

Meanwhile, further conversations with the parents of the index case uncovered a travel history revealing that the three-year-old had visited Cuba, where her grandparents lived, the week before becoming sick and while there had attended some sort of large gathering. Sara Valdez, Public

Exhibit 11-2. Community Descriptions

Sparsely populated and predominantly rural (fewer than thirteen persons per square mile), New Mexico was the nation's fifth largest state. Communities were separated by deserts and by mountains that ranged in height from 2,800 to 13,000 feet. In some parts of the state, a person could drive for ninety miles without seeing another human being. The Rio Grande, one of the Southwest's most important waterways, ran from the northern part of the state to the southern part.

More than 1.6 million people lived in New Mexico. The median age was 32; 50 percent of the population was Anglo, 40 percent Hispanic, and 9 percent Native American. The Native American population in the state was dispersed among twenty pueblos that included the Jicarillo Apaches, the Mescalero Apaches, and 90,000 Navajos. The Native American population differed from the state's non–Native American population in such vital statistic indicators as lower prenatal care, lower birth weight, and leading causes of death. The life expectancy of whites and Hispanics in New Mexico was higher than the United States as a whole; however, for African Americans and Native Americans it was lower.

New Mexico was an economically poor state, ranking forty-fourth in per capita income. Socioeconomic indicators revealed that 46 percent of Native Americans lived at or below the poverty level, as compared with 17 percent for the state as a whole. Medicaid benefits were received by 250,000 New Mexicans.

The Navajo Nation was a large reservation established in 1880 that spanned much of the Four Corners region (so named because the borders of four different states—Utah, Colorado, Arizona, and New Mexico—met there). With more than 200,000 members, the Navajo was the largest Indian tribe in the United States. The Navajo people experienced a great deal of change during the twentieth century, but many of their population were still tending livestock and engaging in traditional crafts such as rug weaving or silver smithing. The younger generation, however, tended to look for employment off the reservation and often commuted long distances to reach the hospitals, schools, or businesses where they worked. Dwellings consisted of traditional wood hogans as well as newer cinder block and wood frame houses and trailers. Because of the openness of the landscape, the usual infrastructure of natural gas, running water, electricity, and telephones was still in the developmental stage. It was not unusual to enter a home where only electricity was available to the family.

Cuba was somewhat of an anomaly in an otherwise rapidly growing Sandoval County that also contained the communities of Torreon, Ojo Encino, and Counselors. The county adjoined Albuquerque, the largest city in New Mexico. State Highway 44, Cuba's main street, was the link between Albuquerque and Farmington, the two major business areas in northern New Mexico. Although the overall population of the county had increased 82 percent since the 1990 census, the community of Cuba went from a population of 760 to 733. Cuba, originally known as Naciemento, was a farming and ranching center for 200 years. Many ranches were scattered throughout the area, including the "checkerboard," which was a geographical region west of Cuba that presented a patchwork of privately owned and reservation land. With no major industry, the primary occupations were federal, state, and county related. The town was a refueling stop for tourists and truckers. The entire area was situated in the western foothills of the Jemez mountains and attracted hunters, campers, hikers, archaeologists, and anthropologists.

A grade school, middle school, high school, and small Catholic elementary school served the educational needs in Cuba. Many students were bused in from the surrounding communities. A new, large senior center in town served as a senior meal site. Many residents of outlying areas came to Cuba for grocery shopping and medical care. This area included sections of the Jicarillo Apache reservation.

Health care facilities in the Cuba area included Presbyterian Medical Services (PMS) clinic, Naciemento Health Care clinic, and a volunteer ambulance service. PMS operated a primary care facility and provided an emergency room and stabilization service for transfer to Albuquerque or Farmington when higher medical technology was needed. It was served by rotating staff medical doctors out of Albuquerque.

(Continued)

Exhibit 11-2. Continued

The Naciemento Health Care Foundation, a not-for-profit community organization, was staffed by two physicians and a part-time nurse. In addition, the organization provided office space for the New Mexico Public Health Department's public health nurse. The Cuba Public Health Office was a single-wide trailer provided through a contract with the Naciemento Foundation. The office had a fax machine, two incoming and outgoing telephone lines, and a small, slow copy machine. The office was adjacent to the Naciemento Health Center.

As State Highway 44 passed through Cuba and headed north to Farmington, it went through the small community of Counselors at the northern border of Sandoval County. This settlement had an evangelical mission, a day school, and a boarding school that served many children from the Navajo Reservation.

Ojo Encino and Torreon were about thirty miles southwest of Cuba and eighty miles east of the nearest Indian Health Service hospital. The two communities were located about one-and-a-half hours from Santa Fe or Albuquerque. They were more realistically described as geographic areas rather than full-fledged towns. Geographically, the two communities differed mostly in terrain. Ojo tended to be flatter and with sandier soil, whereas Torreon had more of a rocky terrain, with small plateaus dotting the greater part of the community. Both communities were reached by a paved road out of Cuba; however, once past the main community, dirt roads became the norm. The clusters of homes in which most of the population lived were called "camps" and were often separated by miles of dirt roads, best traveled in a pickup truck or a four wheel drive vehicle. Basic electronic communication was hindered by the scarcity of telephones or fax machines and an almost nonexistent cellular phone system.

Ojo Encino and Torreon had a combined population of about 4,500. Family members in many homes spanned the age range from infants to senior citizens. Although younger adults and children were likely to speak both the traditional Navajo language and English, elders usually spoke and understood only Navajo. Income came from a variety of sources, such as senior supplemental income, self-employment, and live-stock proceeds. Younger adults, if employed in neighboring towns and cities, often returned home late in the evening, sometimes only on weekends, or during school breaks or the holiday season.

The traditional Navajo philosophy concerning life encompassed an older, pre-European religious and social system. This philosophy included concepts of health and illness and a value system that led to such expectations as sharing material resources such as income, pickup trucks, and child-rearing duties among family members. It also included a number of religious events called ceremonies. Traditionally many young women continued to live in their parents' camps after marriage. Grandparents were enlisted to help care for children because of the employment of parents in nearby cities. Older family members might be the only adults at home during the work day and often assumed an informal guardian-like role for their grandchildren.

The meningococcal outbreak occurred in five communities—Cuba, Counselors, Ojo Encino, Torreon, and Pueblo Pintado—located in the Four Corners area.

Health Nursing Director at the Crownpoint Medical Facility (IHS), called to let Navarro know the status of the ongoing contact investigation in Ojo Encino. The large extended family of the thirteen-year-old had been given Rifampin. No connection with the first case had been uncovered.

On Wednesday, March 8, Dr. George Hegland, who was on day call for the NMDOH Division of Epidemiology, was called by UNMH lab with culture results on the thirteen-year-old boy. *Neisseria meningitidis* was growing on his CSF culture. The sample was being sent to the state lab for serotyping. In addition, Dr. Hegland received a call from IHS in Crownpoint on another suspected meningitis case. A thirty-two-year-old pregnant woman who was in the Ojo Encino area had been delivered at a neighbor's home the previous night. She was now showing signs and symptoms of meningitis and had been airlifted to UNMH that day. A spinal tap had been done and showed Gram-negative diplococci. The lab in Crownpoint had also found serum positive for Type C *Neisseria meningitidis* by counterimmunoelectrophoresis. The isolate was being sent to the state lab. Sara Valdez already had IHS public health nurses following up on prophylaxis of family members.

It was beginning to look suspicious. The large geographic area and the visiting habits of the native people were making contact investigation difficult. There was still no firm link between the cases, and they were still thought to be isolated incidents.

Meanwhile, measles and a case of botulism were occupying a large portion of the divisions' time. A teleconference between Dr. Hegland and IHS physicians in Albuquerque and Crownpoint on Wednesday evening focused on getting a measles vaccine campaign up and running on the Navajo Reservation. There was only brief mention of the two recent meningitis cases.

The State Epidemiology nurse on call received a telephone call from a physician at the Cuba Clinic. He was sending two patients to UNMH with fever, maculopapular rashes, headaches, and other signs and symptoms compatible with meningococcal disease. One patient, an eight-year-old Native American female, was airlifted to UNMH. Another patient, a seventeen-year-old Native American male, was sent to UNMH by ground ambulance. His sister, who also reported fever, back pain, and a stiff neck, was coming in to the Cuba Clinic as soon as possible.

What to Do?

Dr. Cooperman's immediate reaction to this latest news was disbelief, followed by apprehension. The north-central area of New Mexico, beginning at the boundary of the small village of San Ysidro, sixty miles north of Albuquerque, was dominated by State Highway 44. The road was a well-traveled major link between the state's largest city, Albuquerque, and its fourth largest, San Juan, with a population of 100,000. The communities between Albuquerque and San Juan were tiny, scattered, and lacking in many basic services. Many families still carried in their own water. Many homes were without electricity or telephone service. Residents traveled long distances for food and medical care, often over rutted and muddy roads. There was often no transportation available.

"If this is a community outbreak," Dr. Cooperman thought, "it will not be easy to get information, staff, and services to the area." Cellular phone service was very limited in this area, as were fax machines. IHS vehicles were equipped with two-way radios, but they did not interface with state communications. In terms of local state-employed staff, the Cuba area was home to one full-time public health nurse, one full-time clerk who spoke Spanish, and a full-time WIC clerk who spoke Navajo. The public health office was housed in a white single-wide trailer just off the main street.

Because they knew of the fear that gripped northwest New Mexico during the *Hantavirus* outbreak in 1993 and the subsequent incidents of racial stereotyping that developed, the conference call participants were concerned not only about the health of the people in the region but also about their well-being as a community. The "measles" call turned into a "meningitis" call. The discussion of the emerging meningitis situation continued. Public Health Division Director Marge Dayton and Dr. Simon Friedman, Chief Medical Officer for the state, joined the discussion, as had Harriet Bradley, Director of Public Health Nursing for the northwest area. Secretary of Health David Navia had been notified and joined the call shortly thereafter.

As the conversation progressed, Dr. Cooperman's sense of concern deepened because the disease seemed to be spreading so rapidly. She commented, "We really need to make our decisions quickly. The area is remote and seems to be where the outbreak is occurring." She felt that the Indian Health Service had most of the responsibility for the area but that the roles and responsibilities were far from clear. She knew about the follow-up and prophylaxis on the cases that were in Albuquerque, where Public Health had jurisdiction, but she did not know the status of the cases in the IHS areas that had been referred. She listened anxiously to the alternatives that were being discussed and began to think about the implications for swift action that each presented.

Attempting to Reach Consensus

Efforts were made to include IHS in the conference call, but it was after 5:00 p.m., and key staff could not be reached. The absence of Jack Estes, the Chief Epidemiologist for IHS, was an important factor as the discussion progressed. Without his input, there were distinct gaps in information that could influence major decisions. The group tried to decide: Considering his background and training in epidemiology, would he support intense contact investigations or mass immunizations or both? Furthermore, they questioned how well plans made by the group would fit into the context of IHS philosophy and resources. So far, the cases involved several families and several schools, most in Estes's jurisdiction. What public health intervention would he recommend?

Secretary Navia was very new to his responsibilities at the State Health Department. After being notified of the rapid developments of Thursday afternoon, he listened carefully to the discussion. As he listened, he could not help reflecting that he was hearing a group of excellent professionals doing what they did best. He thought about the area of the state that was involved. It was a very rural area, and he did not know who the contacts were at the community level. He was concerned about whether the community would really understand the difference between a cluster outbreak and a community-wide outbreak. In addition, he wondered whether the health professionals could locate the actual

source of the outbreak. As head of the department, he knew he could challenge the decisions of the participants in the conference call, but he was not going to second-guess their medical and epidemiological expertise.

The Centers for Disease Control and Prevention (CDC) in Atlanta was contacted to consult on the outbreak. Dr. Jason Dever took the call. He shared his experience in community outbreaks and institutional (point source) outbreaks. The current situation was unusual for a community outbreak in light of the rapidity of new case occurrences. The cases seemed much too scattered for it to be an institutional outbreak.

Everyone on the call seemed to struggle with the uncertainty. There was still no clear picture of what was happening. IHS had begun the investigation of the third case, but it had not been completed. It was not clear what the "Cuba Connection" was. Everyone participating in the call, including the CDC representative, was amazed at the rapidity of the evolution of the cases. Dr. Cooperman said, "This is not the usual behavior for sporadic meningococcal cases when aggressive contact investigation and chemoprophylaxis of exposed close contacts contains the spread. The usual measures are not working this time, and the cases are piling up faster than the contact investigation is able to proceed—especially given the cultural, geographical, and language barriers." Many of the other participants voiced their agreement.

Dr. Cooperman was gripped by the responsibility of having to protect the public against a frequently lethal and rapidly spreading organism when the usual public health weapons seemed to be failing. She questioned, "Are we dealing with an extremely susceptible population? An incredibly virulent organism with a high attack rate? Are there some environmental circumstances, events, or cultural behaviors that allowed for the rapidity of the spread? Are we going to be able to answer these questions in a timely manner to prevent new cases? What impact would the previous *Hantavirus* experience have on the area? Would people panic? Would people trust that the right decision would be made? Would residents of the area be willing to cooperate in the case investigations given their previous experience?" Dr. Cooperman further thought, "There is little time to decide on a coherent, rational, and feasible public health response—but the trust and goodwill of the people will depend on it." Then she was back to the questions: "What is the right public health response under the circumstances? Would vaccination work?"

Dr. Dever of the CDC was noncommittal when the possible need for a vaccine effort was suggested. "Whenever there have been community outbreaks, immunization strategies seem to work in stopping the outbreak, but it isn't clear if that is a result of the vaccine or the natural progression of the event. I can understand why you might want to try it, but I'm not sure if that's the solution," he stated.

Dr. Underwood from the University of New Mexico Hospital (UNMH) joined the call and stated, "I have examined the most recent cases, and there is no question in my mind that the diagnosis in all three new cases is meningococcal infection." Suddenly and rapidly, the case count climbed from three to six!

Decision Time

As Chief Medical Officer, Simon Friedman would be the lead person in making the final decisions. Dr. Friedman, a pediatrician with twenty-five years of leadership experience in public health practice, was not new to this type of complex public health judgment. He remembered that the experiences of this same community during the *Hantavirus* outbreak had weakened the trust that the community had for the public health system. He wondered whether, in the time since the *Hantavirus* experience, enough work had been done not only to rebuild the confidence of the communities for the public health system but also to strengthen the relationships between the many organizations and medical professionals involved in caring for this rural multicultural population.

His background had taught him that difficult decisions were part of public health practice and that trusting professional and community relationships should be in place before such decisions had to be made. As he listened and participated in the conference call discussion, Dr. Friedman realized that the judgment to treat this occurrence as a point source outbreak or a community-wide outbreak would be the primary decision. A cascade of other necessary decisions would follow from this primary judgment.

It was 7:30 p.m. The conference call had lasted more than ninety minutes thus far. Dr. Friedman leaned back in his chair. Racing through his mind were the medical, financial, and sociocultural implications of his decision. He thought, "What do we need to do if this is a point source outbreak? What would we do differently if this is considered a community-wide outbreak?" Manpower issues, transportation, and communication were among the considerations.

Then Dr. Friedman thought about press relations. He realized, "Not only do we have to do a much better job interfacing with the press than was done during the *Hantavirus* outbreak, but we have to have a good solid rationale for our decisions. Whatever intervention strategies we choose, we had better be able to explain them in a culturally sensitive, scientifically credible, and politically supportable way." Decisions needed to be made very soon. Dr. Friedman could sense that the discussion was over and that the judgments were now his.

Glossary

CDC—Centers for Disease Control and Prevention

DEEP—Division of Epidemiology, Evaluation and Planning (in NMDOH)

EMS—Emergency Medical Services

IHS—Indian Health Service

NMDOH—New Mexico Department of Health

NNDOH—Navajo Nation Department of Health

OMI—Office of the Medical Investigator

PHD—Public Health Division (in NMDOH)
SJRMC—San Juan Regional Medical Center
SLD—Scientific Laboratory Division (in NMDOH)
UNMH—University of New Mexico Hospital
UNMHSC—University of New Mexico Health
Science Center

Note

1. Kenneth A. Brown, *Four Corners: History, Land, and People of the Desert Southwest* (New York: HarperCollins, 1995), p. 3.

C. W. Williams Community Health Center

The Metrolina Health Center was started by Dr. Charles Warren "C. W." Williams and several medical colleagues with a $25,000 grant from the Department of Health and Human Services. Concerned about the health needs of the poor and wanting to make the world a better place for those less fortunate, Dr. Williams, Charlotte's first African American to serve on the surgical staff of Charlotte Memorial Hospital (Charlotte's largest hospital), enlisted the aid of Dr. John Murphy, a local dentist; Peggy Beckwith, director of the Sickle Cell Association; and health planner Bob Ellis to create a health facility for the unserved and underserved population of Mecklenburg County, North Carolina. The health facility received its corporate status in 1980. Following Dr. Williams's death in 1982, when the health facility was still in its infancy, the Metrolina Comprehensive Health Center was renamed the C. W. Williams Health Center.

Michelle Marrs commented:

We're celebrating our fifteenth year of operation at C. W. Williams, and I'm celebrating my first full year as CEO. I'm feeling really good about a lot of things—we are fully staffed for the first time in two years, and we are a significant player in a pilot pro-

gram by North Carolina to manage the health care of Medicaid patients in Mecklenburg County (Charlotte area) through private HMOs. We're the only organization that's approved to serve Medicaid recipients that's not an HMO. We have a contract for primary care case management. We're used to providing care for the Medicaid population, and we're used to providing health education. It's part of our original mission [see Exhibit 12-1] and has been since the beginning of C. W. Williams.

I've been in health care for quite awhile but things are really changing rapidly now. The center might be forced to align with one of the two hospitals because of managed-care changes. Although we don't want to take away the patient's choice, it might happen. In order for me to do all that I should be doing externally, I need more help internally. I believe we should have a director of finance. We have a great opportunity to buy another location so that we can serve more patients, but this is a relatively unstable time in health care. Buying another facility would be a stretch financially, but the location would be perfect. The asking price does seem high, though. . . .

Exhibit 12-2 contains a biographical sketch of Ms. Marrs.

This case was prepared by Linda E. Swayne, University of North Carolina at Charlotte, and Peter M. Ginter, University of Alabama at Birmingham. It is intended as a basis for classroom discussion rather than to illustrate effective or ineffective handling of an administrative situation. Used with permission from Linda E. Swayne.

Exhibit 12-1. C. W. Williams Health Center Mission, Vision, and Values Statements

Mission

To promote a healthier future for our community by consistently providing excellent, accessible health care with pride, compassion, and respect.

Values

- Respect each individual, patient, and staff as well as our community as a valued entity that must be treasured.
- Consistently provide the highest quality patient care with pride and compassion.
- Partner with other organizations to respond to the social, health, and economic development needs of our community.
- Operate in an efficient, well-staffed, comfortable environment as an autonomous and financially sound organization.

Vision

Committed to the pioneering vision of Dr. Charles Warren Williams, Charlotte's first Black surgeon, we will move into the twenty-first century promoting a healthier and brighter future for our community. This means:

C. W. Williams Health Center will offer personal, high-quality, affordable, comprehensive health services that improve the quality of life for all.

- C. W. Williams Health Center, while partnering with other health care organizations, will expand its high-quality health services into areas of need. No longer will patients be required to travel long distances to receive the medical care they deserve. C. W. Williams Health Center will come to them!
- C. W. Williams Health Center will be well managed using state-of-the-art technology, accelerating into the twenty-first century as a leading provider of comprehensive community-based health services.
- C. W. Williams Health Center will be viewed as Mecklenburg County's premier community health agency, providing care with RESPECT:

  - **R**eliable health care

  - **E**fficient operations

  - **S**upportive staff

  - **P**ersonal care

  - **E**ffective systems

  - **C**lean environments

  - **T**imely services

Exhibit 12-2. Michelle Marrs, Chief Executive Officer of C. W. Williams Health Center

Michelle Marrs had over twenty years' experience working in a variety of health care settings and delivery systems. On earning her BS degree, she began her career as a community health educator working in the prevention of alcoholism and substance abuse among youth and women. In 1976, she pursued graduate education at the Harvard School of Public Health and the Graduate School of Education, earning a master's of education with a concentration in administration, planning, and social policy. She worked for the U.S. Public Health Service, Division of Health Services Delivery; for the University of Massachusetts Medical Center as director of the Patient Care Studies Department and administrator of the Radiation Oncology Department; for the Mattapan Community Health Center (a comprehensive community-based primary care health facility in Boston) as director; and as medical office administrator for Kaiser Permanente. Marrs was appointed chief executive officer of the C. W. Williams Health Center in November, 1994.

Community Health Centers[1]

When the nation's resources were mobilized during the early 1960s to fight the War on Poverty, it was discovered that poor health and lack of basic medical care were major obstacles to the educational and job training progress of the poor. A system of preventive and comprehensive medical care was necessary to battle poverty. A new health care model for poor communities was started in 1963 through the vision and efforts of two New England physicians—Count Geiger and Jack Gibson of the Tufts Medical School—to open the first two neighborhood health centers, located in Mound Bayou (in rural Mississippi) and in a Boston housing project.

In 1966, an amendment to the Economic Opportunity Act formally established the Comprehensive Health Center Program. By 1971, a total of 150 health centers had been established. By 1990, more than 540 community and migrant health centers at 1,400 service sites had received federal grants totaling $547 million to supplement their budgets of $1.3 billion. By 1996, the numbers had increased to 700 centers at 2,400 delivery sites providing service to more than 9 million people.

Community health centers had a public health perspective; however, they were similar to private practices staffed by physicians, nurses, and allied health professionals. They differed from typical medical offices in that they offered a broader range of services, such as social services and health education. Health centers removed the financial and nonfinancial barriers to health care. In addition, health centers were owned by the community and operated by a local volunteer governing board. Federally funded health centers were required to have patients as a majority of the governing board. The use of patients to govern was a major factor in keeping the centers responsive to patients and generating acceptance by them. In response to the increasing complexity of health care delivery, many board members took advantage of training opportunities through their state and national associations to better manage the facility.

Community Health Centers Provide Care for the Medically Underserved

Federally subsidized health centers were required by law to serve populations that were identified by the Public Health Service as medically underserved. Half of the medically underserved population lived in rural areas where there were few medical resources. The other half was located in economically depressed inner-city communities where individuals lived in poverty, lacked health insurance, or had special needs such as homelessness, AIDS, or substance abuse. Approximately 70 percent of health center patients were

Exhibit 12-3. Ethnicity of Urban and Rural Health Center Patients

Urban Health Center Patients (%)		Rural Health Center Patients (%)	
African American/Black	37.0	African American/Black	19.6
White/Non-Hispanic	29.9	White/Non-Hispanic	49.3
Native American	0.8	Native American	1.1
Asian/Pacific Islander	3.2	Asian/Pacific Islander	2.9
Hispanic/Latino	27.2	Hispanic/Latino	26.5
Other	1.9	Other	0.6

Exhibit 12-4. Insurance Status of U.S. Health Center Patients, C. W. Williams Health Center Patients, the U.S. Population, and the North Carolina Population

	Health Center Patients (%)	U.S. Population (%)	North Carolina Population (%)	C. W. Williams Health Center Patients (%)
Uninsured	42.9	13.4	14	21
Private insurance	14.0	63.2	64	10
Public insurance	43.0	23.4	22	69

minorities in urban areas, whereas 50 percent were white/non-Hispanics in rural areas (see Exhibit 12-3).

Typically, nearly 43 percent of health center patients neither had private health insurance nor qualified for public health insurance (Medicaid or Medicare). That compared to 13.4 percent of the U.S. population that was uninsured (see Exhibit 12-4). More than 80 percent of health center patients had incomes below the federal poverty level ($28,700 for a family of four in 1994). Most of the remaining 20 percent were between 100 percent and 200 percent of the federal poverty level.

Community Health Centers Are Cost-Effective

Numerous national studies had indicated that the kind of ongoing primary care management provided by community health centers resulted in significantly lowered costs for inpatient hospital care and specialty care. Because illnesses were diagnosed and treated at an earlier stage, more expensive care interventions often were not needed. Hospital admission rates were 22 to 67 percent lower for health center patients than for community residents. A study of six New York City and

New York State health centers found that Medicaid beneficiaries were 22 to 30 percent less costly to treat than those not served by health centers.[2] A Washington State study found that the average cost to Medicaid per hospital bill was $49 for health center patients versus $74 for commercial sector patients.[3] Indigent patients at health centers were less likely to make emergency room visits—a reduction of 13 percent overall and 38 percent for pediatric care. In addition, defensive medicine (the practice of ordering every and any diagnostic tests to avoid malpractice claims) was less frequently used. Community health center physicians had some of the lowest medical malpractice loss ratios in the nation.

Not only were community health centers cost-efficient, but patients also were highly satisfied with the care received. A total of 96 percent were satisfied or very satisfied with the care they received, and 97 percent indicated they would recommend the health center to their friends and families.[4]

Movement to Managed Care

In 1990, a little more than 2 million Medicaid beneficiaries were enrolled in managed care plans; in 1993, the number had increased to 8 million; and in 1995, more than 11 million Medicaid beneficiaries were enrolled. Medicaid beneficiaries and other low-income Americans had higher rates of illness and disability than others, and thus accumulated significantly higher costs of medical care.[5]

C. W. Williams Health Center

C. W. Williams was beginning to recognize the impact of managed care. Like much of the South, the Carolinas had been slow to accept managed care. The major reasons seemed to be the rural nature of many Southern states; markets that were not as attractive to major managed care organizations; dominant insurors that continued to provide fee for service, ensuring choice of physicians and hos-

pitals; and medical inflation that accelerated more slowly than in other areas. Major changes began to occur, however, beginning in 1993. By 1996, managed care was being implemented in many areas at an accelerated pace.

Challenges for C. W. Williams

Michelle reported:

One of my greatest challenges has been how to handle the changes imposed by the shift from a primarily fee-for-service to a managed care environment. Local physicians who in the past had the flexibility, loyalty, and availability to assist C. W. Williams by providing part-time assistance or volunteer efforts during the physician shortage are now employed by managed-care organizations or involved in contractual relationships that prohibit them from working with us. The few remaining primary care solo or small group practices are struggling for survival themselves and seldom are available to provide patient sessions or assist with our hospital call-rotation schedule. The rigorous call-rotation schedule of a small primary care facility like C. W. Williams is frequently unattractive to available physicians seeking opportunities, even when a market-competitive compensation package is offered. Many of these physician recruitment and retention issues are being driven by the rapid changes brought on by the impact of managed care in the local community. It is a real challenge to recruit physicians to provide the necessary access to medical care for our patients.

My next greatest challenge is investment in technology to facilitate this transition to managed care. Technology is expensive, yet I know it is crucial to our survival and success. We also need more space, but I don't know if this is a good time for expansion.

One of the pressing and perhaps most difficult efforts has been the careful and strategic consideration of the need to affiliate to some degree with one of the two area hospitals in order to more fully integrate and broaden the range of services to patients of our center. Although a decision has not been made at this juncture, the organization has made significant strides to comprehend the needs of this community, consider the pros and cons of either choice, and continue providing the best care possible under some very difficult circumstances.

Hospital Affiliation

Traditionally, the patients of C. W. Williams Health Center who needed hospitalization were admitted to Charlotte Memorial Hospital, a large regional hospital that was designated at the Trauma I level—one of five designated by the state of North Carolina to handle major trauma cases twenty-four hours a day, seven days per week (full staffing), as well as to perform research in the area of trauma. Uncompensated inpatient care was financed by the county. Charlotte Memorial became Carolinas Medical Center (CMC) in 1984, when it began a program to develop a totally integrated system. In 1995, C. W. Williams provided Carolinas Medical Center with more than 3,000 patient bed days; however, the patients usually were seen by their regular C. W. Williams physicians. As Carolinas Medical Center (CMC) purchased physician practices (more than 300 doctors were employed by the system) and purchased or managed many of the surrounding community hospitals, some C. W. Williams patients became concerned that CMC would take over C. W. Williams and that their community health center would no longer exist.

According to Michelle:

My preference is that our patients have a choice of where they would prefer to go for hospitalization. Our older patients expect to go to Carolinas Medical, but many of our middle-aged patients have expressed a preference for Presbyterian. Both hospitals have indicated an interest in our patients. We may not really have a choice, however. We recently were sent information that reported the twelve largest hospitals in the state, including the teaching hospitals—Duke, University of North Carolina at Chapel Hill, Carolinas Medical Center, and East Carolina—have formed a consortium and will contract with the state to pay for Medicaid patients. At the same time, all twenty of the health centers in the state—including us at C. W. Williams—are cooperating to develop a health maintenance organiza-

Exhibit 12-5. C. W. Williams Health Center Services

Primary care and preventive services
Diagnostic laboratory
Diagnostic X-ray (basic)
Pharmacy
EMS (crash cart and CPR-trained staff)
Family planning
Immunizations (MD-directed as well as open clinic—no relationship required)
Prenatal care and gynecology
Health education
Parenting education
Translation services
Substance abuse counseling
Nutrition counseling
Diagnostic testing
    HIV testing
    Mammogram
    Pap smears
    TB testing
    Vision/hearing testing
    Lead testing
    Pregnancy testing
    Drug screening

tion. We expect to gain approval for the HMO by July, 1997. Since 60 percent of our patients are Medicaid, if the state contracts with the new consortium, then we will be required to send our patients to Carolinas Medical Center.

Services

C. W. Williams Health Center provided primary and preventive health services including medical, radiology, laboratory, pharmacy, subspecialty, and inpatient managed care; health education/promotion; community outreach; and transportation to care (Exhibit 12-5 lists all services). The center was strongly linked to the Charlotte community, and it worked with other public and private health services to coordinate resources for effective patient care. No one was denied care because of an inability to pay. A little more than 20 percent of the patients at C. W. Williams were un-insured.

The full-time staff included five physicians, two physician assistants (PAs), two nurses, one X-ray technician, one pharmacist, and a staff of twenty-eight. Of the five physicians, one was an internist, two were in family practice, and two were pediatricians. The PAs "floated" to work wherever help was most needed. With the help of one assistant, the pharmacist filled more than 20,000 prescriptions annually.

Patients at C. W. Williams

All first-time patients at C. W. Williams were asked what type of insurance they had. If they had some type of insurance—private, Medicare, or Medicaid—an appointment was scheduled im-mediately. New patients without insurance were asked if they would be interested in applying for the C. W. Williams discount program (the dis-count could amount to as much as 100 percent, but every person was asked to pay something). The discount was based on income and the num-ber of people in the household. If the response was "No," the patient was informed that payment was expected at the time services were rendered. Visa, Mastercard, cash, and personal check (with two forms of identification) were accepted. At C. W. Williams, all health care was made affordable.

C. W. Williams made reminder calls to the pa-tient's home (or to a neighbor's or relative's tele-phone) several days prior to the appointment. When patients arrived at the center, they provided their name to the nurse at the front reception desk and then took a seat in a large waiting room. The pharmacy window was near the front door for the convenience of patients who were simply picking up prescriptions. The reception desk, pharmacy, and waiting room occupied the first floor.

When the patient's name was called, he or she was taken by elevator to the second floor, where there were ten examination rooms. After seeing the physician, physician assistant, or nurse, the pa-tient was escorted back down the elevator to the pharmacy if a prescription was needed and then to the reception desk to pay. Pharmaceuticals were discounted, and a special program by Pfizer Phar-maceuticals provided more than $60,000 worth of drugs in 1995 for medically indigent patients.

The center's patient population was 63 percent female (see Exhibit 12-6). Nearly 80 percent of pa-tients were African Americans, 18 percent were white, and 2 percent were other minorities. Pa-tients were quite satisfied with the services pro-vided, as indicated in patient surveys conducted by the center. Paralleling national studies, 97 per-cent of C. W. Williams patients would recommend the center to family or friends. (Selected service indicators from the patient satisfaction study ap-pear in Exhibit 12-7.)

C. W. Williams Organization

The center was managed by a board of direc-tors, responsible for developing policy and hiring the CEO.

Board of Directors

The federal government required that all com-munity health centers have a board of directors that was made up of at least 51 percent patients or citizens who lived in the community. The board chairman of C. W. Williams, Mr. Daniel Dooley, was a center patient. C. W. Williams had a board of fifteen, all of whom were African Americans and four of whom were patients and out of the workforce. Two members of the board were man-agers/directors from the Public Health Depart-ment (which was under the management of CMC). There were two other health profession-als—a nurse and a physician. Other board mem-bers included a CPA, a financial planner, an insur-ance agent, a vice president for human resources, an executive in a search firm, and a former profes-sor of economics. A majority of the board had not had much exposure to the changes occurring in the health care industry (aside from their own personal situations), nor were they trained in stra-tegic management.

Exhibit 12-6. C. W. Williams Health Center Patients by Age and Sex

	1991	1992	1993	1994	1995
Females					
< 1	343	408	263	198	101
1–4	434	552	692	647	417
5–11	322	572	494	641	658
12–14	376	197	150	148	124
15–17	361	168	146	121	92
18–19	264	152	85	82	67
20–34	749	1,250	967	964	712
35–44	869	617	479	532	467
45–64	583	567	617	658	658
65+	400	488	531	527	524
Total females	4,701	4,971	4,424	4,518	3,820
Males					
< 1	367	471	328	199	119
1–4	439	516	707	625	410
5–11	440	644	598	846	738
12–14	171	175	128	120	104
15–17	180	133	79	76	155
18–19	126	67	28	23	69
20–34	296	389	219	187	126
35–44	313	296	182	205	132
45–64	229	316	273	294	235
65+	151	248	190	190	181
Total males	2,712	3,255	2,732	2,765	2,269
Total	7,413	8,226	7,156	7,283	6,089

SOURCE: C. W. Williams documents.

Exhibit 12-7. Patient Satisfaction Study

Rank	Selected Service Indicators	Mean Score
1	Helpfulness/attitudes of medical staff	3.82
2	Clean/comfortable/convenient facility	3.65
3	Relationship with physician/nurse	3.58
4	Quality of health services	3.28
5	Ability to satisfy all medical needs	3.20
6	Helpfulness/attitudes of nonmedical staff	2.72

SOURCE: C. W. Williams documents.

NOTE: Score of 4.0 is highest agreement with the statement.

Exhibit 12-8. Metrolina Comprehensive Health Center, Inc. dba C. W. Williams Health Center

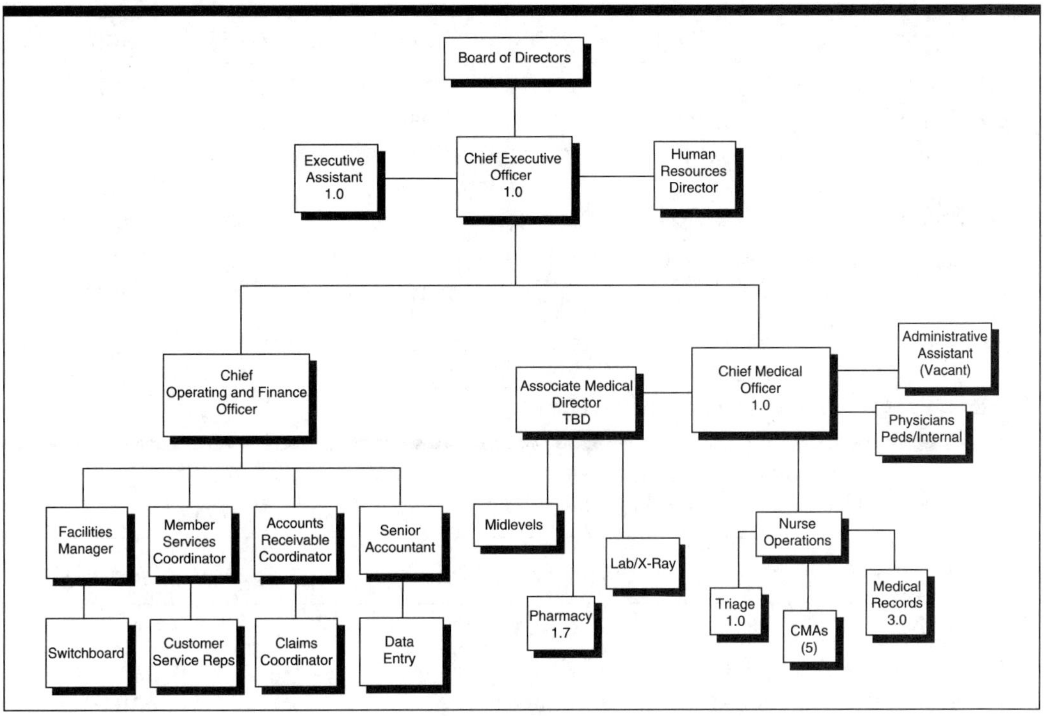

Staff

The center was operated by CEO Michelle Marrs, who had an operations officer and medical director reporting to her (see Exhibit 12-8 for an organization chart).

Recently, the director of finance, who had worked at the center for more than ten years, had resigned. "She was offered another position within C. W. Williams," said Michelle, "but she declined to take it. Frankly, I have to have someone with greater expertise in finance. With capitation on the horizon, we need to do some very critical planning to better manage our finances and make sure we are receiving as much reimbursement from Washington as we are entitled."

There were some disagreements between the board and Ms. Marrs over responsibilities. Employees frequently appealed to the chairman and other members of the board when they felt that they had not been treated fairly. Michelle preferred the board to be more involved in setting strategic direction for C. W. Williams. "A two-year strategic plan was developed late in 1995 that has not been moved along, embraced, and further developed," she said. "Committees have not met on a regular basis to actualize stated objectives."

C. W. Williams Is Financially Strong

The center received an increasing amount of federal grant money for the first ten years of its operation as the number of patients grew, but that funding had leveled off as most government allocations had been reduced (see Exhibit 12-9). Although the amount collected from Medicare was increasing, the amount collected compared to the full charge was decreasing. (See Exhibits 12-10 through 12-14 for details of the financial situation.)

Exhibit 12-9. C. W. Williams Funding Sources

Funding Source	1991	1992	1993	1994	1995
Grant (federal)	$ 740,000	$ 666,524	$ 689,361	$ 720,584	$ 720,584
Medicare	152,042	157,891	258,104	260,389	301,444
Medicaid	381,109	453,712	641,069	562,380	456,043
Third-party pay	25,673	14,128	84,347	90,253	51,799
Uninsured self-pay	300,748	441,508	174,992	262,817	338,272
Grant (miscellaneous)	0	0	0	11,500	48,000
Total	$1,599,572	$1,733,763	$1,847,873	$1,907,923	$1,916,142

Exhibit 12-10. Funding Accounts Receivable

	1994		1995	
	Full Charge	Amount Collected	Full Charge	Amount Collected
Medicare	$436,853	$260,389	$369,306	$301,444
Medicaid	$914,212	$562,380	$725,175	$456,043
Insured	$ 99,202	$ 90,253	$ 61,021	$ 51,799
Patient fees	$899,055	$262,817	$754,864	$338,272

Carolina ACCESS: A Pilot Program

In fiscal year 1994 (July 1, 1994 to June 30, 1995), North Carolina served more than 950,000 Medicaid recipients at a cost of more than $3.5 billion. The aged, blind, and disabled accounted for 26 percent of the eligibles and 65 percent of the expenditures. Families and children accounted for 74 percent of the eligibles and 35 percent of the expenditures. Services were heavily concentrated in two areas: inpatient hospital (accounting for 20 percent of expenses) and nursing facility/intermediate care/mentally retarded services (accounting for 34 percent of expenses). Mecklenburg County had the highest number of eligibles within the state, at 50,849 people, representing 7 percent of the state's Medicaid population.

What started out in 1986 as a contract with Kaiser Permanente to provide medical services for recipients of Aid to Families With Dependent Children in four counties became a complex mixture of three models of managed care. Carolina ACCESS was North Carolina Medicaid's primary care case management model of managed care. It began a pilot program named "Health Care Connections" in Mecklenburg County on June 1, 1996.

Health Care Connections

The state of North Carolina wanted to move 42,000 Mecklenburg County Medicaid recipients into managed care. The state contracted with six health plans and C. W. Williams, as a federally

Exhibit 12-11. C. W. Williams Health Center Balance Sheets

	1992–1993	1993–1994	1994–1995	1995–1996
ASSETS				
Current Assets				
Cash	$ 280,550	$ 335,258	$ 339,459	$ 132,925
Certificates of deposit	23,413	24,496	25,446	529,826
Accounts receivable (net)	213,815	285,934	202,865	160,230
Accounts receivable (other)	5,661	4,721	2,936	10,069
Security deposits	1,847	97	-0-	-0-
Notes receivable	-0-	-0-	29,825	10,403
Inventory	26,191	23,777	30,217	26,844
Prepaid loans	12,087	21,605	9,722	11,159
Investments	269	269	269	51,628
Total current assets	563,833	696,157	640,739	933,084
Property and Equipment				
Land	10,000	10,000	10,000	10,000
Building	311,039	311,039	311,039	311,039
Building renovations	904,434	904,434	909,754	915,949
Equipment	282,333	312,892	328,063	387,178
Less depreciation	(393,392)	(452,432)	(523,384)	(597,284)
Total property and equipment	1,114,414	1,085,933	1,035,472	1,026,882
Total Assets	$1,678,247	$1,782,090	$1,676,211	$1,959,966
LIABILITIES AND NET ASSETS				
Liabilities				
Accounts payable	$ 11,066	$ 31,582	$ 13,136	$ 34,039
Vacation expense accounts	36,694	42,857	19,457	28,144
Deferred revenue	42,641	37,910	43,400	59,433
Total liabilities	90,401	112,349	75,993	121,616
Net Assets				
Unrestricted	1,587,846	1,669,741	1,600,218	1,838,350
Temporary restricted	-0-	-0-	-0-	-0-
Total net assets	1,587,846	1,669,741	1,600,218	1,838,350
Total Liabilities and Net Assets	$1,678,247	$1,782,090	$1,676,211	$1,959,966

qualified health center, to serve the Mecklenburg County Medicaid population. Because one organization was dropped from the program, Medicaid recipients were to choose one of six different plans for their health care (see Exhibit 12-15).

An integral part of the selection process was the use of a health benefits advisor to assist families in choosing the appropriate plan. By law, none of the organizations was permitted to promote its plan to Medicaid recipients. Rather, the Public Consulting Group of Charlotte was awarded the contract to be an independent enrollment counselor to assist Medicaid recipients in their choices of health care options.

Exhibit 12-12. Statement of Support, Revenue, Expenses, and Change in Fund Balances

	1992–1993	1993–1994	1994–1995	1995–1996
CONTRIBUTED SUPPORT AND REVENUE				
Contributed	$ 720,712	$ 720,584	$ 732,584	$ 768,584
Earned Revenue				
Patient fees	1,213,919	1,186,497	1,183,904	1,129,030
Medicare	-0-	-0-	-0-	465,248
Contributions	-0-	-0-	-0-	5,676
Interest income	7,228	9,666	12,567	14,115
Dividend income	-0-	-0-	-0-	2,387
Rental income	-0-	-0-	-0-	1,980
Miscellaneous income	5,962	5,941	4,772	11,055
Total earned	1,227,109	1,202,104	1,201,243	1,629,491
Total contributed support and revenue	1,947,821	1,922,688	1,933,827	2,398,075
Expenses				
Program	1,782,312	1,840,447	2,002,633	2,157,768
Other	442	349	217	2,166
Total expenses	1,782,754	1,840,796	2,002,850	2,159,934
Increase (decrease) in net assets	165,062	81,892	(69,523)	238,141
Net assets (beginning of year)	1,310,155	1,587,849	1,669,741	1,600,218
Adjustment	112,629[a]	-0-	-0-	-0-
Net assets (end of year)	$1,587,846	$1,669,741	$1,600,218	$1,838,359

a. Federal grant funds earned but not drawn down in prior years were not recognized as revenue. The error had no effect on net income for fiscal year ended March 31, 1992.

"More than 33,000 of the Medicaid recipients were women and children," said Michelle Marrs. "Sixty percent of the group had no medical relationship. Slightly over 50 percent of C. W. Williams patients are Medicaid recipients." (See Exhibits 12-16 and 12-17 for C. W. Williams users by pay source and number of visits.)

Michelle said:

We have about 8,000 patients coming to us for about 30,000 visits. Approximately half of the people who currently come to us for health care will be required to choose a health plan. The state decided that an independent agency had to sign people up so that there would be no 'bounty hunting' for enrollees. In the first month, about 2,300 Medicaid recipients enrolled in the pilot program. Almost half

of the people who signed up chose Kaiser Foundation Health Plan. It has a history of serving Medicaid patients. We received the next highest number of enrollees, because we too have a history of serving this market. We had 402 enrollees during that first month. Of those, only 38 were previous patients. What we don't know yet is whether we have lost any patients to other programs. The lack of up-to-date information is frustrating. We need a better information system.

We decided that we could provide care for up to 8,000 Medicaid patients at C. W. Williams. I embrace managed care for a number of reasons: patients must choose a primary care provider, patients will be encouraged to take an active role in their health care, and there will be less duplication of medical services and costs. In the past, some doctors have shied away from Medicaid patients be-

Exhibit 12-13. Statement of Functional Expenditures, Fiscal Year Ended March 31

	1992–1993	1993–1994	1994–1995	1995–1996
Personnel				
Salaries	937,119	1,016,194	1,102,373	1,181,639
Benefits	190,300	210,228	210,674	211,705
Total	$1,127,419	$1,226,422	$1,313,047	$1,393,344
Other				
Accounting	5,250	5,985	6,397	7,200
Bank charges	840	300	213	1,001
Building maintenance	38,842	54,132	49,586	53,828
Consultants	26,674	2,733	39,565	44,923[a]
Contract MDs	-0-	-0-	-0-	87,159
Dues/publications/conferences	17,371	21,655	22,066	24,258
Equipment maintenance	28,732	27,365	30,402	27,352
Insurance	15,182	3,146	3,215	3,292
Legal fees	688	2,774	3,652	3,582
Marketing	6,358	1,958	5,734	15,730
Patient services	28,959	28,222	35,397	43,815
Pharmacy	271,542	237,761	225,762	188,061
Physician recruiting	14,171	32,929	56,173	21,395
Postage	8,435	11,622	10,019	14,182
Printing	729	963	2,405	9,696
Supplies	73,020	62,828	72,977	84,064
Telephone	16,755	17,967	20,914	25,002
Travel-board	2,713	1,202	4,977	3,476
Travel-staff	13,889	14,576	12,631	15,978
Utilities	15,782	18,305	16,548	16,536
Total other	585,932	546,423	618,633	690,530
Total personnel and other	1,713,351	1,772,845	1,931,680	2,083,874
Depreciation	(68,966)	(67,604)	(70,952)	(73,891)
Total expenses	$1,782,317	$1,840,449	$2,002,632	$2,157,765

a. Includes contracted medical director.

cause they didn't want to be bothered with the paperwork, the medical services weren't fully compensated, and Medicaid patients tended to have numerous health problems.

There are seven different companies that applied and were given authority to provide health care for Medicaid recipients in Mecklenburg County. Although I understand one had to withdraw, we are the only one that is not a health maintenance organization—an HMO. Although we don't provide hospitalization, we do provide for patients' care whether they need an office visit or to be hospitalized. Our physicians provide care while the patient is in the hospital.

Medicaid beneficiaries have to be recertified every six months. We are three months into the sign-up process or approximately halfway. Kaiser has enrolled the highest number, about one-third of the beneficiaries [see Exhibit 12-18]. We have enrolled over 12 percent. The independent enroll-

Exhibit 12-14. C. W. Williams Health Center Statement of Cash Flows, Fiscal Year Ended March 31

	1992–1993	1993–1994	1994–1995	1995–1996
NET CASH FLOW FROM OPERATIONS				
Increase in Net Assets	$165,062	$ 81,892	$(69,523)	$238,141
Noncash Income Expense (Depreciation)	68,966	67,604	70,952	73,891
Increase in Deposits	(1,750)	1,750	-0-	-0-
Decrease in Receivables	(86,620)	(71,179)	55,028	65,328
(Increase) in Prepaid Expenses	(2,277)	(9,518)	11,980	(1,437)
(Increase) Decrease in Inventory	(4,105)	2,414	(6,440)	3,373
Increase in Payables	14,094	20,516	(18,445)	20,903
Increase (Decrease) in Vacation Expense Accrual	(8,583)	6,163	(23,400)	8,688
(Increase) in Notes Receivable	-0-	-0-	-0-	(10,403)
Increase in Deferred Revenue	(2,992)	(4,731)	5,490	16,032
Net Cash Flow From Operations	141,795	94,911	25,642	414,516
Cash Flow From Investing (Purchase Fixed Assets)	(52,547)	(39,120)	(20,491)	(65,311)
Purchase Marketable Securities	-0-	-0-	-0-	(51,359)
Net Cash Used by Investments	(52,547)	(39,120)	(20,491)	(116,670)
Net Cash From Financing Activities	112,629	-0-	-0-	-0-
Increase in Cash	201,877	55,791	5,151	297,846
Cash + Cash Equivalents				
Beginning of Year April 1	130,274	332,151	387,942	393,093
End of Year March 31	332,151	387,942	393,093	690,939

ment counselor is responsible for helping Medicaid recipients enroll during the initial twelve months. I expect the numbers to dwindle for the last six months of that time period. Changes will come primarily from new patients to the area and patients who are unhappy with their initial choice.

Medicaid patients were going to be a challenge for managed care. Because many of them were used to going to the emergency room for care, they were not in the habit of making or keeping appointments. Some facilities overbooked appointments to try to utilize medical staff efficiently; however, the practice caused very long waits at times. Other complicating factors included lack of telephones for contacting patients for reminder calls or physician follow-ups, lack of

transportation, the number of patients at high risk as a result of poverty or lifestyle factors, and patients who did not follow doctors' orders.

Health Connection Enrollment

Medicaid recipients were required to be recertified every six months in the state of North Carolina. During this process, a time was allocated for the Public Consulting Group of Charlotte to make a presentation about the managed care choices available. The presentation included

- A discussion of managed care and HMOs, including how they were different and the same from previous Medicaid practices

Exhibit 12-15. Health Care Connections Plan Choices

Plan Name	Type	Hospital Affiliation
Atlantic Health Plans	HMO	Carolinas Medical Center, University Hospital, Mercy Hospital, Mercy South, Union Regional Medical, Kings Mountain Hospital
Kaiser Permanente	HMO	Presbyterian Hospital, Presbyterian Hospital-Matthews, Presbyterian Orthopedic, Presbyterian Specialty Hospital
Maxicare North Carolina, Inc.	HMO	Presbyterian Hospital, Presbyterian Hospital-Matthews, Presbyterian Orthopedic, Presbyterian Specialty Hospital
Optimum Choice/Mid-Atlantic Medical	HMO	Presbyterian Hospital, Presbyterian Hospital-Matthews, Presbyterian Orthopedic, Presbyterian Specialty Hospital
The Wellness Plan of NC, Inc.	HMO	Carolinas Medical Center, University Hospital, Mercy Hospital, Mercy South, Union Regional Medical, Kings Mountain Hospital
C. W. Williams Health Center	Partially federally funded, community health center	Carolinas Medical Center, University Hospital, Mercy Hospital, Mercy South, Union Regional Medical, Kings Mountain Hospital or Presbyterian Hospital, Presbyterian Hospital-Matthews, Presbyterian Orthopedic, Presbyterian Specialty Hospital

- Benefits of Health Care Connections, such as having a medical home, a twenty-four-hour, seven-day-a-week hotline to ask questions about medical care, physician choice, and plan choice
- Methods to choose a plan based on wanting to use a doctor that the patient had used before, hospital choice (some plans were associated with a specific hospital), and location (for easy access)

Medicaid recipients who did not choose a plan that day had ten working days to call in on the hotline to choose a plan. If they had not done so by that deadline, they were randomly assigned to a plan. Public Consulting Group's health benefits advisors made the presentations and then assisted each individual in determining what choice he or she would like to make and filling out the paper-

work. More than 80 percent of the Medicaid recipients who went through the recertification process and heard the presentation decided on site. Most others called back on the hotline after more carefully studying the information. About 3 percent were randomly assigned because they did not select a plan.

New Medicaid recipients were provided individualized presentations because they tended to be new to the community, had recently developed a health problem, or were pregnant. Because they might have less information than those who had been "in the system" for some time, it took a more detailed explanation from the health benefits advisor.

The information was presented in a fair, factual, and useful manner for session attendees. For the first several months, the advisors attempted to thoroughly explain the difference between an

Exhibit 12-16. Users by Pay Source

Source	Percentage of Users	Number of Users	Income to C. W. Williams ($)	Number of Encounters
1994–1995				
Medicare	13%	791	301,444	2,392
Medicaid	56%	3,410	456,043	10,305
Full pay	10%	609	318,424	1,840
Uninsured	21%	1,279	42,421	3,865
Total 1994–1995		6,089	1,118,332	18,402
1993–1994				
Medicare	12%	1,037	195,352	2,880
Medicaid	53%	4,579	585,446	12,720
Full pay	11%	950	178,525	2,640
Uninsured	24%	2,074	101,569	5,760
Total 1993–1994		8,640	1,060,892	24,000
1992–1993				
Medicare	10%	853	189,927	2,304
Medicaid	36%	3,072	401,355	8,294
Full pay	10%	853	158,473	2,304
Uninsured	44%	3,755	186,708	10,138
Total 1992–1993		8,533	936,463	23,040
1991–1992				
Medicare	20%	1,614	162,980	4,032
Medicaid	30%	2,419	312,680	6,048
Full pay	10%	806	157,101	2,016
Uninsured	40%	3,225	159,855	8,064
Total 1991–1992		8,064	792,616	20,160

HMO and a "partially federally funded community health center," but they decided it was too confusing to the audience and did not really make a difference in patients' health care. For the past month they had explained "managed care" more carefully and touched lightly on HMOs. C. W. Williams was presented as one of the choices, although some of the advisors mentioned that it was the only choice that had evening and weekend hours for appointments.

Strategic Plan for C. W. Williams

With the help of Michelle Marrs, the C. W. Williams Board of Directors was beginning to de-

velop a strategic plan. (Exhibit 12-19 provides the SWOT analysis that was developed.)

According to Michelle:

Part of our strategic plan was to go to the people—make it easier for our patients to visit C. W. Williams by establishing satellite clinics. We recently became aware of a building that is for sale that would meet our needs. The owner would like to sell to us. He's older and likes the idea that the building will "do some good for people," but he's asking $479,000. The location is near a large number of Medicaid beneficiaries plus a middle-class area of minority patients that could add to our insured population. I just don't know if we should take the risk to buy the building. We own our current build-

Exhibit 12-17. C. W. Williams Health Center Patient Visits

Primary care visits	
Internal medicine	8,248
Family practice	4,573
Pediatrics	2,643
Gynecology	236
Midlevel practitioners	3,609
Total	19,309
Subspecialty/ancillary service visits	
Podiatry	82
Mammography	101
Immunizations	1,766
Perinatal	429
X-ray	1,152
Dental	17
Pharmacy prescriptions	20,868
Hospital	1,762
Laboratory	13,103
Health education	412
Other medical specialists	1,032
Total	40,724

Exhibit 12-18. ACCESS Enrollment Data for the Week Ended September 6, 1996

	Atlantic	Kaiser Permanente	Maxi-care	Optimum Choice	Wellness Plan	C. W. Williams	Total
Week totals	229	347	66	114	189	124	1,069
Month-to-date	229	347	66	114	189	124	1,069
Year-to-date	3,708	5,384	1,164	1,507	2,238	2,016	16,017
Project-to-date	3,708	5,384	1,164	1,507	2,238	2,016	16,017

ing and have no debt. We are running out of space at C. W. Williams. We have two examination rooms for each physician and all patients have to wait on the first floor and then be called to the second floor when a room becomes free. I know that ideally for the greatest efficiency we should have three exam rooms for each doctor.

We have had an architect look at the proposed facility. He estimated that it would take about $500,000 for remodeling. According to the tax records, the building and land are worth about $250,000. Since we don't yet know how many patients we will actually receive from Health Care Connection or how many of our patients will

Exhibit 12-19. C. W. Williams Health Center SWOT Analysis

Strengths	*Weaknesses*
Community-based business	Need for deputy director
Primary care provider with walk-in component	Lack of RN/triage director
	Staffing and staffing pattern
Large patient base	Managed-care readiness
Fast, discounted pharmacy	Number of providers
Cash reserve	Recruitment and retention
Laboratory/X-ray	Limited referrals
Clean facility in good location	Limited services
Satellites	No social worker/nutritionist/health educator
Good reputation with community and funders	No on-site Medicaid eligibility
	Weak relationship with community MDs
Resources for disabled patients	Limited hours of operation
Strong leadership/management	Transportation is a problem for many patients
Growth potential	Organizational structure
Property owned with good parking	Management information systems
Excellent quality of care	Market share at risk of erosion
Culturally sensitive staff	Staff orientation to managed care
Nice environment	
Dedicated board and staff	

Opportunities	*Threats*
Many in the community are uninsured and have multiple medical care needs	Uncertain financial future of health care in general
A number of universities are in located in the Charlotte area	Health care reform
Health care reform	Competition form other health care providers for the medically underserved
Oversupply of physicians means that many will not set up private practices or be able to join just any practice	Loss of patients as they choose HMOs other than C. W. Williams
Managed care	Managed care
Charlotte market is growing and prosperous	Reimbursement restructuring
	Shortage of health care professionals

choose an HMO, it's hard to decide if we should take the risk.

What To Do

"At the end of the week I sometimes wonder what I've accomplished," Michelle stated. "I seem to spend a lot of time putting out fires when I should be concentrating on developing a strategic plan and writing more grants."

Notes

1. This section is adapted from Mickey Goodson, *A Quick History,* an undated National Association of Community Health Centers Publication.

2. *Utilization and Costs to Medicaid of AFDC Recipients in New York Served and Not Served by Community Health Centers* (Columbia, MD: Center for Health Policy Studies, June, 1994).

3. *Using Medicaid Fee-for-Service Data to Develop Community Health Center Policy* (Seattle: Washington Association of Community Health Centers and Group Health Cooperative of Puget Sound, 1994).

4. *Key Points: A National Survey of Patient Experiences in Community and Migrant Health Centers* (New York: Commonwealth Fund, 1994).

5. *Health Insurance of Minorities in the U.S.*, report by the Agency for Health Care Policy and Research (Rockville, MD: U.S. Department of Health and Human Services, 1992); *Overview of Entitlement Programs Under the Jurisdiction of the Ways and Means Committee* (Green Book), U.S. House of Representatives, 1994.

Building for the Future of Public Health in Alabama

The second hand of the official clock in the Alabama House of Representatives swept with an inexorable force. Friends of Alabama's Department of Public Health were fighting desperately to save the bill that would authorize a $45 million bond issue for the building and renovation of every outdated public health facility across the state. It had come down to a final vote, on the last day, in the final hours of the session. It was a popular measure, because almost every legislator was getting one or more new buildings in his or her district. There was no doubt of the bill's passage—if it could be brought to a vote. Finally, the maneuvering came to a close. The ayes and nays were called. The bill passed.

Applause erupted in the gallery among the department staff who had worked for the measure. There was jubilation among the legislators on the floor. One, the representative from Pike County, waved to the senior public health staff watching in the gallery, seeking their attention. He then took their picture with an imaginary camera. They knew what he meant. When asked earlier for his support, he had instantly pledged his vote on the playful condition that his picture was taken for the papers at the ground-breaking and grand opening. "You got it, friend," thought Earl Fox, the State Health Officer. "A picture or two is little enough reward for the support."

The Legislature-Approved Bonds Fail

The state and county staff were thrilled at the prospect of new buildings. The state's Department of Public Health operated in all sixty-seven counties of the state through more than 140 separate facilities. The facilities served as public health clinics, a base of operations for home health staff, and as offices for department personnel providing nonclinical services. Most of the facilities were severely inadequate and required improvement or replacement. Most were built under the federal Hill-Burton program; the average age of the state's facilities was thirty-six years. Generally, they were poorly maintained and outdated for provision of modern medical care. This shortcoming was particularly critical in Alabama, where the public health system was an important part of the health care safety net. During 1995, the department provided more than 1 million clinic visits for

This case was prepared by Rueben E. Davidson, Alabama Department of Public Health; Stuart A. Capper, University of Alabama at Birmingham; and Mahmud Hassan, Rutgers University. It is intended as a basis for classroom discussion rather than to illustrate effective or ineffective handling of an administrative situation. Used with permission from Rueben E. Davidson.

hundreds of thousands of patients in a variety of programs. For example, half of all pregnant women in Alabama received some level of prenatal care in public health clinics, and more than half of the state's children received immunizations from the department.

Every bond issue required two fundamental ingredients: an investor willing to take risks (usually minimal risks) and an issuer with a convincing revenue stream to repay the investment. The more secure the revenue stream, the better would be the bond rating and the lower would be the interest rate on the bonds. The source of revenue for the repayment of the public health bond issue was to be a tax placed on hazardous waste deposited at the landfill located in Emelle, Alabama. The Legislature created a two-tiered tax system with a higher rate for out-of-state waste and lower rate for in-state waste. This differential tax structure was challenged immediately in court and ultimately ruled to be unconstitutional. During the protracted litigation, the public health bonds could not be sold, and after the litigation was resolved and a single tax rate was established, insufficient waste tonnage was being deposited at Emelle to provide sufficient tax revenue for timely repayment of the bonds. Thus, it became clear that this bond—the bond to be used to renovate numerous public health facilities in the state— would not be issued.

Alabama Public Health Facilities in Crisis

Just as the repayment source had failed, so were public health facilities in Alabama. The problem of inadequate buildings in disrepair, coupled with gross overcrowding, became even worse as the department experienced tremendous growth in clinical and home health programs. The number of employees grew from about 1,800 in 1989 to more than 5,000 in 1995. Of the 140 separate facilities operated in the state, 85 were county-owned and 55 were leased. To accommodate this growth, county health departments rented space on the private market and were paying in excess of $1.2

million a year, primarily to house home health and environmental health staff. Acquired on an ad hoc basis, the space was poorly designed in most cases and was less than ideal in meeting the department's mission.

By the time it became clear that the bond issue would not be sold, Dr. Donald E. Williamson had replaced Dr. Fox as State Health Officer. After several additional failed attempts to find reliable, tax-based revenue for repayment of bonds, a new approach was needed. Dr. Williamson met with Governor Folsom's Chief of Staff to discuss another option—one that had never before been used by a state agency for statewide public health facility construction. It previously had been used by local health care authorities for hospital construction, but never by a state agency in a statewide, public health construction program.

Another Option Pursued

Alabama law allowed for the creation of public finance authorities specifically for construction of health care facilities such as hospitals, nursing homes, public health facilities, and so on. The law required that a board be established in a county of the state. The board was authorized to sell tax-exempt bonds and construct buildings not only in the county in which the board was incorporated but also in any other county of the state. The bonds could be marketed based on a pledge of rent payments from the local health department to the public health finance authority to repay the debt service. (A copy of the law allowing creation of such authorities is labeled Exhibit 13-1.)

This approach seemed particularly attractive for several reasons:

1. The Department of Public Health had an operating budget in excess of $370 million and no debt. The estimated debt service of about $2 million was less than half of one percent of the total operations budget.

2. The department's funding base had, over the past decade, moved to a "cost-based" system rather than state and local governmental appropriations (Exhibit 13-2). This cost-based system

(text continues on page 360)

Exhibit 13-1. Alabama Enabling Legislation

Article 11.
Health Care Authorities.

§§22-21-310. Short title.

This article shall be known and may be cited as "The Health Care Authorities Act of 1982."

(Acts 1982, No. 82-418, p. 629, §1.)

§§22-21-311. Definitions.

(a) The following words and phrases used in this article, and others evidently intended as the equivalent thereof, shall, in the absence of clear implication herein otherwise, be given the following respective interpretations herein:

(1) APPLICANT. A natural person who files a written application with the governing body of a county or municipality, or two or more thereof, in accordance with the provisions of Section 22-21-313.

(2) AUTHORITY. A public corporation organized, and any public hospital corporation reincorporated, pursuant to the provisions hereof.

(3) AUTHORIZING RESOLUTION. The resolution adopted by the governing body of an authorizing subdivision, in accordance with the provisions of Section 22-21-313 or Section 22-21-341, that authorizes the incorporation of an authority or the reincorporation of a public hospital corporation.

(4) AUTHORIZING SUBDIVISION. Each county and municipality with the governing body of which an application for the incorporation of an authority hereunder or for the reincorporation of a public hospital corporation hereunder is filed.

(5) BOARD. The board of directors of an authority.

(6) CODE. The Code of Alabama 1975 and all amendments thereto and, with respect to any particular title, chapter, article, division, section or other portion thereof, any act of the Legislature or other code preceding such portion of the code or subsequently replacing the same.

(7) COUNTY. Any county in the state.

(8) COUPON. Any interest coupon evidencing an installment of interest payable with respect to a security.

(9) DIRECTOR. A member of a board.

(10) FEDERAL SECURITIES. Debt securities that are direct obligations of the United States of America for the payment of which the full faith and credit of the United States of America is pledged, or debt securities issued by a person controlled or supervised by and acting as an instrumentality of the United States of America, the payment of the principal of and interest on which is fully and unconditionally guaranteed by the United States of America.

(11) FISCAL YEAR. A fiscal year of the authorizing subdivision.

(12) GOVERNING BODY. With respect to a county, its county commission or other like governing body, and with respect to a municipality, its city or town council, board of commissioners or other like governing body.

(13) HEALTH CARE FACILITIES. Generally, any one or more buildings or facilities which serve to promote the public health, either by providing places or facilities for the diagnosis, treatment, care, cure or convalescence of sick, injured, physically disabled or handicapped, mentally ill, retarded or disturbed persons, or for the prevention of sickness and disease, or for the care, treatment and rehabilitation of alcoholics, or for the care of elderly persons, or for research with respect to any of the foregoing, including, without limiting the generality of the foregoing:

    a. Public hospitals of all types, public clinics, sanitoria, public health centers and related public health facilities, such as medical or dental facilities, laboratories, out-patient departments, educational facilities,

(Continued)

Exhibit 13-1. Continued

nurses' homes and nurses' training facilities, dormitories or residences for hospital personnel or students, other employee-related facilities, central service facilities operated in connection with public hospitals and other facilities (such as, for example, gift and flower shops, cafe and cafeteria facilities and the like) ancillary to public hospitals;

b. Retirement homes, nursing homes, convalescent homes, apartment buildings, dormitory or domiciliary facilities, residences or special care facilities for the housing and care of elderly persons or other persons requiring special care;

c. Appurtenant buildings and other facilities:

1. To provide offices for persons engaged in the diagnosis, treatment, care or cure of diseased, sick or injured persons, or in preventive medicine, or in the practice of dentistry; or

2. To house or service equipment used for the diagnosis, treatment, care or cure of diseased, sick or injured persons, or in preventive medicine, or in the practice of dentistry, or the records of such diagnosis, treatment, care, cure or practice or research with respect to any of the foregoing;

d. Parking areas, parking decks, facilities, buildings and structures appurtenant to any of the foregoing;

e. Ambulance, helicopter and other similar facilities and services for the transportation of sick or injured persons; and

f. Machinery, equipment, furniture and fixtures useful or desirable in the operation of any of the foregoing.

(14) HOSPITAL TAX. Any tax which may be levied for the benefit of an authority or any health care facilities owned or operated by it or the proceeds of which may have been appropriated, allocated or apportioned to such authority, or to or for the benefit of any such health care facilities, by the legislature or by the governing body of a county or municipality.

(15) INCORPORATORS. The natural persons forming an authority pursuant to the provisions of this article.

(16) INDENTURE. A mortgage, mortgage indenture, mortgage and trust indenture or trust indenture executed by an authority as security for any of its securities.

(17) LEGISLATURE. The Legislature of the state.

(18) MUNICIPALITY. An incorporated city or town of the state.

(19) PRINCIPAL OFFICE. The place at which the certificate of incorporation of an authority and amendments thereto, the bylaws and the minutes of the proceedings of the board are kept.

(20) PUBLIC HOSPITAL CORPORATION. Any public authority, public corporation or public association or entity organized on a local or regional basis by or with the consent of any county or municipality (or any two or more thereof) and having the power to own or operate any health care facilities, including (without limitation) any public corporation or authority heretofore or hereafter organized under the provisions of Article 3, Division 1 of Article 4, Article 5, or Article 6 of this chapter, Section 22-21-5, or Chapter 95 of Title 11, but excluding the state, any state institution of higher learning owning or operating health care facilities or any other state (as distinguished from local or regional) agency owning or operating health care facilities.

(21) SECURITIES. Bonds, notes, warrants, certificates of indebtedness or other evidences of indebtedness, including (without limiting the generality of the foregoing) notes issued in anticipation of the sale of any of the foregoing.

(22) STATE. The State of Alabama.

(b) The terms "herein," "hereby," "hereunder," "hereof," and other equivalent words refer to this article as an entirety and not solely to the particular section or portion hereof in which any such word is used. The definitions set forth herein shall be deemed applicable whether the words defined are used in the singular or plural. Whenever used herein any pronoun or pronouns shall be deemed to include both singular and plural and to cover all genders.

(Continued)

Exhibit 13-1. Continued

(Acts 1982, No. 82-418, p. 629, §2.)

§§22-21-312. Legislative findings and intent.

The Legislature hereby finds and declares:

(1) That publicly-owned (as distinguished from investor-owned and community-nonprofit) hospitals and other health care facilities furnish a substantial part of the indigent and reduced-rate care and other health care services furnished to residents of the state by hospitals and other health care facilities generally;

(2) That as a result of current significant fiscal and budgetary limitations or restrictions, the state and the various counties and municipalities therein are no longer able to provide, from taxes and other general fund moneys, all the revenues and funds necessary to operate such publicly-owned hospitals and other health care facilities adequately and efficiently; and

(3) That to enable such publicly-owned hospitals and other health care facilities to continue to operate adequately and efficiently, it is necessary that the entities and agencies operating them have significantly greater powers with respect to health care facilities than now vested in various public hospital or health-care authorities and corporations and the ability to provide a corporate structure somewhat more flexible than those now provided for in existing laws relating to the public hospital and health-care authorities.

It is therefore the intent of the Legislature by the passage of this article to promote the public health of the people of the state (1) by authorizing the several counties and municipalities in the state effectively to form public corporations whose corporate purpose shall be to acquire, own and operate health care facilities, and (2) by permitting, with the consent of the counties or municipalities (or both) authorizing their formation, existing public hospital corporations to reincorporate hereunder. To that end, this article invests each public corporation so organized or reincorporated hereunder with all powers that may be necessary to enable it to accomplish its corporate purposes and shall be liberally construed in conformity with said intent.

(Acts 1982, No. 82-418, p. 629, §3.)

§§22-21-313. Application for incorporation of authority; authorizing resolution.

(a) In order to incorporate an authority, any number of natural persons, not less than three, shall first file a written application with the governing body of any county or municipality, or any two or more thereof, which application shall:

(1) Recite the name of each county and municipality with the governing body of which such application is being filed;

(2) Contain a statement that the applicants propose to incorporate an authority pursuant to the provisions of this article;

(3) State that each of the applicants is a duly qualified elector of the authorizing subdivision (or, if there is more than one, at least one thereof); and

(4) Request that the governing body of such authorizing subdivision adopt a resolution declaring that it is wise, expedient and necessary that the proposed authority be formed, approving its certificate of incorporation and authorizing the applicants to proceed to form the proposed authority by filing for record a certificate of incorporation in accordance with the provisions of Section 22-21-314.

Every such application shall be accompanied by the form of certificate of incorporation of the proposed authority and by such other supporting documents as the applicants may consider appropriate.

(b) As promptly as may be practicable after the filing of the aforesaid application with it in accordance with the preceding provisions of this section, the governing body of each authorizing subdivision with which the application was filed shall review the contents of the application and the accompanying form of certificate of incorporation and shall adopt a resolution either

(Continued)

Exhibit 13-1. Continued

(1) Denying the application; or

(2) Declaring that it is wise, expedient and necessary that the proposed authority be formed, approving the form of its certificate of incorporation and authorizing the applicants to proceed to form the proposed authority by filing for record such a certificate of incorporation in accordance with the provisions of Section 22-21-314.

While it shall not be necessary that any such resolution be published in any newspaper or posted, the governing body of each authorizing subdivision with which the application is filed shall cause a copy of the application (and accompanying documents) to be included in the aforesaid resolution or otherwise spread upon or made a part of the minutes of the meeting thereof at which final action thereon is taken. Except as otherwise provided in Section 22-21-341, no authority shall be formed hereunder unless the application required by this section shall be made and unless an authorizing resolution for which provision is made in this section shall be adopted by each authorizing subdivision.

(Acts 1982, No. 82-418, p. 629, §4.)

§§22-21-314. Certificate of incorporation—Filing; form and contents; recordation.

(a) Within 40 days following the adoption of the authorizing resolution (or, if there is more than one, the last adopted thereof), the applicants shall proceed to incorporate an authority by filing for record, in the office of the judge of probate of the county in which the principal office of the authority is to be located, a certificate of incorporation which shall comply in form and substance with the requirements of this section, shall be in the form and executed in the manner herein provided and shall also be in the form theretofore approved by the governing body of each authorizing subdivision.

(b) In addition to any other provisions required by this article to be included therein, the certificate of incorporation of an authority shall state:

(1) The names of the incorporators, together with the address of the residence of each thereof, and that each of them is a duly qualified elector of the authorizing subdivision (or, if there is more than one, at least one thereof);

(2) The name of the authority, which may be a name indicating in a general way the area proposed to be served by the authority and shall include the words "Health Care Authority" (e.g., "The . . . Health Care Authority," or "The Health Care Authority of . . . ," the blank space to be filled in with the name of one or more of the authorizing subdivisions or other geographically descriptive word or words, such descriptive word or words not, however, to preclude the authority from locating health care facilities or otherwise exercising its powers in other geographical areas), unless the Secretary of State shall determine that such name is identical to the name of another corporation organized under the laws of the state or so nearly similar thereto as to lead to confusion and uncertainty, in which case the incorporators may insert additional identifying words so as to eliminate said duplication or similarity or adopt some other similar name that is available;

(3) The period for the duration of the authority (if the duration is to be perpetual, subject to the provisions of Section 22-21-339, that fact shall be stated);

(4) The name of each authorizing subdivision, together with the date on which the governing body thereof adopted an authorizing resolution;

(5) The location of the principal office of the authority, which shall be within the boundaries of the authorizing subdivision (or, if more than one, at least one thereof);

(6) That the authority is organized pursuant to the provisions of this article;

(7) If the exercise by the authority of any of its powers hereunder is to be in any way prohibited, limited or conditioned, a statement of the terms of such prohibition, limitation or condition;

(8) If the authority is to have the extraordinary power set out in Section 22-21-319, a statement to that effect;

(9) The number of directors, which shall be an odd number not less than three, the duration of their respective terms of office (which shall not be in excess of six years), and (subject to the provisions of Section 22-21-316) the manner of their election or appointment;

(Continued)

Exhibit 13-1. Continued

(10) Any provisions, not inconsistent with Section 22-21-339, relating to the vesting of title to its assets and properties upon its dissolution; and

(11) Any other matters relating to the authority that the incorporators may choose to insert and that are not inconsistent with this article or with the laws of the state.

(c) The certificate of incorporation shall be signed and acknowledged by each of the incorporators before an officer authorized by the laws of the state to take acknowledgements to deeds.

(d) When the certificate of incorporation is filed for record, there shall be attached to it:

(1) A certified copy of each authorizing resolution; and

(2) A certificate by the Secretary of State that the name proposed for the authority is not identical to that of any other corporation organized under the laws of the state or so nearly similar thereto as to lead to confusion and uncertainty.

(e) Upon the filing for record of the certificate of incorporation and the documents required by subsection (d) of this section to be attached thereto, the authority shall come into existence and shall constitute a public corporation under the name set forth in its certificate of incorporation. The said judge of probate shall thereupon record the certificate of incorporation in an appropriate book in his office.

(Acts 1982, No. 82-418, p. 629, §5.)

§§22-21-315. Certificate of incorporation—Amendment; application; approving resolution; filing and recordation of certificate.

(a) The certificate of incorporation of any authority incorporated under the provisions of this article, as well as that of any public hospital corporation reincorporated hereunder, may at any time and from time to time be amended, but only in the manner provided in this section. The board shall first adopt a resolution proposing an amendment to the certificate of incorporation of the authority, which amendment shall be set forth in full in the said resolution and which may include any matters that might have been included in an original certificate of incorporation hereunder.

(b) After the adoption by the board of a resolution proposing an amendment to the certificate of incorporation, the chairman and the secretary of the authority shall sign and file, with the governing body of each authorizing subdivision, a written application in the name and on behalf of the authority, under its seal, requesting such governing body to adopt a resolution approving the proposed amendment, and accompanied by a certified copy of the said resolution adopted by the board proposing the amendment to the certificate of incorporation, together with such documents in support of the application as the chairman may consider appropriate. As promptly as may be practicable after the filing of the application with the governing body of an authorizing subdivision as aforesaid, such governing body shall review the application and shall adopt a resolution either denying the application or approving and authorizing the proposed amendment. While it shall not be necessary that any such resolution be published in any newspaper or posted, the governing body of each authorizing subdivision with which any such application is filed shall cause a copy of the application and all accompanying documents to be included in the aforesaid resolution or otherwise spread upon or made a part of the minutes of the meeting of such governing body at which final action upon such application is taken. The certificate of incorporation of an authority may be amended only after the filing of such an application therefor and the adoption by the governing body of each authorizing subdivision of an approving resolution.

(c) Within 40 days following the adoption of a resolution approving the proposed amendment by the governing body of the authorizing subdivision (or, if there is more than one, the last adopted of such approving resolutions), the chairman and the secretary of the authority shall sign and file for record in the office of the judge of probate of the county in which the certificate of incorporation of the authority was filed a certificate in the name and on behalf of the authority, under its seal, reciting the adoption of said respective resolutions by the board and by the governing body of each authorizing subdivision and setting forth the proposed amendment. The said judge of probate shall thereupon record such certificate in an appropriate book in his office. When such certificate has been so filed and recorded, such amendment shall become effective, and the certificate of incorporation shall thereupon be amended to the extent provided in such amendment.

(Continued)

Exhibit 13-1. Continued

(Acts 1982, No. 82-418, p. 629, §6.)

§§22-21-316. Board of directors; qualifications; election or appointment; terms; vacancies; reimbursement for expenses; quorum; regular, special and called meetings; waiver of notice; record of proceedings; use as evidence; removal from office.

(a) Each authority shall have a board of directors composed of the number of directors provided in the certificate of incorporation, as most recently amended. Unless provided to the contrary in its certificate of incorporation, all powers of the authority shall be exercised, and the authority shall be governed, by the board or pursuant to its authorization. Subject to the provisions of subdivision (9) of subsection (b) of Section 22-21-314, the board shall consist of directors having such qualifications, being elected or appointed by such person or persons (including, without limitation, the board itself, the governing body or bodies of one or more authorizing subdivisions or other counties and municipalities, and other entities or organizations) and in such manner, and serving for such terms of office, all as shall be specified in the certificate of incorporation of the authority; provided however, that no fewer than a majority of the directors shall be elected by the governing body or bodies of one or more of the authorizing subdivisions and the certificate of incorporation of each authority must contain provisions having this effect.

(b) If, at the expiration of any term of office of any director, a successor thereto shall not have been elected or appointed, then the director whose term of office shall have expired shall continue to hold office until his successor shall be so elected or appointed. If at any time there should be a vacancy on the board, whether by death, resignation, incapacity, disqualification or otherwise, a successor director to serve for the unexpired term applicable to such vacancy shall be elected or appointed by the person or persons who elected or appointed the predecessor director. Each election or appointment of a director, whether for a full term or to complete an unexpired term, shall be made not earlier than 30 days prior to the date on which such director is to take office as such. Any director, irrespective of by whom elected or appointed, shall be eligible for reelection or reappointment.

(c) Each director shall serve as such without compensation but shall be reimbursed for expenses actually incurred by him in and about the performance of his duties. A majority of the directors shall constitute a quorum for the transaction of business, but any meeting of the board may be adjourned from time to time by a majority of the directors present or may be so adjourned by a single director if such director is the only director present at such meeting. No vacancy in the membership of the board shall impair the right of a quorum to exercise all the powers and perform all the duties of the board. The board shall hold regular meetings at such times as may be provided in the bylaws of the authority, may hold other meetings at any time and from time to time upon such notice as may be required by the bylaws of the authority, and must upon call of the chairman of the authority or a majority of the total number of directors, hold a special meeting, none of which meetings shall be subject to the provisions of Section 13A-14-2 or other similar law. Whenever any notice is required by the bylaws of the authority to be given of any meeting of the board, a waiver thereof in writing, signed (whether before or after such meeting) by the person or persons entitled to such notice, shall be the equivalent to the giving of such notice. Any matter on which the board is authorized to act may be acted upon at any regular, special or called meeting. At the request of any director, the vote on any question before the board shall be taken by yeas and nays and entered upon the record. All resolutions adopted by the board shall constitute actions of the authority, and all proceedings of the board shall be reduced to writing and signed by the secretary of the authority and shall be recorded in a well-bound book. Copies of such proceedings, when certified by the secretary of the authority, under the seal of the authority, shall be received in all courts as prima facie evidence of the matters and things therein certified.

(d) Any director may be impeached and removed from office in the same manner and on the same grounds provided in Section 175 of the Constitution of Alabama of 1901 and the general laws of the state for impeachment and removal of the officers mentioned in said Section 175.

(Acts 1982, No. 82-418, p. 629, §7.)

§§22-21-317. Officers; election; terms; duties.

The officers of an authority shall consist of a chairman, a vice-chairman, a secretary, a treasurer and such other officers as the board shall deem necessary or desirable. The chairman and the vice-chairman of the authority shall be elected by the board from its membership but neither the secretary, the treasurer nor any of the other officers of the authority need be a director. The offices of secretary and treasurer may, but need not be, held by the same person. The chairman and the vice-chairman of the authority shall be elected by the board for terms of not exceeding three years each, and the secretary, the

(Continued)

Exhibit 13-1. Continued

treasurer and the other officers of the authority shall be elected by the board for such terms as it deems advisable. The duties of the chairman, vice-chairman, secretary and treasurer shall be such as are customarily performed by such officers and as may be prescribed by the board. The duties of any other officers of the authority shall be such as are from time to time prescribed by the board.

(Acts 1982, No. 82-418, p. 629, §8.)

§§22-21-318. Powers of authority.

(a) In addition to all other powers granted elsewhere in this article, and subject to the express provisions of its certificate of incorporation, an authority shall have the following powers, together with all powers incidental thereto or necessary to the discharge thereof in corporate form:

(1) To have succession by its corporate name for the duration of time, which may be in perpetuity, specified in its certificate of incorporation or until dissolved as provided in Section 22-21-339;

(2) To sue and be sued in its own name in civil suits and actions, and to defend suits and actions against it, including suits and actions ex delicto and ex contractu, subject, however, to the provisions of Chapter 93 of Title 11, which chapter is hereby made applicable to the authority;

(3) To adopt and make use of a corporate seal and to alter the same at pleasure;

(4) To adopt, alter, amend and repeal bylaws, regulations and rules, not inconsistent with the provisions of this article or its certificate of incorporation, for the regulation and conduct of its affairs and business;

(5) To acquire, construct, reconstruct, equip, enlarge, expand, alter, repair, improve, maintain, equip, furnish and operate health care facilities at such place or places, within and without the boundaries of its authorizing subdivisions and within and without the state, as it considers necessary or advisable;

(6) To lease or otherwise make available any health care facilities or other of its properties and assets to such persons, firms, partnerships, associations or corporations and on such terms as the board deems to be appropriate, to charge and collect rent or other fees or charges therefor and to terminate any such lease or other agreement upon the failure of the lessee or other party thereto to comply with any of its obligations thereunder;

(7) To receive, acquire, take and hold (whether by purchase, gift, transfer, foreclosure, lease, devise, option or otherwise) real and personal property of every description, or any interest therein, and to manage, improve and dispose of the same by any form of legal conveyance or transfer; provided however, that the authority shall not, without the prior approval of the governing body of each authorizing subdivision, have the power to dispose of (i) substantially all its assets, or (ii) any health care facilities the disposition of which would materially and significantly reduce or impair the level of hospital or health care services rendered by the authority; and provided further, that the foregoing proviso shall not be construed to require the prior approval of any such governing body for the mortgage or pledge of all or substantially all its assets or of any of its health care facilities, for the foreclosure of any such mortgage or pledge or for any sale or other disposition thereunder;

(8) To mortgage, pledge or otherwise convey its property and its revenues from any source;

(9) To borrow money in order to provide funds for any lawful corporate function, use or purpose and, in evidence of such borrowing, to sell and issue interest-bearing securities in the manner provided and subject to the limitations set forth hereinafter;

(10) To pledge for payment of any of its securities any revenues (including proceeds from any hospital tax to which it may be entitled) and to mortgage or pledge any or all of its health care facilities or other assets or properties or any part or parts thereof, whether then owned or thereafter acquired, as security for the payment of the principal of and the interest and premium, if any, on any securities so issued and any agreements made in connection therewith;

(11) To provide instruction and training for, and to contract for the instruction and training of, nurses, technicians and other technical, professional and paramedical personnel;

(Continued)

Exhibit 13-1. Continued

(12) To select and appoint medical and dental staff members and others licensed to practice the healing arts and to delineate and define the privileges granted each such individual;

(13) To affiliate with, and to contract to provide training and clinical experience for students of, other institutions;

(14) To contract for the operation of any department, section, equipment or holdings of the authority, and to enter into agreements with any person, firm or corporation for the management by said person, firm or corporation on behalf of the authority of any of its properties or for the more efficient or economical performance of clerical, accounting, administrative and other functions relating to its health care facilities;

(15) To establish, collect and alter charges for services rendered and supplies furnished by it;

(16) To make all needful or appropriate rules and regulations for the conduct of any health care facilities and other properties owned or operated by it and to alter such rules and regulations;

(17) To provide for such insurance as the business of the authority may require;

(18) To receive and accept from any source aid or contributions in the form of money, property, labor or other things of value, to be held, used and applied to carry out the purposes of this article, subject to any lawful condition upon which any such aid or contributions may be given or made;

(19) To cooperate with the State Board of Health and the State Department of Mental Health and to make contracts with either of said agencies respecting the operation of any health care facilities or other properties owned or operated by it, whether as an agent for either or both of said agencies or otherwise;

(20) To enter into contracts with, to accept aid, loans and grants from, to cooperate with and to do any and all things not specifically prohibited by this article or the Constitution of the state that may be necessary in order to avail itself of the aid and cooperation of the United States of America, the state, any county or municipality, or any agency, instrumentality or political subdivision of any of the foregoing in furtherance of the purposes of this article; to give such assurances, contractual or otherwise, to or for the benefit of any of the foregoing as may be required in connection with, or as conditions precedent to the receipt of, any such aid, loan or grant; and to take such action not in violation of law as may be necessary in order to qualify the authority to receive funds appropriated by any of the foregoing;

(21) To give such assurances, contractual or otherwise, and to make such commitments and agreements as may be necessary or desirable to preclude the exercise of any rights of recovery with respect to, or the forfeiture of title to, any of its health care facilities or other property or any health care facilities or other property proposed to be acquired by it;

(22) To make and alter rules and regulations for the treatment of indigent patients;

(23) To assume any obligations of any entity that conveys and transfers to the authority any health care facilities or other property, or interest therein, provided that such obligations appertain to the health care facilities, property or interest so conveyed and transferred to the authority;

(24) To assume, establish, fund and maintain retirement, pension or other employee benefit plans for its employees;

(25) To appoint, employ, contract with, and provide for the compensation of, such employees and agents, including but not limited to, architects, attorneys, consultants, engineers, accountants, financial experts, fiscal agents and such other advisers, consultants and agents as the business of the authority may require;

(26) To invest, in any trust fund established under and subject to the general laws of the state for investment or self-insurance purposes with investment authority as may be authorized by law for such trusts, any funds of the authority available therefor;

(27) To the extent permitted by its contracts with the holders of its securities, to purchase securities out of any of its funds or moneys available therefor and to hold, cancel or resell such securities;

(28) To make any expenditure of any moneys under its control that would, if the authority were generally subject to State Corporate Income Taxation, be considered an ordinary and necessary expense of the authority within the

(Continued)

Exhibit 13-1. Continued

meaning of Section 40-18-35 and applicable regulations thereunder, and without limiting the generality of the fore-going, to expend its moneys for the recruitment of employees and physicians, dentists and other health care professionals and for the promotion of employee morale and well-being; provided however, that nothing herein contained shall be construed to permit the authority (i) to increase the compensation of any of its officers or employees on a retroactive basis, (ii) to pay any extra compensation to any of its officers or employees for services theretofore rendered, (iii) to furnish free or below-cost office space to any nonhospital-based physician, dentist or other health care professional for use in his private practice, or (iv) to guarantee the income of any nonhospital-based physician, dentist or other health care professional in his private practice;

(29) To provide scholarships for students in training for work in the duties peculiar to health care;

(30) To enter into affiliation, cooperation, territorial, management or other similar agreements with other institutions (public or private) for the sharing, division, allocation or exclusive furnishing of services, referral of patients, management of facilities and other similar activities;

(31) To exercise all powers granted hereunder in such manner as it may determine to be consistent with the purposes of this article, notwithstanding that as a consequence of such exercise of such powers it engages in activities that may be deemed "anticompetitive" within the contemplation of the antitrust laws of the state or of the United States; and

(32) To enter into such contracts, agreements, leases and other instruments, and to take such other actions, as may be necessary or convenient to accomplish any purpose for which the authority was organized or to exercise any power expressly granted hereunder.

(b) The Legislature hereby declares:

(1) That any expenditure permitted by the provisions of subdivision (28) of the preceding subsection (a) of this section to be made by or on behalf of an authority shall be deemed an expenditure of operating and maintaining public hospitals and public health facilities for a public purpose; and

(2) That no expenditure permitted by the provisions of said subdivision (28) to be made by or on behalf of an authority shall be considered to be a lending of credit or a granting of public money or thing of value to or in aid of any individual, association or corporation within the meaning of any constitutional or statutory provision.

Nothing herein contained shall be construed as prohibiting or rendering unlawful any otherwise lawful expenditure made by or on behalf of an authority, solely because such expenditure is not expressly permitted by the terms of said subdivision (28).

(c) As a basis for the power granted in subdivision (31) of the preceding subsection (a), the legislature hereby:

(1) Recognizes and contemplates that the nature and scope of the powers conferred on authorities hereunder are such as may compel each authority, in the course of exercising its other powers or by virtue of such exercise of such powers, to engage in activities that may be characterized as "anticompetitive" within the contemplation of the antitrust laws of the state or of the United States; and

(2) Determines, as an expression of the public policy of the state with respect to the displacement of competition in the field of health care, that each authority, when exercising its powers hereunder with respect to the operation and management of health care facilities, acts as an agency or instrumentality of its authorizing subdivisions and as a political subdivision of the state.

(d) Nothing herein contained shall be construed as granting to an authority the power to levy any taxes.

(Acts 1982, No. 82-418, p. 629, §9.)

§§22-21-319. Extraordinary power of authority.

If and only if its certificate of incorporation or an appropriate amendment thereto (both of which must, under the terms of this article, be approved by the governing body of each authorizing subdivision) shall expressly so provide, an authority shall have, in addition to all other powers granted elsewhere in this article, the same power of eminent domain as is vested

(Continued)

Exhibit 13-1. Continued

by law in any authorizing subdivision, in the same manner and under the same conditions as are provided by law for the exercise of the power of eminent domain by such authorizing subdivision; provided however, that under no circumstances may an authority exercise the power of eminent domain for the purposes of providing office facilities for any physician, dentist or other health care professional primarily for use in his private practice.

(Acts 1982, No. 82-418, p. 629, §10.)

§§22-21-320. Securities of authority.

Securities of an authority may be executed and delivered by it at any time and from time to time, shall be in such form and denominations and of such tenor and maturity or maturities not exceeding 40 years from their date, shall bear such rate or rates of interest (which may be fixed or which may float or vary based on some index or other standard deemed appropriate by the board), shall be payable and evidenced in such manner, may contain provisions for redemption prior to maturity and may contain other provisions not inconsistent with this article, all as may be provided by the resolution of the board authorizing the same or by the indenture whereunder such securities are authorized to be issued. Each such security having a specified maturity date more than 10 years after its date shall be made subject to redemption at the option of the authority at the end of the tenth year after its date, and on any interest payment date thereafter, under such terms and conditions as may be provided in the resolution authorizing the same or the indenture under which issued. Any borrowing may be effected by the issuance and sale of securities at either public or private sale in such manner, at such price or prices, at such time or times and on such other terms and conditions as may be determined by the board to be most advantageous to the authority.

(Acts 1982, No. 82-418, p. 629, §11.)

§§22-21-321. Refunding securities.

(a) An authority may at any time and from time to time sell and issue its refunding securities for the purpose of refunding the principal of and interest on any then outstanding securities of the authority, whether or not such securities shall have matured or be redeemable at the option of the authority at the time of such refunding, and for the payment of any expenses incurred in connection with such refunding and any premium or other sum necessary to be paid to redeem or retire the securities so to be refunded; provided however, that the principal amount of securities that the authority may at any time issue for refunding purposes shall not exceed the sum of the following:

(1) The outstanding principal or face amount of the securities refunded thereby;

(2) The unpaid interest accrued or to accrue thereon to their respective maturities (or, in the event the securities to be refunded, or any part thereof, are to be retired prior to their respective maturities, the interest accrued or to accrue thereon to the date or dates on which they are to be retired);

(3) Any premium or other sum necessary to be paid in order to redeem or retire the securities to be refunded (but only if such securities are in fact to be redeemed or retired prior to their respective maturities); and

(4) The expenses estimated to be incurred in connection with such refunding.

The authority may also at any time and from time to time sell and issue its securities for the combined purpose of so refunding any of its securities and of obtaining funds for any other purpose for which it is authorized by this article to sell and issue securities, in which event the provisions of this article relating to refunding securities shall apply only to those of such securities issued for refunding purposes.

(b) The principal proceeds derived by the authority from the sale of any refunding securities shall be used only for the payment of the principal of and the interest (and premium) on the securities being refunded and for payment of the expenses referred to in the preceding subdivision (4) of subsection (a) of this section; provided, that if in the judgment of the board such is necessary or desirable to effect an advantageous refunding, a portion of said proceeds may be used for payment of principal of and interest on such refunding securities themselves and the remainder of said proceeds for payment of the securities being refunded and of said expenses; and provided further, that any portion of said proceeds that shall at the time not be needed therefor, may be invested in such investments as are specified in Section 22-21-332.

(Continued)

Exhibit 13-1. Continued

(c) Any such refunding may be effected either by sale of refunding securities and the application of the proceeds thereof as provided in subsection (b) of this section, or by exchange of the refunding securities for the securities or coupons to be refunded thereby, or by any combination thereof; provided, that the holders of any securities or coupons so to be refunded shall not be compelled without their consent to surrender their securities or coupons for payment or exchange prior to the date on which they may be paid or redeemed by call of the authority under their respective provisions. All provisions of this article pertaining to securities of the authority that are not inconsistent with the provisions of this section shall, to the extent applicable, also apply to refunding securities issued by the authority and to securities issued by the authority for both refunding and other purposes.

(Acts 1982, No. 82-418, p. 629, §12.)

§§22-21-322. Execution of securities.

All securities of an authority shall be signed in the name and behalf of the authority by its chairman or vice-chairman, and the seal of the authority shall be affixed thereto and attested by its secretary or an assistant secretary; provided, that a facsimile of the signature of one, but not both, of the officers whose signature will appear on such securities may be imprinted or otherwise reproduced on any thereof in lieu of his manually signing the same; and provided further, that a facsimile of the seal of the authority may be imprinted, or otherwise reproduced, on any such securities in lieu of being manually affixed thereto. Any coupons applicable to any securities of the authority shall be signed either manually by, or with a facsimile of the signature of, the chairman or the vice-chairman of the authority. If after any such securities or coupons shall be so signed, whether manually or by facsimile, any such officer shall, for any reason, vacate his office, the securities and coupons so signed may nevertheless be delivered at any time thereafter as the act and deed of the authority.

(Acts 1982, No. 82-418, p. 629, §13.)

§§22-21-323. Source of payment; security.

(a) Securities issued by an authority shall not be general obligations of the authority but shall be payable solely out of the revenues from any health care facilities or other properties or assets (including, without limitation, proceeds from such securities, investment income and insurance and condemnation proceeds) owned or operated by it and the proceeds of any hospital tax appropriated, apportioned or allocated to it or for its benefit, or any portion of either thereof, all as may be provided or specified in the resolution of the board authorizing such securities or the indenture under which issued. The principal of and interest (and premium, if any) on any securities issued by the authority shall be secured by a pledge of the revenues or taxes (or both) out of which the same are payable and may be secured by a trust indenture evidencing such pledge or by a foreclosable mortgage, mortgage indenture or mortgage and trust indenture conveying as security for such securities all or any part of its property.

(b) Any indenture executed on behalf of the authority and any resolution of the board authorizing the issuance of securities may contain such agreements as the board may deem advisable respecting the operation and maintenance of the properties of the authority, the application and use of any revenues (including hospital tax proceeds) out of which any such securities are payable, the rights or duties of the parties to such instrument or the parties for the benefit of whom such instrument is made and the rights and remedies of such parties in the event of default, and may also contain provisions restricting the individual rights of action of the holders of any such securities. Any such indenture may be filed in the office of the judge of probate of any county in which any of the property, real, personal or mixed, subject to the lien thereof is, or is anticipated to be, located, and the lien of such indenture shall, with respect to all personal property and fixtures subject thereto (including after-acquired property) and notwithstanding any contrary provisions of, and without compliance with, the Alabama Uniform Commercial Code (Title 7), be valid and binding against all parties having claims of any kind against the authority, irrespective of whether the parties have actual notice thereof, from the time such indenture is so filed. Any such pledge of any such revenues (including hospital tax proceeds) shall be valid and binding from the time it is made, and the revenues (including hospital tax proceeds) so pledged and thereafter received by the authority shall immediately become subject to the lien of such pledge without any physical delivery thereof or further act. The lien of such pledge shall, notwithstanding any contrary provisions of the Alabama Uniform Commercial Code (Title 7), and without compliance with the provisions thereof, be valid and binding against all parties having claims of any kind against the authority, irre-

Exhibit 13-1. Continued

spective of whether the parties have actual notice thereof, from the time there is filed in the office of the judge of probate of the county in which the principal office of the authority is located a notice stating the date on which the resolution authorizing the issuance of the securities was adopted by the board, the principal amount of the securities issued, a brief description of the revenues (including any hospital tax proceeds) so pledged and a brief description of any property the revenues from which are so pledged. Issuance by any authority of one or more series of securities for one or more purposes shall not preclude it from issuing other securities, but the resolution or indenture whereunder any subsequent securities may be issued shall recognize and protect any prior pledge or mortgage made for the benefit of any prior issue of securities unless in the proceedings authorizing such prior issue the right was reserved to issue subsequent securities on a parity with such prior issue. The trustee under any indenture may be a trust company or bank having trust powers, whether located within or without the state, and may be selected by the board without regard to the provisions of Chapter 25 of Title 36.

(Acts 1982, No. 82-418, p. 629, §14.)

§§22-21-324. Use of proceeds.

(a) The principal proceeds derived from any borrowing made by an authority shall be used solely for the purpose or purposes for which such borrowing was authorized to be made. If any securities are issued for the purpose of financing costs of acquiring, constructing, improving, enlarging and equipping health care facilities, such costs shall be deemed to include the following:

(1) The cost of any land forming a part of such health care facilities;

(2) The cost of the labor, materials and supplies used in any such construction, improvement or enlargement, including architectural and engineering fees and the cost of preparing contract documents advertising for bids;

(3) The purchase price of, and the cost of installing, equipment for such health care facilities;

(4) The cost of landscaping the lands forming a part of such health care facilities and of constructing and installing roads, sidewalks, curbs, gutters, utilities and parking places in connection therewith;

(5) Legal, accounting, publishing, printing, fiscal and recording fees and expenses incurred in connection with the authorization, sale and issuance of the securities issued in connection with such health care facilities; bond discount, commission or other financing charges; fees and expenses of financial advisers and planning and management consultants; the cost of any feasibility studies deemed necessary or advisable in connection with the issuance and sale of such securities; the amount of any debt service reserve that the board deems necessary or advisable to be funded out of the proceeds from the sale of such securities; and such other expenses as shall be necessary or incident to such borrowing;

(6) Interest on such securities for a reasonable period prior to the commencement of the construction and equipment of such health care facilities, or of any improvements or additions being financed (in whole or in part) out of the proceeds from the sale of such securities, and during the period estimated to be required for such construction and equipment and for a period of not more than two years after the completion of such construction and equipment;

(7) The reimbursement to itself, or to its general fund or any one or more of its other funds, to any authorizing subdivision or other county or municipality, and to any public hospital corporation or other public agency, authority or body, of any funds advanced, to or for the benefit of the authority or any health care facilities owned by it, in anticipation of the issuance of securities by the authority, including the amount of any interest paid or incurred on any borrowings made for the purpose of obtaining funds to advance to or for the benefit of the authority or such health care facilities; and

(8) The amount of such reserves for the payment of debt service on any such securities and for the maintenance, repair, replacement, improvement and enlargement of any of its health care facilities and other properties as the board shall deem advisable.

(b) Any portion of the principal proceeds derived from any such borrowing not needed for any of the purposes for which such borrowing was authorized to be made shall be applied and used:

(1) For retirement of the securities issued in evidence of such borrowing;

(2) For payment of the interest thereon;

(Continued)

Exhibit 13-1. Continued

(3) For payment into one or more special funds created for payment of principal or interest, or both, or for the creation of reserves for the payment of debt service or for maintenance, repair, replacement, improvement or enlargement; or

(4) For any combination thereof, all as shall be specified in the indenture under which such securities are issued or in the resolution of the board authorizing any such borrowing.

(Acts 1982, No. 82-418, p. 629, §15.)

§§22-21-325. **Obligations not debt of state, county or municipality.**

All agreements and obligations undertaken, and all securities issued, by an authority shall be solely and exclusively an obligation of the authority and shall not create an obligation or debt of the state, any authorizing subdivision or any other county or municipality within the meaning of any constitutional or statutory provision. The faith and credit of the state, any authorizing subdivision or any other county or municipality shall never be pledged for the payment of any securities issued by an authority; nor shall the state, any authorizing subdivision or any other county or municipality be liable in any manner for the payment of the principal of or interest on any securities of an authority or for the performance of any pledge, mortgage, obligation or agreement of any kind whatsoever that may be undertaken by an authority.

(Acts 1982, No. 82-418, p. 629, §16.)

§§**Section 22-21-326. Securities issued under article as legal investments.**

Securities issued under the provisions of this article are hereby made legal investments for savings banks and insurance companies organized under the laws of the state. Unless otherwise directed by the court having jurisdiction thereof or the document that is the source of authority, a trustee, executor, administrator, guardian or one acting in any other fiduciary capacity may, in addition to any other investment powers conferred by law and with the exercise of reasonable business prudence, invest trust funds in securities of an authority. The governing body of any authorizing subdivision (or any county or municipality in which any health care facilities of an authority may be situated) is authorized, in its discretion, to invest in securities of such authority any idle or surplus money held in its treasury which is not otherwise earmarked or pledged.

(Acts 1982, No. 82-418, p. 629, §17.)

§§22-21-327. **Securities and coupons as negotiable instruments.**

Securities issued by an authority, while not registered, shall be construed to be negotiable instruments although payable solely from a specified or limited source. All coupons applicable to any securities issued by an authority, while the applicable securities are not registered as to both principal and interest, shall likewise be construed to be negotiable instruments although payable solely from a specified or limited source.

(Acts 1982, No. 82-418, p. 629, §18.)

§§22-21-328. **Exemption from usury and interest laws.**

An authority shall be exempt from all laws of the state governing usury or prescribing or limiting interest rates, including, but without limitation to, the provisions of Chapter 8 of Title 8.

(Acts 1982, No. 82-418, p. 629, §19.)

§§22-21-329. **Notice of issuance of securities; limitation on actions to contest.**

Any resolution authorizing any securities under this article may contain a recital that they are issued pursuant to the provisions of this article, which recital shall be conclusive evidence that such securities have been duly authorized pursuant to the provisions of this article, notwithstanding the provisions of any other law now in force or hereafter enacted or

(Continued)

Exhibit 13-1. Continued

amended. Upon the adoption by the board of any resolution providing for the issuance of securities, the authority may, in its discretion, cause to be published, once a week for two consecutive weeks, in a newspaper then published in the county in which the principal office of the authority is located, or, if there is no such newspaper, then in a daily newspaper published in the state, a notice in substantially the following form, with any appropriate changes, to the extent applicable and with the blanks being properly filled in:

"_____, a public corporation and instrumentality under the laws of the state of Alabama, has authorized the issuance of $_____ principal amount of securities of the said authority to be dated _____, for purposes authorized in Act No. 82-418 enacted at the 1982 Regular Session of the legislature of Alabama. Any action or proceeding questioning the validity of the said securities, or the pledge [and any indenture] to secure the same, must be commenced within 20 days after the first publication of this notice."

Any action or proceeding in any court to set aside or question the validity of the proceedings for the issuance of the securities referred to in said notice or to contest the validity of any such securities, the validity of any pledge made therefor or the validity of any indenture with respect thereto must be commenced within 20 days after the first publication of such notice. After the expiration of the said period, no right of action or defense questioning or attacking the validity of the said proceedings, the said securities, any pledge herein authorized, or such indenture shall be asserted, nor shall the validity of the said proceedings, securities, pledge or indenture be open to question in any court on any ground whatsoever except in an action commenced within said period.

(Acts 1982, No. 82-418, p. 629, §20.)

§§22-21-330. Lease agreements with authorizing subdivision; terms; renewal options; special pledge as security for payment of rental, etc.; use of vacant space.

(a) Each authority and any authorizing subdivision are hereby respectively authorized to enter into one or more lease agreements with each other whereunder any health care facilities situated within (or within 10 miles of) such authorizing subdivision or any part thereof shall be leased by the authority to such authorizing subdivision, but if and only if such authorizing subdivision is then permitted by law to operate such health care facilities, to issue its bonds, warrants, notes or other securities therefor and to pledge for the benefit of any such securities its full faith and credit. No such lease agreement shall be for a term longer than the then current fiscal year in which it is made. Any such lease agreement may, however, contain a grant to such authorizing subdivision of successive options to renew such lease agreement, on the conditions specified therein, for additional terms, but no such additional term shall be for a period longer than the fiscal year in which such renewal shall be made. Such lease agreement may contain provisions as to the method by which such renewal may be effected.

(b) The obligation on the part of such authorizing subdivision to pay the rental required to be paid and to perform the agreements on its part required to be performed during any fiscal year during which such lease agreement is in effect shall constitute a general obligation of such authorizing subdivision, which is authorized to pledge its full faith and credit for the payment of such rental and the performance of such agreements; provided, that the rental required to be paid and the agreements required to be performed by such authorizing subdivision under such lease agreement during any fiscal year during which such lease agreement is in effect shall be payable solely out of the current revenues of such authorizing subdivision for such fiscal year.

(c) As additional security for the payment of the rental required to be paid and for performance of the agreements on the part of such authorizing subdivision required to be performed during the first or initial term of any lease agreement made by the authority with such authorizing subdivision, such authorizing subdivision is authorized to pledge specially so much of the following revenues and tax proceeds as may be necessary to pay the rental and to perform the agreements which are required in said lease agreement to be paid and performed during the said initial term:

(1) The revenues that may be received by such authorizing subdivision during the said initial term from the operation of the health care facilities covered by the said lease agreement remaining after the payment of all reasonable expenses during the said initial term for the operation and maintenance of the said health care facilities; and

(2) The proceeds that may be received by such authorizing subdivision during the said initial term from any tax or taxes, the proceeds of which the authorizing subdivision is authorized, in Section 11-81-16, to pledge for the benefit of bonds of such authorizing subdivision.

(Continued)

Exhibit 13-1. Continued

Whenever a lease agreement containing such a special pledge is renewed under its terms for an additional term, such special pledge shall be deemed effective for such additional term without the necessity of a new pledge being made or a new lease agreement being entered into for that purpose, and the exercise of the option to renew shall be construed as a renewal also of the said special pledge; provided, that said special pledge shall be applicable only to the aforesaid pledged revenues that are received by such authorizing subdivision during the fiscal year for which the lease agreement is renewed. Each such special pledge that shall be so effected by renewal of said lease agreement for an additional term shall be deemed to relate to, and to have been made as of, the date on which such lease agreement was made and shall take precedence over any pledge of said pledged revenues which might be made by such authorizing subdivision and over any claim which might arise against the said pledged revenues between the date on which such lease agreement was made and the first day of the additional term for which such lease agreement shall be so renewed. Any pledge of revenues made by such authorizing subdivision as aforesaid under the provisions of any contract made by it subsequent to the date of the lease agreement containing such special pledge shall be subordinate to the special pledge contained in such lease agreement.

(d) In any instance where a lease agreement contains a pledge of any tax proceeds, such authorizing subdivision shall during each fiscal year that such lease agreement shall be in effect:

(1) Levy the tax or taxes so pledged; and

(2) Use so much of the proceeds therefrom as may be necessary to pay the rentals and perform the agreements on the part of such authorizing subdivision which are required in such lease agreement to be paid and performed during such fiscal year.

(e) Any lease agreement may contain such covenants as shall not be inconsistent with this article. The rental required to be paid and the agreements required to be performed by such authorizing subdivision under the provisions of such lease agreement shall never create an indebtedness of such authorizing subdivision within the meaning of any constitutional or statutory limitation or provision. If any space available for rent in any health care facilities which shall have been leased, in whole or in part, to such authorizing subdivision should become vacant after acquisition or construction of such health care facilities by the authority, then until such time as all such vacant space therein shall have been filled or rented, neither such authorizing subdivision nor any officer, department or agency thereof, shall thereafter enter into any rental agreement, or renew any then existing rental agreement, for other space in or about such authorizing subdivision to be used for the same purposes for which such vacant space in such health care facilities is capable of being used.

(Acts 1982, No. 82-418, p. 629, §21.)

§§22-21-331. Remedies for default in payment of securities or performance of lease agreement.

(a) If there should be any default in the payment of the principal of or interest on any securities issued under this article, then the holder of any such securities and any coupons applicable thereto (subject to any provision of the resolution or indenture under which such securities were issued restricting the individual rights of action of any such holders or vesting such rights exclusively in a trustee), and the trustee under any indenture, or any one or more of them:

(1) May, by mandamus, injunction or other proceedings, compel performance of all duties of the directors and officers of the authority with respect to the use of funds for the payment of such securities and for the performance of the agreements of the authority contained in the proceedings under which they were issued;

(2) Shall be entitled to a judgment against the authority for the principal of and interest on the securities so in default;

(3) May, in the event such securities are secured by a mortgage on or security interest in any physical properties of the authority, foreclose such mortgage or pledge, exercise any powers of sale contained therein or exercise any possessory or other similar rights as are provided for in the resolution or indenture under which such securities were issued;

(4) Regardless of the sufficiency of the security for the securities in default and as a matter of right, shall be entitled to the appointment of a receiver:

a. To make lease agreements respecting any health care facilities or other properties out of whose revenues the securities so in default are payable and fix and collect rents therefor; and

(Continued)

Exhibit 13-1. Continued

b. To operate, administer and maintain such health care facilities and other properties, with all powers of a receiver in the exercise of any of said functions.

The income derived from any lease agreement made, and any operation of such health care facilities and other properties carried on, by any such receiver shall be expended in accordance with the provisions of the proceedings under which the securities were authorized to be issued and the orders of the court by which such receiver is appointed.

(b) If there should be any default by the authorizing subdivision in the payment of any installment of rent or in the performance of any agreement required to be made or performed by it under the provisions of any lease agreement described in Section 22-21-330, the authority and the trustee under any indenture, or either of them:

(1) May, by mandamus, injunction or other proceedings, compel performance by the officials of the authorizing subdivision of their duties respecting the payment of the rentals required to be paid and performance of the agreements on the part of the authorizing subdivision required to be performed under any such lease agreement; and

(2) Shall be entitled to a judgment against the authorizing subdivision for all monetary payments required to be made by the authorizing subdivision under the provisions of such lease agreement with respect to which the authorizing subdivision is then in default.

(c) The remedies specified in this section shall be cumulative to all other remedies which may otherwise be available, by law or contract, for the benefit of the holders of the securities and the coupons applicable thereto.

(Acts 1982, No. 82-418, p. 629, §22.)

§§22-21-332. Investment of funds.

(a) To the extent permitted by the contracts of the authority with the holders of its securities and if not otherwise specifically prohibited by any other provision of this article, the authority may invest any portion of the principal proceeds derived from the sale of any of its securities which is not then needed for any of the purposes for which such securities were authorized to be issued, the moneys held in any special fund created pursuant to any resolution or indenture authorizing or securing any of its securities, and any other moneys of the authority not then needed by it, in any of the following:

(1) Federal securities;

(2) Any debt securities that are direct obligations of any agency of the United States of America;

(3) Interest-bearing bank time deposits and interest-bearing bank certificates of deposit; and

(4) Interest-bearing time deposits and interest-bearing certificates of deposit of any federally chartered savings and loan association.

(b) Any securities, time deposits or certificates of deposit in which any such investment is made may, at any time and from time to time, be sold or otherwise converted into cash. The income derived from any such investments shall be disbursed on order of the board for any purpose for which the authority may lawfully expend funds.

(Acts 1982, No. 82-418, p. 629, §23.)

§§22-21-333. Exemptions from taxation.

All properties of an authority, whether real, personal or mixed, and the income therefrom, all securities issued by an authority and the coupons applicable thereto and the income therefrom, and all indentures and other instruments executed as security therefor, all leases made pursuant to the provisions of this article and all revenues derived from any such leases, and all deeds and other documents executed by or delivered to an authority shall be exempt from any and all taxation by the state, or by any county, municipality or other political subdivision of the state, including, but without limitation to, license and excise taxes imposed in respect of the privilege of engaging in any of the activities in which an authority may engage. An authority shall not be obligated to pay or allow any fees, taxes or costs to the judge of probate of any county in respect of its incorporation, the amendment of its certificate of incorporation or the recording of any document. Further, the gross proceeds of the sale of any property used in the construction and equipment of any health care facilities for an authority,

(Continued)

Exhibit 13-1. Continued

regardless of whether such sale is to such authority or any contractor or agent thereof, shall be exempt from the sales tax imposed by Article 1 of Chapter 23 of Title 40 and from all other sales and similar excise taxes now or hereafter levied on or with respect to the gross proceeds of any such sale by the state or any county, municipality or other political subdivision or instrumentality of any thereof; and any property used in the construction and equipment of any health care facilities for an authority, regardless of whether such property has been purchased by the authority or any contractor or agent thereof, shall be exempt from the use tax imposed by Article 2 of Chapter 23 of Title 40 and all other use and similar excise taxes now or hereafter levied on or with respect to any such property by the state or any county, municipality or other political subdivision or instrumentality of any thereof.

(Acts 1982, No. 82-418, p. 629, §24.)

§§22-21-334. **Nonapplicability of Ethics Act.**

The provisions of Chapter 25 of Title 36 shall, any provision thereof to the contrary notwithstanding, not apply to any authority, the members of its board or any of its officers or employees.

(Acts 1982, No. 82-418, p. 629, §25.)

§§22-21-335. **Nonapplicability of competitive bid laws.**

The provisions of Articles 2 and 3 of Chapter 16 of Title 41 shall not apply to any authority, the members of its board or any of its officers or employees.

(Acts 1982, No. 82-418, p. 629, §26.)

§§22-21-336. **Transfer of funds and assets to authority.**

Any municipality or county, any public hospital corporation and any other public agency, authority or body are hereby authorized to transfer and convey to any authority, with or without consideration:

(1) Any health care facilities and other properties, real or personal, and all funds and assets, tangible or intangible, relative to the ownership or operation of any such health care facilities that may be owned by such municipality, county, public hospital corporation or other public agency, authority or body, as the case may be, or that may be jointly owned by any two or more thereof, including, without limiting the generality of the foregoing, any certificates of need, assurances of need or other similar rights appertaining or ancillary thereto, irrespective of whether they have been exercised; and

(2) Any funds owned or controlled by such municipality, county, public hospital corporation or other public agency, authority or body, as the case may be, or jointly by any two or more thereof, that may have been raised or allocated for any of the purposes for which such authority shall have been organized, whether or not such property is considered necessary for the conduct of the governmental or public functions (if any) of such municipality, county, public hospital corporation or other public agency, authority or body.

Such transfer or conveyance shall be authorized by an ordinance or resolution duly adopted by the governing body of such municipality or county or by the board of directors or other governing body of such public hospital corporation or other public agency, authority or body, as the case may be, and it shall not be necessary, any provision of law to the contrary notwithstanding, to obtain any certificate of need, assurance of need or other similar permit for any such transfer or conveyance. In the event of the transfer of any health care facilities to the authority, any hospital tax proceeds, other tax proceeds and other revenues apportioned or allocated to or for the benefit of the prior owner or operator of such health care facilities or for patient care at such health care facilities shall thereafter be paid to the authority.

(Acts 1982, No. 82-418, p. 629, §27.)

§§22-21-337. **Disposition of earnings of authority.**

An authority shall be a public corporation or authority and no part of its net earnings remaining after payment of its expenses shall inure to the benefit of any individual, firm or corporation, except that in the event the board shall determine

(Continued)

Exhibit 13-1. Continued

that sufficient provision has been made for the full payment of the expenses, securities and other obligations of the authority, then any portion, as determined by the board, of the net earnings of the authority thereafter accruing may, in the discretion of the board, be paid to one or more of its authorizing subdivisions.

(Acts 1982, No. 82-418, p. 629, §28.)

§§22-21-338. Authority as designated agency for purposes of Division 2 of Article 4 of this chapter.

An authority shall constitute a "hospital corporation" as that term is used in Division 2 of Article 4 of this chapter; and any county otherwise authorized to do so may designate any authority having the power to own and operate health care facilities situated in such county as the agency of such county to acquire, construct, equip, operate and maintain public hospital facilities in such county, in the manner and with the consequences specified in said Division 2. Such authority shall, if so designated, receive the proceeds from any special public hospital tax referred to in said Division 2. Further, the reincorporation hereunder of any public hospital corporation that has theretofore been designated as the agency of a county to acquire, construct, equip, operate and maintain public hospital facilities in such county shall in no way impair or invalidate such designation, and such reincorporated public hospital corporation shall continue as such (with the consequences specified in said Division 2) just as if it had not been reincorporated hereunder. Nothing in this section shall, however, be construed in any manner to limit any rights or powers otherwise conferred upon an authority pursuant to any other provision of this article.

(Acts 1982, No. 82-418, p. 629, §29.)

§§22-21-339. Dissolution of authority.

At any time when the authority does not have any securities outstanding, and when there shall be no other obligations assumed by the authority that are then outstanding, the board may adopt a resolution, which shall be duly entered upon its minutes, declaring that the authority shall be dissolved. Upon the filing for record of a certified copy of said resolution in the office of the judge of probate in which the certificate of incorporation of the authority was filed, the authority shall thereupon stand dissolved, and in the event that it owned any assets or property at the time of its dissolution, the title to all its assets and property shall, subject to any constitutional provision or inhibition to the contrary, thereupon vest in one or more counties or municipalities in such manner and interests as may be provided in the said certificate of incorporation; provided however, that if the said certificate of incorporation contains no provision respecting the vesting of title to the assets and property of the authority, title to all such assets and property shall, subject to any constitutional provision or inhibition to the contrary, thereupon vest in its authorizing subdivisions as tenants in common.

(Acts 1982, No. 82-418, p. 629, §30.)

§§22-21-340. Multiple corporations permitted.

Neither the formation or dissolution of one authority hereunder nor the reincorporation hereunder of a public hospital corporation shall prevent the subsequent incorporation hereunder of another authority or the subsequent reincorporation hereunder of another public hospital corporation pursuant to authority granted by one or more of the same authorizing subdivisions. Further, any county may authorize the incorporation of an authority hereunder notwithstanding the existence in such county of a public hospital corporation designated as the agency of such county with respect to public hospital facilities therein pursuant to the provisions of Division 2 of Article 4 of this chapter.

(Acts 1982, No. 82-418, p. 629, §31.)

§§22-21-341. Reincorporation of existing corporations.

Any public hospital corporation may be reincorporated under this article, avail itself of all rights, powers and privileges and become subject to all duties, obligations and responsibilities conferred or imposed by this article, in the following manner:

(Continued)

Exhibit 13-1. Continued

(1) The board of directors or other governing body of such public hospital corporation shall adopt a resolution stating that it proposes and applies for permission to reincorporate hereunder and containing a form of proposed certificate of reincorporation, which such certificate of reincorporation shall include, with the necessary changes in detail, the information required to be included in a certificate of incorporation described in Section 22-21-314 other than that referred to in subdivision (b) (1) thereof.

(2) Such public hospital corporation shall as promptly as practicable thereafter file a certified copy of such resolution with the governing body of each county or municipality that authorized the formation of such public hospital corporation (and, with respect to any public hospital corporation organized under the provisions of Article 6 of this chapter, the governing body of any other municipality that is then a "member" thereof); and each such county and municipality shall be deemed an "authorizing subdivision" with respect to any such public hospital corporation reincorporated hereunder.

(3) The governing body of each authorizing subdivision shall, as promptly as may be practicable after the filing of said certified resolution, review and act upon the said resolution and application in the manner, with the necessary changes in detail, prescribed in Section 22-21-313.

(4) The chairman (or other principal officer) and the secretary of such public hospital corporation shall thereupon sign and acknowledge a certificate of reincorporation, in the form included in the resolution referred to in subdivision (1) of this section, and cause it to be filed for record in the office specified in Section 22-21-314.

(5) Thereupon, such certificate of reincorporation shall be filed and recorded by the judge of probate as provided in Section 22-21-314, and the existence of such public hospital corporation as an authority under this article shall begin upon the filing of such certificate of reincorporation as provided for in this section.

No such reincorporation shall in any manner affect the rights of creditors or the rights or liabilities of the public hospital corporation existing at the time of such reincorporation or shall (any provision of law to the contrary notwithstanding) necessitate the obtaining by such reincorporated public hospital corporation or the reissuance of any certificate of need, assurance of need or other similar permit. With respect to any public hospital corporation reincorporated hereunder, any reference herein to a certificate of incorporation thereof shall also include and refer to its certificate of reincorporation.

(Acts 1982, No. 82-418, p. 629, §32.)

§§22-21-342. Provisions of article exclusive.

Any authority organized under the provisions of this article (as well as any public hospital corporation reincorporated hereunder) shall, insofar as the subject matter of this article is concerned, be governed exclusively by the provisions of this article, which shall not be construed in pari materia with any other statute.

(Acts 1982, No. 82-418, p. 629, §33.)

§§22-21-343. Cumulative effect of article.

This article shall not be construed as a restriction or limitation upon any power, right or remedy which any county, municipality or public hospital corporation now in existence or hereafter formed may have in the absence of this article. The provisions of this article are cumulative and shall not be deemed to repeal existing laws, except to the extent such laws are clearly inconsistent with the provisions of this article.

(Acts 1982, No. 82-418, p. 629, §34.)

§§22-21-344. Use of proceeds from hospital taxes.

Nothing in this article shall be construed to permit the use, by or for the benefit of any authority, of the proceeds of any hospital tax for any purpose, at any place, or in connection with any health care facilities, not permitted or described in the constitutional, statutory or other provision of law authorizing the imposition, levy and collection of such hospital tax or the use of the proceeds therefrom. In order to assure the lawful disposition of such hospital tax proceeds, the board may require the deposit thereof into special funds or accounts established for that purpose and the accounting therefor in such manner as the board may deem necessary.

(Acts 1982, No. 82-418, p. 629, §35.)

Exhibit 13-2. Public Health Funding History

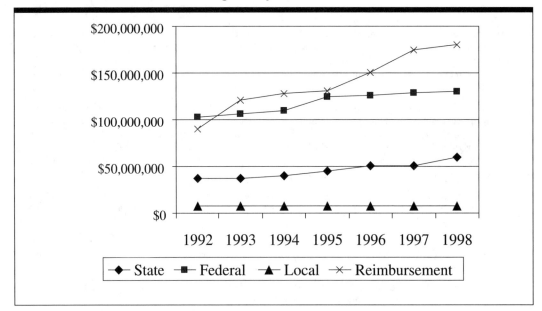

applied to federal grants and to reimbursable programs operated by the department. By 1996, the cost-based portion of the department's financial structure had grown to more than 80 percent systemwide (Exhibit 13-3). The cost of the bond issue could be built into the cost reports for these programs, and the resulting increase in reimbursement could be used to repay the bonds.

3. The department was prepared to make a significant cash contribution to the building program to minimize borrowing.

Public health had two basic areas where significant reimbursements were available—federal grants and reimbursable programs. Federal grants accounted for about 38 percent of the total operations. These grants enabled the department to pay for facilities through "indirect cost" reimbursement. In addition, home health and clinic services provided another large source of reimbursement for facilities. Exhibit 13-4 provides a breakout of the sources of those funds.

Exhibit 13-5 lists major public health clinic services for 1992 and 1996. In the clinics, these services dropped by about 5 percent. Home health,

the other clinical program that was fully funded by Medicaid and Medicare, had experienced considerable growth over the past five years. As shown in Exhibit 13-6, the visits increased from 1.3 to almost 2 million visits in five years.

Federal grant funds were likely to remain stable because of the performance of the programs and resultant strong, bipartisan political support. According to Dr. Williamson,

> We expect continued small declines in our clinical programs due to recent initiatives of Medicaid to move toward managed care, which will adversely affect clinic volumes in some counties. In home health, we expect continued long-term growth with an aging state population and continued strength of home health services in general. We do not expect continued explosive growth as in past years. None of these trends appear to jeopardize the long-term viability of a bond issue.

Management believed that a bond program through a conduit issuer would be attractive to the securities marketplace for the following reasons:

Exhibit 13-3. 1996 Public Health Department Funding by Source

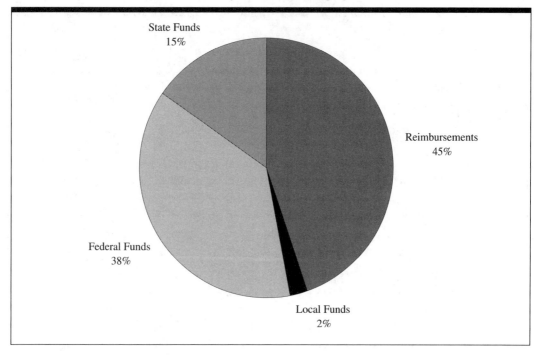

Exhibit 13-4. Sources of Funds, Fiscal Year 1998 Agency Budget Request

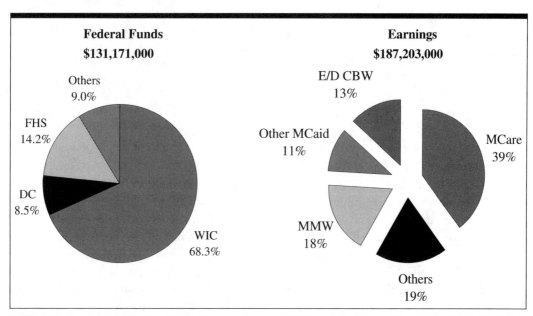

NOTE: FHS = Family Health Services; WIC = Women, Infants, and Children; DC = Disease Control; E/D CBW = Elderly/Disabled Community-Based Waiver; MCare = Medicare; MMW = Medicaid Maternity Waiver; and Other MCaid = Other Medicaid.

Exhibit 13-5. Clinic-Based Services

Service	Fiscal Year 1992 Visits	Fiscal Year 1996 Visits	Change
Family planning	168,647	176,224	7,577
Maternity	169,791	123,757	(46,034)
Child health	151,515	105,793	(45,722)
Women, Infants, and Children	651,094	728,105	77,011
Child primary care	110,578	87,233	(23,345)
Adult care	53,524	28,420	(25,104)
Hypertension	58,264	69,350	11,086
Tuberculosis	140,421	125,461	(14,960)
Sexually transmitted diseases	57,783	45,285	(12,498)
Immunization only	113,676	128,117	14,441
Total	1,675,293	1,617,745	(57,548)

- The department's diversified funding base
- The department's ability to build the increased cost of the bond issue into cost-based programs
- The small cost of the issue compared to the overall budget
- The department carried no debt

The Alabama Public Health Care Authority Is Created

In November, 1995, the State Committee of Public Health (essentially the Board of Directors for the State Department of Public Health) unanimously approved the creation of a public corporation, the Alabama Public Health Care Authority (APHCA), to construct county health department buildings. Monroe County, Alabama, was chosen as the locality for incorporation. Because the board needed to be composed of a majority of residents from the county in which it was incorporated, it consisted of four local employees and the Finance Director of the Monroe County Health Department, as well as the State Health Officer, Dr. Williamson (who served as Chairman), and the State Finance Director, Ed Davidson.

Dr. Williamson pulled together a team of top aides to assist him in the development of the bond program. They included Melvin Marraman and Kathy Vincent (his two Staff Assistants) and Ed Davidson, his Finance Director. The team estimated a total need to be met by the bond authority of about $60 million. Early in the process, it was decided to split the issue into two phases.

"There is no way I can support borrowing the full funding out of the gate," said Dr. Williamson. "We need to make it at least two phases in order to gear up and also to see what happens in the health care marketplace."

"I agree," responded Davidson. He continued, "And the phased approach should be easier to sell to the bond insurors as prudent management of the program. We will need their support to get the best bond ratings and thus lower interest rates."

Marraman added, "We've got to get the county health departments to invest in these facilities. Over the years, they have set aside money to improve or rebuild their buildings, but they will never be able to accumulate enough to meet the need. Even if they could accumulate a substantial fund to meet this need, it would be too tempting to the Legislature to cut our funding in the midst of

Exhibit 13-6. Home Health Visit Growth

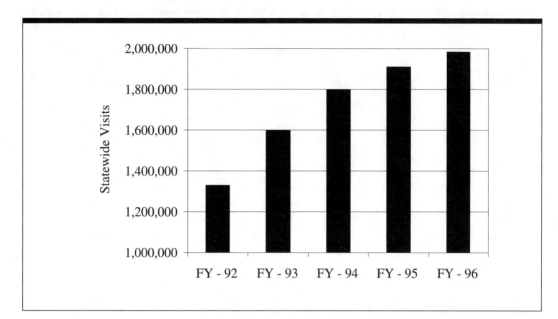

the financial crises suffered periodically by the state because of the state's heavy reliance on sales tax revenue. Whenever sales tax revenues are below projections, the building fund monies have to be used on operations."

"Medicaid is moving quickly to managed care, and we are seeing our clinic volumes drop," added Vincent. "Seeing the future is never an easy job, and it is particularly difficult for us in this environment."

Based on these concerns, a first phase of approximately $30 million was planned to enable the department to develop operational methodologies and to provide time for pending changes in the health system to mature. If this bond issue was financially and operationally successful, a subsequent bond issue would be undertaken allowing the Department to meet the total building needs of the agency within a five- to six-year window.

Priority Setting

Because the building program was to be conducted in two phases, the projects would have to be prioritized. Phase I projects were selected in cooperation with local staff, keeping several factors in mind. The highest priority should be given to those counties that had the greatest building needs. In general, these were counties in which facilities were undersized for their current volume of business or had severe structural problems that could not easily be remedied.

Other factors were equally important. Any funds spent on land would not be available to spend on bricks and mortar. Thus, county governments or city governments that were willing to donate land to the public health care authority for construction of a facility had to receive a higher priority than counties that were unwilling to make such a commitment. Finally, although few county health departments would have sufficient local health department funds to finance construction completely, many counties had some funds available to partially fund their construction needs. Thus, the decision as to which counties received priority for the first $30 million bond issue ultimately was based upon three factors: need, ability to acquire land, and funds available to put into the program.

Exhibit 13-7. Phase I Project Building Sizes and Budget Requirements

County	Facility Size	Project Budget ($)
Bibb	8,948	800,000
Chilton	16,000	1,500,000
Choctaw	11,893	1,300,000
Escambia	21,525	700,000
Jackson	18,120	1,700,000
Lamar	7,595	1,200,000
Lawrence	15,305	1,700,000
Macon	5,000	1,000,000
Marengo	12,116	1,300,000
Marion	14,303	1,500,000
Monroe	17,639	1,700,000
Perry	9,000	1,100,000
Sumter	11,299	1,200,000
Calhoun	25,000	2,500,000
Chambers	16,500	1,500,000
Clay	10,000	1,000,000
Dallas	29,405	3,000,000
Shelby	17,280	1,700,000
Talladega	13,000	1,300,000
Warehouse		2,000,000
Estimated project cost		29,700,000
Plus reserves and other		5,740,695
Equals total cost		35,440,695

Ten counties had adequate, modern facilities. Twelve county health departments had set aside enough cash for their projects or, in several of the counties, the county government provided loans (to be repaid through rent) to the county health department to build the project. To meet the needs of the remaining counties, the financing strategy was to build in two phases, require counties to donate the land, provide local funding where it could be afforded, and build local projects in total where funds were available (Exhibit 13-7). With a strategy developed, the Department approached financial advisors and began the detailed planning required to make the bond issue a reality.

Bond Amount and Terms

The $30 million bond issue amount was based on estimates of funding requirements for about half of the building need. It quickly became evident that more funding would be required than at first envisioned by the steering committee. To support bond proceeds of $30 million, an additional $5.1 million would be required to establish a debt service and capitalized interest fund. Exhibits 13-8 and 13-9 provide an analysis of the sources and uses of cash for the bond issue for Phase I and Phase II.

"Like my Daddy says, be careful what you pray for, you just may get it," laughed Marraman as the

Exhibit 13-8.

CONSOLIDATED PROJECT BUDGET
SOURCES AND USES OF CASH
ALABAMA PUBLIC HEALTH CARE AUTHORITY

	Phase I ($)	Phase II ($)	Total ($)
Sources of Cash			
Bond Proceeds	30,000,000	28,129,121	58,129,121
Funds Transfers			
Debt Service Reserve Fund	2,235,760	2,095,620	4,331,380
County Construction Fund	4,520,016	0	4,520,016
State Construction Fund	1,000,000	0	1,000,000
Proceeds from Investment of Funds			
Construction Proceed Fund	3,458,393	2,500,000	5,958,393
Debt Service Reserve Fund	389,022	350,000	739,022
Capitalized Interest Fund	206,515	200,000	406,515
Total Cash Available	41,809,706	33,274,741	75,084,447
Uses of Cash			
Construction of County Facilities	35,540,695	28,129,121	63,669,816
Underwriting	240,000	200,000	440,000
Cost of Issuance	140,000	110,169	250,169
Insurance	195,566	153,895	349,461
Establish Debt Service Reserve Fund	2,235,760	2,095,620	4,331,380
Capitalized Interest	2,913,470	2,292,665	5,206,135
Other Costs	544,215	293,271	837,486
Total Uses of Cash	41,809,706	33,274,741	75,084,447

team reconvened to discuss the bond issue yet one more time.

"You've got that right," agreed Dr. Williamson. "The Governor, the State Committee, and the new APHCA board have given us the green light, and now we have to make this deal work."

"I'm surprised at how much cash is required to complete the transaction," added Vincent.

"I know what you mean," said Davidson. "By the time you take care of the required reserves, pay the lawyers and advisors, and fund the capitalized interest, the overhead on the deal really adds up." He continued, "I'm really concerned about the choice of term on the bonds. If we go 20 years we pay a lot less interest, but the depreciation on the facilities will take much longer. Perhaps we should try to match the cash demanded by the debt service to our ability to charge the depreciation and interest on the cost reports."

Exhibit 13-9. Alabama Department of Public Health Building Program: APHCA Funded and Locally Funded

	Number of Projects	Total Cost[a]	Local Funds Available[a]	Authority Funds Required[a]
APHCA funded projects				
Phase I	20	29.8	3.9	25.9
Phase II	28	30.6	3.0	25.6
Total	48	60.4	6.9	51.5
Locally funded projects	12			
Total projects	60			

a. Dollar amounts shown in millions.

A decision on the term of the bonds had to be made. The lowest long-term cost would require the shortest term; however, an early payoff would cause a mismatch between the depreciation charged to grants and reimbursable programs. Davidson concluded, "In other words, we need to make sure that our cash payout matches, to the extent possible, the depreciation schedule. I've put together a graphic analysis of the data to aid us in making this decision." (See Exhibit 13-10.) The team left to finalize plans for the bonds.

Making the Decision

"Important decisions have been made to get to this point," Dr. Williamson thought as he sat for a quiet moment in the now empty conference room. "We have decided to complete the building program in two phases and to invest departmental funds. We have operational, economic, and financial reasons for this course. The health care system in Alabama is changing, and with it, the public health system. Over the past two years, clinic volumes in maternity, well child, and adult care have fallen dramatically. Medicaid's effort at managed care could accelerate that trend. Will public health's role in the provision of clinical services

change in the future? What impact will that have on the building program?"

He continued mulling over the issue. "Revenues from home health services play a vital role in our financing plan, but the cost-based reimbursement system may change to a prospective payment system over the next few years. Will that adversely affect the Department's ability to repay the bonds? How could such an effect be minimized?"

Another concern was the ability of staff to carry out such an ambitious project. He thought, "The department does not have a staff with the training or experience to manage a statewide building program. Can such an effort be organized to obtain economies of scale and ensure that the buildings are completed on time and on budget to meet the bond requirements?"

Dr. Williamson's final concern was that in Alabama's past, the legal, financial, architectural, and construction work associated with bond issues had been highly politicized. He pondered, "How can the department insulate the bond issue from these forces and ensure that decisions are based on prudent management of the program and not unduly influenced by politics? The Act under which the Public Health Care Authority was organized specifically exempts the public corporation from state ethics and competitive bid laws. How can I

Exhibit 13-10. Comparison of Depreciation Charged to Debt Service Public Health Bond Issue

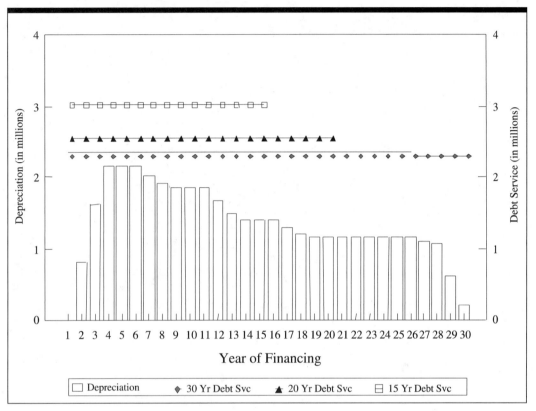

institutionalize ethical standards in the current and future operations of the Authority?"

Although he had concerns, Dr. Williamson knew that the possibilities for progress presented by the bond issue were enormous; however, careful analysis of the risks for the department in this complex and rapidly changing environment was essential. The team had analyzed everything its members could think of. It was time for a final "go" or "no go" decision.

Possible Bioterrorism in New Hampshire

A Public Health Response

It was Wednesday morning, April 21, 1999. Dr. Dan Blumenfeld, the State Epidemiologist for the New Hampshire Department of Health and Human Services, was sitting in a meeting at the offices of the state hospital association. The meeting had been called to discuss the state requirements for the collection of vital records data. Shortly after the meeting began, Dr. Blumenfeld received a telephone call from his secretary. She informed him that Dr. Ned Fairman of the U.S. Centers for Disease Control and Prevention (CDC) in Atlanta, Georgia, was trying to get in touch with him. Dr. Fairman had asked that Dr. Blumenfeld return the call as soon as possible.

Dr. Blumenfeld stepped out of the meeting to return the call. He thought this call was unusual. Typically, the state would call CDC. He wondered, "Why is CDC calling me? And why do I need to call back so quickly?"

Dr. Blumenfeld was able to reach Dr. Fairman right away, and what he was told caught New Hampshire's senior epidemiologist by surprise. "Dan, there may be a bioterrorism event in process in the state of New Hampshire," Dr. Fairman began. He went on to tell Dr. Blumenfeld that the FBI had contacted CDC, and he shared with Dr. Blumenfeld the information from the FBI. Both epidemiologists knew that a lot of additional information was needed before any actions could be taken. They agreed to work expeditiously and to keep each other informed.

The telephone conversation alarmed Dr. Blumenfeld. He left the meeting quickly and headed back to his office. He thought, "I can't believe it. If this is really the first bioterrorism event in the United States, why did it have to be my state? Why would a bioterrorist pick New Hampshire?" He also wondered exactly where this was happen-

This case was prepared by Stuart A. Capper, University of Alabama at Birmingham and the Centers for Disease Control and Prevention. It is intended as a basis for classroom discussion rather than to illustrate effective or ineffective handling of an administrative situation. The author is indebted to Dr. James Lando and trainees of the Epidemiology Program Office, CDC; Dr. David Ashford of the National Center for Infectious Diseases, CDC; and officials of the New Hampshire, Massachusetts, and Boston Departments of Public Health for their assistance in preparation of this case. Used with permission from Stuart A. Capper.

ing. "Are there people in other public health jurisdictions that need to be notified?" He also realized he did not know how big a threat this really was.

During the trip back to his office, Dr. Blumenfeld thought about the fact that he was very short on professional staff. The position of Chief of Communicable Disease Control in his agency was vacant. In addition, his CDC Epidemic Intelligence Service (EIS) officer, Dr. Samantha Winston, was at an EIS conference in Atlanta. He needed a lot more information, and he knew he needed some help.

When he reached his office, Dr. Blumenfeld immediately called the local FBI office. The local agent informed Dr. Blumenfeld that he was unfamiliar with this situation or bioterrorism in general and that he would have to contact the regional office. Later that afternoon, a special agent from the regional FBI office contacted Dr. Blumenfeld. He was more aware of the current situation and bioterrorism. Dr. Blumenfeld thought about the fact that Ned Fairman had told him that it was the FBI that had alerted CDC in the first place. Dr. Blumenfeld wondered why he was the last to know, but he would worry about the communication problems later.

Dr. Blumenfeld's biggest concern at the moment was getting more information on the potential threat, so he called the senior public health nurse in his organization and the city health nurse at the Nashua, New Hampshire City Health Department. During that conference call, he informed them of the situation and what he had learned from Dr. Fairman.

Information From Dr. Fairman's Briefing of Dr. Blumenfeld

According to the information Dr. Fairman related to Dr. Blumenfeld, on March 25, 1999, a thirty-eight-year-old Costa Rican woman who lived in New Hampshire had gone to the emergency room of City Hospital in Nashua, New Hampshire, complaining of fever, chills, headache, muscle pain, and weakness. Initially, she was sent home

with a diagnosis of influenza-like symptoms. She returned to the hospital the following day after her symptoms became more severe, and she was admitted. Her initial presenting symptom of muscle aches diminished over the first two days. On the third day of hospitalization, her respiratory status began to deteriorate rapidly, necessitating mechanical ventilation.

On April 15, after three weeks of respiratory support, the patient was transferred to Park Hospital in Boston, Massachusetts. A slide agglutination test for anti-*Brucella* antibodies, using paired sera drawn on March 29 and April 15, was performed at Park Hospital. The acute serum sample drawn on March 29 at City Hospital showed a titer of 1:20, and the second serum drawn at Park had a titer of 1:320. (See Exhibit 14-1 for information on brucellosis.)

Hospital personnel interviewed family members, who reported no history of traditional risk factors for *Brucella* exposure (e.g., relevant food, infected animal contact, or travel history). Although the rapid respiratory deterioration was not typical for *Brucella* infection, the findings from the slide agglutination test met the surveillance case definition for brucellosis. Based on these results, a tentative diagnosis of brucellosis was made on April 16, 1996. The suspected brucellosis case was reported to the Boston Public Health Commission (BPHC) on the same day.

The following day, April 17, relatives of the patient informed a medical resident at Park Hospital that the patient's boyfriend had a laboratory and kept microbiological materials at the patient's apartment in New Hampshire. The family wanted to know if the materials could be associated with her illness. They identified the boyfriend as a marine biologist from Saudi Arabia who had a previous affiliation with a local university. The medical resident asked the family to bring the suspicious materials to the hospital so that they could be tested.

Dr. Fairman also said that he had heard that the boyfriend had gone to the hospital in New Hampshire before the patient was transferred and had attempted to remove jewelry the patient

Exhibit 14-1. About Brucellosis

Brucellosis (also known as undulant fever, Bang's disease, Mediterranean fever, and Malta fever) is a zoonotic disease (disease of animals transmissible to humans) caused by an organism of the genus *Brucella*. *Brucellae* are small, nonmotile (unable to move on its own), nonsporulating (non–spore forming), aerobic (oxygen metabolizing), gram-negative (unable to hold the purple dye when stained by Gram's method) coccobacilli (variable shaped bacterium).

Historically, *Brucellae* that infect mammals are classified into six subspecies of *Brucella melitensis*. These bacteria are passed primarily among animals, and they cause disease in many different vertebrates. Various *Brucella* species affect sheep, goats, cattle, deer, elk, pigs, dogs, and several other animals. Each species has a different likelihood of infecting certain domestic animal species. Humans become infected by coming in contact with animals or animal products that are contaminated with these bacteria.

Epidemiology

Humans are generally infected in one of three ways: eating or drinking something that is contaminated with *Brucella*, breathing in the organism (inhalation), or having the bacteria enter the body through skin wounds. The most common way to be infected is by eating or drinking contaminated milk products. When sheep, goats, cows, or camels are infected, their milk is contaminated with the bacteria. If the milk is not pasteurized, these bacteria can be transmitted to persons who drink the milk or eat cheeses made from the milk. Inhalation of *Brucella* organisms is not a common route of infection, but it can be important for those working in laboratories where the organism is cultured and could be inhaled by accident. Contamination of skin wounds may be a problem for persons working in slaughterhouses or meat packing plants or for veterinarians. Hunters may be infected through skin wounds or by accidentally ingesting the bacteria after cleaning deer, elk, moose, or wild pigs that they have killed. Direct person-to-person spread of brucellosis is extremely rare. Mothers who are breastfeeding may transmit the infection to their infants. Sexual transmission has been reported.

Brucellosis is not very common in the United States, where 50 to 200 cases occur each year, but it can be very common in some developing countries. Although brucellosis can be found worldwide, it is more common in countries that do not have effective public health and domestic animal health programs. Areas currently listed as high risk are the Mediterranean Basin (Portugal, Spain, southern France, Italy, Greece, Turkey, North Africa), South and Central America, Eastern Europe, Asia, Africa, the Caribbean, and the Middle East.

Clinical Aspects

Brucellosis has an incubation period from five to sixty days. In the acute form (less than eight weeks from illness onset) nonspecific, flu-like symptoms including fever, chills, weakness, profuse sweating when at rest, fatigue, loss of appetite, headache, joint pain, localized inflammation, and nausea are present. Back pain is frequent.

In the chronic form (more than one year from illness onset), symptoms can include chronic fatigue syndrome, arthritis, eye damage, and depressive episodes. Chronic undulant fever is characterized by periods of normal temperature between attacks. Symptoms might persist for years, either continuously or intermittently.

B. melitensis tends to be associated with a more acute, severe, systemic illness than the other *Brucella* species. Infection with *B. melitensis* can lead to bone or joint disease in about 30 percent of patients.

(Continued)

Exhibit 14-1. Continued)

Other sites of infection include the heart, central nervous system, and skin. Endocarditis, a rare complication, accounts for 80 percent of deaths from brucellosis. Central nervous system infection usually manifests as chronic meningoencephalitis (infection of the brain and its covering), but brain hemorrhage also occurs. Naturally occurring brucellosis has a low mortality rate (less than 5 percent).

Diagnosis

A thorough history eliciting details of appropriate exposures is an important part of diagnosis. Confirmation of brucellosis can be achieved by (1) isolation of *Brucella* species from a clinical specimen, (2) fourfold or greater rise in *Brucella* agglutination titer between acute- and convalescent-phase serum specimens obtained greater than or equal to two weeks apart and studies done at the same laboratory, or (3) demonstration by immunofluorescence of *Brucella* species in a clinical specimen. The best tissue sources for culture are blood, bone marrow, or fluid from any lesions. Because the organism potentially grows slowly, cultures of suspected brucellosis patients should be kept for a minimum of twenty-one days. Standard liquid media is adequate for *Brucella* species. For culturing, repeated samples three days apart are recommended. Also, blood tests can be done to detect antibodies against the bacteria (serologic testing). If serologic testing is used, two blood samples should be collected two weeks apart. The agglutination tests remain the standard assays for serologic diagnosis. Brucellosis should be considered in the diagnosis of fever of unknown origin or in chronic fatigue.

Treatment

Brucellosis is treatable by antibiotics, but treatment usually requires combination therapy over a long duration. Therapy with a single drug results in a high relapse rate, so combined antibiotic regimens should be used whenever possible. Doxycycline plus rifampin or streptomycin for six weeks is recommended for uncomplicated disease in adults. There is no available vaccine for the prevention of brucellosis among humans. There are no data on the effectiveness of post-exposure antibiotic prophylaxis in prevention of brucellosis, though it is recommended for accidental exposure to the live cattle vaccine.

---

was wearing. There may have been a scuffle between the boyfriend and a hospital security guard, with the boyfriend fleeing the hospital. "He appears to have left the United States," Dr. Fairman said. "At least no one has been able to locate him."

On Sunday, April 18, the patient's sister arrived at Park Hospital with a cardboard box containing laboratory flasks, Petri dishes, and culture tubes. Several contained an unidentified clear liquid, and some were dated back to the 1980s. The weekend technician in the microbiology laboratory of Park Hospital refused to handle the materials because of the suspicious circumstances, so they were stored in an unlocked utility room of the medical intensive care unit (MICU).

On Monday, April 19, the MICU charge nurse reported the existence of the box of biological materials to the infection control nurse, who then notified the chief of infection control. The infection control nurse also called a pager number that was posted for reporting communicable disease issues to public health authorities. She was not sure if the contact she made was to a state or city public health official. The telephone page was returned, but the responding individual was not very interested in the issue, although he did assure her that he would pass on the information.

Park Hospital's chief of infection control spoke to the chief of the laboratory at the hospital. The chief of the laboratory voiced his concerns. He said that their "objectives were to get the box of biological materials out of the utility room and determine if there was reason for concern about the spread of contagious disease." Because Monday, April 19, was a state holiday, the chief of infection control contacted Dr. Alice Morgan, the Communicable Disease Control Director at the Boston Public Health Commission the following day.

Just before noon on April 20, Dr. Morgan received the call from the Chief of Infection Control at Park Hospital concerning this possible biological threat. The situation was suspicious because of the unusual presentation and rapid deterioration of the patient and because of the laboratory equipment in the patient's apartment. Dr. Morgan tried to contact relatives of the patient to clarify the nature of the biologicals from the apartment, but she was unable to reach any of the patient's family members. While she was trying to reach family members, Dr. Morgan was handed a routine infectious disease surveillance report. To her surprise, that report detailed a second brucellosis case.

The second case originally had been admitted to Park Hospital on April 1 with a three-week history of fevers, chills, and muscle aches. A serologic diagnosis of brucellosis was made on the basis of a single agglutination test result showing an anti-*Brucella* antibody titer of 1:640.

Dr. Morgan called the Assistant Director of Microbiology at Park Hospital to verify the serologic test results on both patients. In addition, she talked with the chief of security at the hospital and the MICU resident about the biologicals. Then she contacted the director of emergency medical services in Boston. She asked if he was aware of any increase in calls, above the normal number, for EMS response to febrile illness. No unusual increase in febrile illness had been noticed, but the EMS director suggested that Dr. Morgan contact

the FBI, which she did late on the afternoon of April 20.

By the following day, Wednesday, April 21, the FBI had notified the Massachusetts State Department of Public Health and CDC. Within CDC, the information was routed quickly to the National Center for Infectious Diseases (NCID). On that same day, Dr. Fairman, Medical Epidemiologist in the NCID Division of Bacterial and Mycotic Diseases, was briefed on the FBI notification.

Dr. Fairman's first thoughts were that this was an unusual presentation of a *Brucella* infection and that the diagnosis needed to be confirmed. In addition, he was concerned about the reports of nefarious activity, and he knew that the biologicals in the apartment could be a public health threat even if they turned out not to be implicated in bioterrorism. Furthermore, he was concerned that this was a true *Brucella* case. He knew that a lot of bioterrorism planning and preparation had been done with the FBI and local emergency response units; however, most of this preparation had been done considering the possibility of a bioterrorism threat from anthrax. He thought, "This might throw a monkey wrench in the works" because these agencies would not be familiar with the infectious characteristics of *Brucella*.

Dr. Fairman knew that activity needed to start quickly from CDC. He wondered how quickly CDC could send epidemiologic assistance into that area of the country. Then he realized that he was not sure that all the local public health agencies were aware of what was occurring. The initial report came from Massachusetts, but the female patient's residence was in New Hampshire. Dr. Fairman picked up the phone and placed a call to the New Hampshire Chief Epidemiologist, Dr. Dan Blumenfeld. Dr. Fairman was only able to reach Dr. Blumenfeld's secretary because Dr. Blumenfeld already was out of the office in a meeting at the State Hospital Association offices. Dr. Blumenfeld returned Dr. Fairman's call very quickly. It was during this telephone conversation that Dr. Fairman gave Dr. Blumenfeld the available information and his thoughts on the possible bioterrorism event in New Hampshire.

Public Health Responses in New Hampshire and Massachusetts

Dr. Blumenfeld finished his briefing of the public health nurses and then asked for their help. He asked his senior public health nurse to contact Park Hospital in Boston and collect crucial information regarding the index case and transfer of the patient. He asked the city public health nurse from Nashua to inform her city health officer and find out about the initial hospitalization at City Hospital. It was about 1:00 p.m.

Dr. Blumenfeld's senior public health nurse quickly got back to him with some potentially disturbing news. "There may be a third brucellosis case," she said. When she had called Nashua City Health Department and begun asking about the known brucellosis case, she was told that one of the health department's part-time laboratory workers also may have been exposed to *Brucella*. They had heard that this lab employee had received prophylaxis for *Brucella* because he had been exposed while processing a sample at a Lowell, Massachusetts, hospital. Dr. Blumenfeld asked his senior public health nurse to contact the Massachusetts Department of Public Health and ask for a check of its records. She was able to confirm quickly that a second case did exist in Massachusetts. A twenty-three-year-old woman had presented to a Hospital in Lowell on January 30 with a one-month history of fever, chills, and muscle aches. A blood culture taken in Lowell on January 31 yielded *Brucella melitensis*. The patient was started on antibiotic treatment and released.

In a relatively short period of time, there appeared to be three cases of brucellosis. Dr. Blumenfeld needed to inform his State Health Officer and the State Medical Director. It was not until later that afternoon that he was able to get in touch with them. He knew there was epidemiologic work to be done in both states, and the question of the biologicals in the New Hampshire apartment was still a major issue. The remainder of the afternoon was spent talking to CDC about getting some additional help with the epidemiologic investigation.

Meanwhile, in Atlanta, Dr. Fairman was trying to round up people and paperwork to initiate the epidemic assistance to the states in this potential bioterrorism event. At the same time, also in Atlanta at the EIS Conference, there was a buzz going around about the potential biological attack in New Hampshire. Dr. Vishu Yeolekar, an EIS officer, heard Dr. Fairman talking to another staff member about paired sera samples being sent in for repeat testing to confirm a diagnosis of brucellosis that might be due to biological attack. Dr. Yeolekar expressed his interest to Dr. Fairman and proceeded to get more information. Initially, Dr. Yeolekar was thinking that the whole thing seemed a bit odd, like a made-for-TV drama. His skepticism was due to the fact that this situation was occurring at the time when major anthrax hoaxes were occurring. He was intrigued, nonetheless. There was talk about sending an EIS officer to New Hampshire to assist, and Dr. Yeolekar thought that he was next in line for such an assignment and wanted to go. Later, while Dr. Fairman was in a conference call with Dr. Blumenfeld, he asked Dr. Yeolekar to find Dr. Samantha Winston, the EIS officer assigned to New Hampshire, who was also in Atlanta for the EIS conference.

When Dr. Yeolekar found Dr. Winston, she was unaware of the situation. A short time later, she and Dr. Yeolekar joined Dr. Fairman in the conference call with Dr. Blumenfeld. "I need you back in New Hampshire as soon as possible, Samantha," Dr. Blumenfeld said. "I would like Vishu to accompany you and come to New Hampshire as well," he concluded. "There is a possibility that an Epi-Aid will be needed in Massachusetts."

Drs. Winston and Yeolekar Head to New Hampshire

Dr. Winston went back to her hotel to pack, and Dr. Yeolekar then began to shuffle through the necessary paperwork so that he could be approved for the trip. Even in these rapidly evolving, potentially emergency situations, there was always concern for appropriate approvals for staff travel because such approvals affected whose budget was charged for the expenses. Dr. Yeolekar told the secretary that he needed travel orders, and they began to prepare the "Epi-1" document that was needed for budget approval. Dr. Fairman reviewed the Epi-1 and forwarded it to the Branch Chief, who approved it. It was then sent to CDC's Epidemiology Program Office (EPO) to see if it met the criteria for declaring it an Epi-Aid. If it did, then EPO's budget would cover the expenses.

With the necessary paperwork and approvals underway, Dr. Yeolekar went home to start packing. As he packed, he thought,

> I'm still skeptical of the bioterrorism aspects of this incident, but the presentation of the initial female patient intrigues me. She was undergoing a rapid respiratory deterioration. This is unusual for *Brucella* because it's usually ingested. However, if it had been aerosolized—and therefore inhaled—that could account for this rapid onset of severe respiratory symptoms. Aerosolizing an agent like *Brucella* is one possible method that a terrorist might use to deliver the attack. . . .

Dr. Winston and Dr. Yeolekar managed to catch the last flight leaving Atlanta, around 7 p.m. They arrived in Manchester, New Hampshire, late on Wednesday night, April 21.

Drs. Blumenfeld, Winston, and Yeolekar spent most of the next day in meetings and making phone calls, primarily to coordinate with the many involved agencies. The Nashua City Health Director had informed the local Nashua fire and police departments, as well as the local Hazardous Materials (HAZMAT) response team, of the situation. These agencies seemed to be very hesitant about what they should be doing and what types of equipment they would need. Although they had received some briefing and information on anthrax threats, they were not really familiar with biological terrorism and specifically unfamiliar with *Brucella*. They wanted to know what they should

do. Dr. Blumenfeld told them they did not need to take any specific actions yet.

Based on all the information that was available, it was clear that this was at least a two-state situation. Dr. Blumenfeld commented,

> There is additional information in Massachusetts that needs to be collected. We need to know more about the two existing cases there. In addition, case ascertainment is important to see if there might be any other cases that haven't yet been identified. Somebody needs to evaluate the medical records of the Massachusetts cases and talk directly with Alice Morgan and others. Because Samantha is the New Hampshire EIS Officer, she will need to work here. Vishu, can you go to Massachusetts?

Dr. Yeolekar called Dr. Fairman to discuss going to Massachusetts and the plan of action. Dr. Fairman informed him that the Massachusetts State Epidemiologist had said he was agreeable to having a CDC EIS Officer come to the state. Dr. Yeolekar quickly left for Massachusetts.

That afternoon, Dr. Blumenfeld held a lengthy conference call that included Dr. Fairman and Jeremy Maxian, Associate Director of the National Center for Infectious Diseases. The issue of the biologicals in the cardboard box at Park Hospital and the apartment in New Hampshire occupied much of the conversation. Dr. Fairman stated, "I am concerned about being able to isolate *Brucella* from the lab equipment. Do you all agree that it would be best if the samples were sent to CDC or the Armed Forces Institute of Pathology? These two organizations have the *Brucella* experts."

The group discussed issues concerning how to obtain the needed samples and who would make the final decision on where the samples would go. Dr. Fairman concluded, "I guess the FBI needs to be consulted. . . ."

The Issue of the Apartment

Later that afternoon, the issue of what to do about the apartment had to be resolved. Dr.

Blumenfeld reported, "The FBI told me that they are not willing to take any legal action. They assess the situation as a low threat."

Despite the FBI view, Jeremy Maxian strongly favored going into the apartment. He said, "I believe that regardless of the lack of evidence on bioterrorism, we have to be certain there is no public health threat from any biologicals that might be present."

Dr. Blumenfeld responded, "The local law enforcement officials are not willing to seek a search warrant for the apartment either. They don't believe they have adequate cause to present to the court. They are basing their decisions on the FBI's threat assessment. If we go in, we would not have any type of law enforcement officials with us on this one. I don't know whether we have the authority as public health officials to enter that apartment. I'll have to check with my health director to see if she's OK with this."

Following the conference call with CDC, Dr. Blumenfeld called the health director. In turn, the health director contacted the department's legal counsel, and they all participated in a conference call. The response gave Dr. Blumenfeld some needed assurance. Counsel said, "We agree that there is a concern of a public health threat here and, based on our reading of the statutes, you can go ahead and enter the apartment."

"Well," thought Dr. Blumenfeld, "I'm surprised and encouraged that counsel was so proactive in his response. They're usually more cautious." Based on his consultation with CDC and his own concerns about what might be in the apartment, Dr. Blumenfeld decided to go ahead and have staff enter the apartment without permission of the occupants.

Dr. Blumenfeld received some additional information from Dr. Yeolekar on the cases from Massachusetts. Dr. Yeolekar was able to obtain basic epidemiologic information about both cases. The first was a sixty-three-year-old Kuwaiti man who was admitted to the hospital on April 1 with a three-week history of fever, chills, and muscle pain. His symptoms had begun while he was on a trip to Saudi Arabia, and he had a history of eating goat meat on that trip.

The second case was a twenty-three-year-old woman who had been seen at a hospital in Lowell, Massachusetts, on January 30. She presented with a one-month history of fever, chills, and muscle pain. She had traveled to Greece in October of the past year and had consumed unpasteurized goat cheese during that trip.

Dr. Blumenfeld, Dr. Winston, and the New Hampshire State Laboratory Director met to plan the entry into the apartment. The first question Dr. Blumenfeld asked was, "Based on the knowledge needed, who should actually go in? There is also the question of personal protective equipment." The Department had only limited types of protective equipment, so this was a concern. Dr. Blumenfeld continued, "There is the possibility that some other type of hazard exists. If the apartment was used by bioterrorists, there could be booby traps." The lab director pointed out that other biological hazards could be present as well. The group discussed what would be done once they were in the apartment. This required carefully thinking through the objective of this operation.

All the careful discussion and consultation led Dr. Blumenfeld to a set of initial decisions. "First," he said, "Samantha and Leigh Ralston from the State Public Health Laboratory will enter the apartment as a team. Samantha is a first-rate physician epidemiologist with EIS training, and Leigh is an outstanding public health laboratory scientist. The epidemiologic skills and the lab skills will both be needed to assess the environment of this apartment."

"Second," he continued, "the objective will be to determine whether there is any type of biological production facility or other obvious biological hazard in the apartment. So, I want the team to go in, observe, and then come out. If additional work is required, we will be in a better position to carefully plan—given the information from the initial inspection. Finally, this should be a low-key operation that would not arouse the attention of the press and hopefully be of little concern to the neighbors." The team agreed with the plan and left to begin preparations.

The next day, Friday, April 23, Dr. Blumenfeld, Dr. Winston, Leigh Ralston, and Fran Peerless, the Nashua Public Health Nurse, met at the fire station with members of the local HAZMAT team, local police, and the FBI. The members of the HAZMAT team offered their services to go in with full body protection suits. Dr. Blumenfeld felt that would arouse too much attention and concern, and he therefore declined the offer, at least until the initial inspection could be made. Furthermore, the entry team and Dr. Blumenfeld decided to ride together in a large black Suburban rather than obvious fire department or police vehicles. Dr. Blumenfeld wanted the initial inspection to be as discreet as possible.

Events at the Apartment— Things Do Not Go as Planned

When they arrived at the apartment building, Drs. Blumenfeld and Winston, along with Ralston, quickly found the apartment manager and explained the situation. The others, including the police who had accompanied them, remained in unmarked vehicles down the street. The apartment manager, with his master keys in hand, led them to the suspect apartment. As they approached the apartment door, Dr. Blumenfeld noticed something that immediately caused concern. On the middle of the apartment door was a large, obvious hazardous materials sticker. Apparently, a member of the HAZMAT team had gone to the apartment the day before and placed the warning sticker on the door.

Dr. Blumenfeld thought to himself, "So much for our discreet inspection." He wondered how many of the neighbors had seen the sticker and what kinds of rumors and fears already were circulating. A second event further increased Dr. Blumenfeld's level of concern: None of the apartment manager's keys would open the apartment.

The apartment manager said, "I remember now. This is actually not an apartment anymore. Several of the apartment units were sold as condominiums, and this was one of them. Since this is a private residence and not an apartment, the locks have been changed, and my master key doesn't work for this unit."

"But don't worry," the apartment manager continued. "The apartments, including this one, are quite easy to break into through the patio sliding glass doors. It takes nothing more than a couple of screwdrivers. I've done this several times when people get locked out. I'd be happy to remove the patio door, and the inspection team could enter that way."

Dr. Blumenfeld was really beginning to worry. An entire series of concerns flashed through his mind. He thought, "We are no longer using a legitimate passkey in the possession of an apartment manager to inspect an apartment. Now we are entering a private residence by breaking in though a patio door. Is there enough of a potential threat to warrant this?" Further, he wondered, "What are the neighbors thinking? What if the press is already aware that something is happening? What will I tell them?" Other questions came to mind as well. "What if there is literally nothing of concern in the unit? How will the public and the press see the Health Department? But what if there is a biological production facility in the condo? Our team had agreed to go in and search but come back out if something was found. What are the appropriate next steps if they do find something highly suspicious? Should they go back in immediately? Only the HAZMAT team members have proper equipment, yet they have little experience with biological contamination. How would that be coordinated? What will the FBI and local police authorities want to do if we do find something of questionable legality?"

Dr. Blumenfeld began to wonder whether they had really thought this through. "Have we considered all the possible outcomes of this inspection—especially in light of the possibility of bioterrorism? I don't think it's likely the team will encounter any booby traps. But what if they do? What should I do if one of the team members is injured during the inspection? Do we have procedures for handling that situation? Should I go ahead with this or not? What are the public health ramifications if we delay?" The responsibility weighed heavily as Dr. Blumenfeld tried to decide what to do.

¡Despierta!

A Physician's Stark Encounter With the Grim Human Toll of a Preventable Public Health Problem

We had just spent a pleasant morning with our three-year-old daughter watching mule deer feed at the edge of a high mountain meadow near Chama, New Mexico. Jesse, a recently retired family friend, had showed us where he'd lived while herding sheep as a youngster in the mountains above Tierra Amarilla. The excursion had been a welcome reprieve from hectic lives—mine as a family physician in Albuquerque, my wife, Krista's, as an OB/GYN.

We headed for home early in the afternoon to avoid night and July Fourth traffic on the winding two-lane highway between Chama and Española, which is northeast of Santa Fe. We did not leave early enough. Twenty miles before Española, a small pickup truck with two intoxicated teenagers had crossed the centerline, slamming into an on-coming station wagon driven by a man with his wife and two young boys inside. No emergency vehicles had arrived. A few people stared helplessly at the mangled vehicles. None of the passengers had been wearing seatbelts.

A Country Jaunt Gone Awry

I pulled off the highway. Krista and I sprinted to the collision while Jesse remained behind with our daughter. Trauma is an inadequate description of the carnage we confronted. Two boys, about seven and eight years old, had been dragged from the station wagon and placed on a blanket. Five or six people looked on, unsure of what to do next. Neither child was breathing, although both still had pulses. I wiped the inside of the mouth of the boy closest to me with the cuff of my long-sleeve shirt and began mouth-to-mouth resuscitation. He was a beautiful child, hardly a scratch on him, but the sweep of his mouth stained my sleeve with blood.

At the time of this accident seven years ago, the death rate in New Mexico for young motor vehicle occupants was more than twice that of the United States as whole. New Mexico led the nation in alcohol-related motor vehicle crash fatalities, with 26.7 deaths per 100,000 population versus a national rate of 15.6. Those grim numbers have improved somewhat since the bloody accident I witnessed, as has motor vehicle fatality nationwide over the past century. But that progress has been uneven in states such as Mississippi, Wyoming, Montana, and New Mexico, which share a combination of risk factors for high motor vehicle fatality rates: miles of rural roads; high speed limits; low per capita income; and lax enforcement of drinking laws, seatbelt use, and speed limits.

The Battle for Two Boys

It was miserably hot. The boy's pupils were fixed and dilated, but his pulse was strong and his skin color pink. My mind was whirling, due to hyperventilation or to the sun. A state trooper arrived and began directing traffic, towering over the boy and me, shielding us from the sun.

Krista was on her knees examining the other child when an orthopedist ran up to offer assistance. They determined that resuscitation was useless. The boy's neck was swollen and bruised, obviously broken. They turned their attention to the small pickup. Both teen occupants were dead, crushed in the collapsed cab. Two open beer cans remained undisturbed in their dashboard holders. Empty beer cans were scattered throughout the cab. The smell of beer permeated the stifling hot summer air.

The opportunity for intervention had passed. Despite laws, seatbelt use is low in New Mexico, while intoxicated drivers are common. More than two-thirds of New Mexicans killed in motor vehicle accidents are not restrained. As many as a quar-

ter of the state's children travel in cars without wearing seatbelts or using child safety seats. Often because of alcohol, New Mexico's highways are some of the nation's most lethal, especially on weekends. The situation is worse on rural highways and Indian reservations. Adult seatbelt use within the Navajo Nation was only 8 percent in 1988, child safety seat use was zero, and the motor vehicle fatality rate was five times the national average, a high proportion related to alcohol. Those dismal statistics only began to change when, in 1988, the Navajo Nation Tribal Council passed a seatbelt law, created educational programs, studied the effect of alcohol on motor vehicle fatality, and provided child restraints at no cost. By 1995, two years after the carnage I saw, Navajo Nation motor vehicle–related fatalities had decreased by 52 percent from 1988, child restraint usage increased from zero to 45 percent, and adult seatbelt use rose from 8 percent to 78 percent. Positive trends, but not good enough.

Yet liquor stores flourish in our small towns, especially close to Indian reservations. The alcohol industry furiously battles all legislation and efforts to address the problem.

Death On All Fronts

Krista and the orthopedist moved on to the station wagon. The boys' mother was propped in a sitting position, her back against the car's front tire. When Krista touched her shoulder she slumped over, dead. Her swollen, bruised face and the oval hole in the windshield suggested the cause of death.

A few feet from me, someone gently pulled a blanket over the boy with the broken neck. The boys' father appeared. He was a large Hispanic man, dazed from the accident. After glancing at me, he pulled the blanket back. His callused hands cradled his son's face. In a mournful wail, he cried over and over, "¡Despierta, mi hijo!" (Wake up!).

The first ambulance dispatched had blown a tire. When the second finally arrived, I had been giving mouth-to-mouth resuscitation for more than an hour. The surviving boy's pulse remained strong but he never moved, and his pupils remained fixed and dilated. I learned later that he died within a few hours of arriving at the Rio Arriba County hospital in Española. I felt utterly helpless. My efforts had not been enough to save the child.

The father's voice of despair on that lonely stretch of highway will never leave me. Would the family have survived if they had been wearing seatbelts? Would stricter enforcement of seatbelt laws make a difference? Should there be more traffic checks for drunk drivers on holidays and weekends? Would stronger penalties discourage intoxicated drivers? The answers are probably yes.

A Bleak Landscape

Rio Arriba County, where the accident occurred, is one of the poorest counties in a state that is one of the poorest states in the nation. Residents of the county have the highest heroin addiction rate in the United States. Our governor, Gary Johnson, was interviewed on *60 Minutes* last spring proposing legalization of heroin, while he vetoes funding for substance (alcohol and drug) abuse prevention and treatment programs.

Almost yearly it seems that a high-profile legislator in New Mexico is prosecuted for driving while intoxicated, usually about the time of the legislative session, near one of the favorite Santa Fe watering holes. The lawmaker arrested most recently had twice the legal limit of alcohol in his blood.

Earlier this year an up-and-coming professional golfer and local Native American hero was arrested and served time for driving while intoxicated, a story that was reported in *Sports Illustrated*. It marked his second conviction. He was embarrassed, promised reform, and assured everyone it would not happen again. His work release program included eighteen holes of golf a day.

It is time for us to awake from our slumber. A person dies every thirteen minutes in a motor ve-

hicle accident on our nation's highways, and many more are injured. Three of every ten Americans will become involved in an alcohol-related car accident during their lifetimes. The carnage from motor vehicle deaths and injuries is a public health problem whose cure requires a change of lifestyle, more effective intervention and education, tougher drinking and driving laws, and stricter law enforcement. Prevention and treatment programs, especially in rural areas, are not available or are not covered by health insurance. The paltry number of slots within inpatient and day treatment programs for substance abuse are not meeting demand, and payment by third-party payors for these services is rare.

What Can Be Done?

A man's agonizing loss of wife and two children and the death of the drunk teenagers who triggered the tragedy might have been prevented. To keep the two intoxicated youths off the roads, we might have had more sobriety checkpoints; we could have lowered the legal blood alcohol limit from 0.1 to 0.08 grams/deciliter and introduced zero tolerance for offenders under twenty-one years old. We might have promptly suspended the driver's licenses of the drunk drivers, had they been stopped before the accident. We might have better enforced seatbelt laws, especially those targeting children.

Espousing a more sweeping view of behavior-related prevention, we might enact laws requiring that physicians more consistently perform screening tests for substance abuse during physical examinations, thus better connecting primary medical care with behavioral health. For example, health plans already use some nationally accepted performance benchmarks to measure a range of health care indicators such as immunization and cancer screening rates. If we want to reduce vehicle-related deaths, it is critical to develop metrics similar to the Health Plan Employer Data and Information Set (HEDIS). This data set was initially formed by a consortium of health plans, large purchasers, and consultants to measure the quality of employer-sponsored medical benefits. The consortium then gave the data set to the National Committee for Quality Assurance (NCQA) for further development and implementation. The NCQA now has 250 organizations (representing 400 health plans) that submit annual HEDIS data. Similar standards should be developed for substance abuse screening and for seatbelt and child seat use among publicly funded patient populations. More broadly, requiring states to meet certain outcome measures based on seatbelt use, alcohol related fatalities, and access to prevention and treatment programs might encourage enforcement of strategies that are already considered effective.

There is reason for optimism. Seatbelt use in the nation jumped from 11 percent in 1981 to 68 percent in 1997, because of better enforcement of seatbelt, child restraint, speed limit, and driving while intoxicated laws; improved road construction; safer vehicles; and education programs. But these steps must applied in a more rigorous, more ubiquitous, and more collective manner—across our state and across the whole country.

For a tormented father on the side of a New Mexican road, policies that "might have" been put in place are not good enough. Despite dramatic improvement over the years, motor vehicle–related deaths remain the leading cause of injury related deaths in the United States. How many more fathers will have to watch their children die on the road before something is done?

"¡Despierta!"

Index

The Act to Establish a National Board of Health of 1879, 112 (exhibit)
The Act Relative to Quarantine of 1796, 112 (exhibit)
The Act for the Relief of Sick and Disabled Seaman of 1798, 112-113 (exhibits)
Action planning:
  alternative actions, 17-18
  financial analysis and, 18
  process of, 19-20
  Skilled Nursing Facilities (SNFs), 80
Administrative disciplines, 9
Administrative law, 119
Africa. *See* Mantookan blood supply; Zambia
Agencies. *See* Government; Organizations
Agency for Health Services Research (AHSR), 114 (exhibit)
Agency for Toxic Substances and Disease Registry (ATSDR), 114 (exhibit)
AIDS (acquired immunodeficiency syndrome), 113 (exhibit), 118
  Nepalese experience of, 156-157, 157-161 (exhibits)
  See also HIV infection
AIDSCAP, 155, 157-161
  assessment of, 164-165, 168, 169-171 (exhibits)
  budget for, 164, 168 (exhibit)
  commercial sex workers (CSWs) and, 159, 161, 169 (exhibit)
  communication program in, 162-164
  condom distribution/use, 161-162, 169 (exhibit)
  creative strategy in, 162-164, 163 (exhibit)
  future of, 168, 170
  knowledge of AIDS, 170 (exhibit)
  media in, 164, 165-167 (exhibits), 171 (exhibit)
  target audiences, 162
  See also Nepal
Air Pollution Control Act of 1955, 113 (exhibit)
Alabama public health services, 339
  Alabama Public Health Care Authority (APHCA), 362-366, 365-367 (exhibits)
  clinic services, 360, 362-363 (exhibits)
  facilities crisis, 340
  legislature-approved bonds, 339-340
  public finance authority, 340, 341-361 (exhibits), 360, 362
  See also Cooper Green Hospital (CGH); Jefferson County, Alabama
Alcohol-related road deaths, 379-382
ALLKIDS program, 207
Alternative public health solutions, 17-18
American Board of Medical Specialties, 124
American Board of Preventive Medicine, 124
American Dental Association, 118
American Medical Association, 118
American Nurses Association (ANA), 124
American Nurses Credentialing Center (ANCC), 95, 124
American Public Health Association, 117
American Red Cross, 118
Anesthesiology, developments in, 90
Antitrust legislation, 90, 103-104

Baby formula, 288
Balanced Budget Act (BBA) of 1997, 80, 207, 211
Bioterrorism, 369-370
  brucellosis, 371-372 (exhibit)

casework information, 370-373
HAZMAT (Hazardous Materials) team, 375, 377
public health response, 374-378
Bioterrorism Preparedness and Response Program,
   127
Blood supply:
   Global Blood Safety (GBS) Project, 135 (exhibit)
   Mantookan blood supply, 133-154 (case study)
Boards of Health, 112 (exhibit), 117
Brucellosis, 371-372 (exhibit)

C. W. Williams Health Center, 319, 323
   Carolina ACCESS Program, 328-334, 333-335
      (exhibits)
   challenges for, 323-324
   community health centers and, 321-323
   cost-effectiveness, 322-323
   financial stability of, 327, 328-332 (exhibits)
   hospital affiliation, 324
   managed care plans, 323
   medically underserved population, 321-322, 322
      (exhibits)
   mission/vision/values statements, 320 (exhibit)
   organizational structure, 325, 327, 327 (exhibit)
   patient population, 325, 326 (exhibits)
   services, 324-325, 324 (exhibit)
   strategic planning/SWOT analysis, 334-336, 336
      (exhibit)
Cadbury Schweppes, 229, 230, 231
Capitated health plan, 78-80, 87-89
Carolina ACCESS Program, 328-334
Case analysis, ix, x, 8
   action planning, 19-20
   alternative solutions, 17-18
   decision-making practice, 3, 6
   goal specificity, 14
   health issues and, 9
   information and, 8
   issue identification, 14-16
   organizational mission and, 12-13
   problem-solving and, 6-7
   process in, 4, 5 (exhibit), 20
   real life vs. hypothetical cases, 4-6
   recommendations and, 18-19, 20
   report presentation, 20
   roles in, 7
   situational analysis, 9-11
   strengths, weaknesses, opportunities, and threats
      (SWOT) analysis, 11-12, 13 (exhibit)
   theoretical perspective development, 17
   See also Issue analysis
Case studies:
   AIDSCAP/Nepal, 155-172

Alabama public health services, 339-367
bioterrorism/New Hampshire, 369-378
C. W. Williams Health Center, 319-337
CDC/Mantookan blood supply, 133-154
Cooper Green Hospital/Community Care Plan, 199-
   220
DeKalb County Board of Health (DCBOH), 289-
   297
ethical issues, 285-288
Indian Health Service (IHS), 265-283
Indiana State Department of Health (ISDH), 173-
   197
meningococcal outbreak/New Mexico, 307-317
motor vehicle-related deaths, 379-382
red tide/Escambia County, Florida, 299-305
UNICEF's oral rehydration program/Zambia, 221-
   236
West Nile Virus outbreak/New York State, 237-264
Centers for Disease Control and Prevention (CDC),
   ix, 114 (exhibit), 136, 153
   background of, 137
   Center for Infectious Diseases organization, 139
      (exhibit)
   Epidemic Intelligence Service (EIS), 125, 134-135
      (exhibits), 137
   Epidemiology Program Office (EPO) organization,
      134 (exhibit)
   information, electronic transmission of, 127
   Mantookan blood supply, 133-154 (case study)
   Meningococcal outbreak response, 315, 316
   organization of, 137-139 (exhibits)
   outside employment/activity and, 138, 141 (exhibit),
      146-148 (exhibit)
   Preventive Medicine Residency (PMR) Program,
      140 (exhibit)
   tuberculosis program, 119
Children's Bureau, 113 (exhibit)
Children's Health Insurance Plans (CHIPS), 207
Clean Air Act (CAA), 111
Clean Water Act (CWA), 111
Clinical Laboratory Improvement Act of 1988, 119
Commercial sex workers (CSWs), 155-157, 157
   (exhibit), 158 (exhibit), 159, 161, 162
Community Care Plan (CCP), 200, 201, 202, 215
   Cooper Green Hospital (CGH) and, 219
   enrollment/utilization, 218, 218 (exhibit)
   funding of, 215-216
   health maintenance organization licensing, 219-220
   marketing efforts, 218-219
   member services, 216-217, 216 (exhibit)
   operating costs, 217
   staffing, 217
Community health. *See* C. W. Williams Health
   Center; U. S. public health system

Comprehensive Environmental Response,
  Competition and Liability Act (CERCLA), 111
Condoms. *See* AIDSCAP; Nepal
Constitutional powers, 118-119
Consultants, 7
Consumer Product Safety Commission, 111
Contact tracing, 120
Contextual issues, 4, 8
  decision factors, 9-10
  market constituents, 10
  organizational characteristics, 10-11
  service categories, 10
Cooper Green Hospital (CGH), 199-201, 201
  (exhibit)
  ALLKIDS program, 207
  Children's Health Insurance Plans (CHIPS), 207
  Community Care Plan (CCP), 202, 215-220, 216
    (exhibit), 218 (exhibit)
  county government/authority and, 209-210
  financial statements, 201, 202-203 (exhibits)
  HealthFirst plan, 201-202, 204 (exhibit)
  hospital operations, 210-211, 213 (exhibit), 214-215
  inpatient statistics, 200-201, 201 (exhibit)
  Jefferson Health System (JHS) and, 201, 209-211,
    213 (exhibit), 215
  managed care and, 205
  Medicare/Medicaid and, 205-207, 206 (exhibit)
  mission/vision/value statements, 201, 204 (exhibit)
  nonphysician providers (NPPs), 207
  outpatient statistics, 211, 214, 214 (exhibit)
  U. S. health care reform, 202, 205-207
  See also Alabama public health services; Jefferson
    County, Alabama
Crowding, 110, 112 (exhibit)
Cryptosporidium, 113 (exhibit)
Current procedural terminology (CPT), 77, 78
  (exhibit), 80

Decision-making, 3
  context of, 4, 8, 9-10
  opportunities vs. threat in, 11-12, 13 (exhibit)
  risk in, 6
  See also Case analysis
DeKalb County Board of Health (DCBOH):
  County demographics, 292-293 (exhibit)
  Director, selection of, 289-290
  management's perceptions of, 294 (exhibit)
  mission/function of, 294 (exhibit)
  programs/initiatives, 291 (exhibit)
  strategic transformation of, 295-297
Demographic factors, 9
Diagnosis related groups (DRGs), 76-77
Diarrheal disease, 221

causes/treatment, 223-226
control constraints, 226-228
deaths from, 224-226, 225 (exhibits)
environmental constraints, 226-227
oral rehydration program, 221
Zambia and, 221-223, 223-224 (exhibits)
See also Oral rehydration salts (ORS); Zambia
Disability insurance, 97
Disease control/eradication, 113 (exhibit), 118, 120
Disease/injury reporting, 120
Drug industry, 95-96
Drug therapies, 113 (exhibit), 121

Ebola virus, 126
Economic issues, 4, 6, 9
  allied health services, 94-95
  drug/medical supply industry, 95-96
  gross domestic product (GDP) statistics, 91-92, 92-
    93 (exhibits)
  hospital sector, 92-93, 96
  nursing home services, 95
  physician services, 93-94
  resource allocation, 96
  spending growth, 87, 88-89 (exhibits), 89
  See also Payor categories; Reimbursement
Education:
  government assistance in, 90, 104
  maternal, 112 (exhibit)
  medical school enrollment, 104, 106
  public health management/leadership and, ix, 4-6
  public health training, 124-125
  risk-free, 3, 6
  scientific/medical knowledge, 87
Employees, 4
  health benefits, 89, 103
  See also Payor categories
Encephalitis, 237-239
Environmental factors. *See* Contextual issues
Environmental health, 111, 114, 120
Environmental Protection Agency (EPA), 12, 111, 115
Epidemic Intelligence Service (EIS), 125, 134-135
    (exhibits), 137 (exhibit)
Epidemics, 120, 125, 126
Epidemiological Program Office (EPO), 134 (exhibit)
Escambia County Health Department. *See* Red tide
Escherichia coli, 113 (exhibit)
Ethics, issues in, 285
  Annie O., 287-288
  baby boy-X, 286-287
  free baby formula, 288
  Institutional Ethics Committees (IECs), 285-286
Evaluation:
  alternative solutions, 18

oral presentations, 52-53

Family Health International (FHI), 157
Federal government. *See* Government; U. S. public
    health system
Federal Insecticide, Fungicide, and Rodenticide Act
    (FIFRA), 111
Federal Mine Safety and Health Act (MSHA), 114
Fee-for-service (FFS), 78, 79, 88, 90
Financial analysis, 18, 55
  activity ratios, 68-70
  age of facility, 73
  balance sheets, 57 (exhibit), 59 (exhibit), 60-62
  capital structure ratios, 66-68
  capitation, 78-80
  cost of capital, 75
  cost of debt, 75-76
  financial statements, 55-58, 56-57 (exhibits), 59
    (exhibit)
  health maintenance organizations (HMOs), 78-80
  income statements, 56 (exhibit), 58-60
  liquidity ratios, 62-65
  Medicare reimbursement, 76-77, 80
  outpatient services, 80
  physician reimbursement, 77-78, 78 (exhibit)
  profitability ratios, 70-73
  prospective payment system (PPS), 76-77
  ratio analysis, 62-73, 74-75
  resource-based relative value scale (RBRVS), 77-78,
    78 (exhibit)
  skilled nursing facilities, 80
  working/net working capital, 74
  See also Economic issues
Food and Drug Administration (FDA), 114 (exhibit)
Food, Drug, and Cosmetic Act (FDCA), 114

Gamma Pharmaceuticals, 229, 230-231
General Board of Health for England, 110
General Pharmaceutical Ltd., 229
Genetic diseases, 126-127
Global Blood Safety (GBS) Project, 135 (exhibit)
Goldfarb vs. Virginia Bar, 90
Government, 55
  health care interventions, 90
  Medicare/ Medicaid, 76-78, 78 (exhibit), 80, 103
  public health activities, 100, 101 (exhibit)
  state police powers, 118
  See also U. S. public health system
Great Britain, 110-111
Group Health Cooperative, 87

Hansen's disease, 109-110
Hantavirus, 113 (exhibit), 126, 307, 314, 316
  See also Meningococcal outbreak/New Mexico
Health Alert Network, 127
Health care. *See* U. S. health care system
Health Care Financing Administration (HCFA), 76,
  80, 86, 114 (exhibit), 119, 206
Health care reform, 189, 190, 192 (exhibit), 202, 205
Health Maintenance Organization (HMO) Act of
  1973, 88-89
Health Maintenance organizations (HMOs), 78-80,
  87-89, 103, 104 (exhibit), 205
Health Plan Employer Data and Information Set
  (HEDIS), 381-382
Health Professions Education Assistance Act of 1963,
  90
Health Resources and Services Administration
  (HRSA), ix, 114 (exhibit)
Healthcare Financial Management Association
  (HFMA), 74
HealthFirst, 201-202, 204 (exhibit)
HealthWatch needs assessment survey, 219
Hemorrhagic fever, 307
High-density living conditions, 110, 112 (exhibit)
Hill-Burton Act for Health Facilities Construction of
  1946, 90, 200, 339
HIV infection, 118
  blood supply and, 133-154 (case study)
  See also AIDSCAP
Hookworm Eradication Project, 116, 118
Hospitals, 92-93
  physician relationship with, 96
  utilization trends, 101-103, 102 (exhibit)
Human Genome Project, 90, 126
Hygienic Laboratory, 112 (exhibit)
Hypothetical cases, 4-6

Immunization, 117, 120
India, 155-157
Indian Health Care Improvement Act of 1976, 268
Indian Health Service (IHS), 97, 114 (exhibit), 265-
  266
  demographics/health factors, 269-272 (exhibits)
  funding, 278-279, 280-282 (exhibits), 283
  historical perspective, 267-268, 268 (exhibits)
  meningococcal outbreak and, 315
  organizational structure of, 272-274, 273-275
    (exhibits)
  personnel, 275-276, 277-278 (exhibits), 278
  programs/initiatives, 274-275, 276-277 (exhibits)
  service population, 269-272
  tribal/community self-determination, 266-267, 283
  tribal contracts/compacts, 278, 279 (exhibit)

Indian Self-Determination and Educational
  Assistance Act of 1975, 266-267, 278
Indiana State Department of Health (ISDH), 173, 176,
  177 (exhibit)
  adaptive strategy formulation, 190-193
  directional strategy formulation, 187
  evaluation, 194-197
  external environmental analysis, 178-180
  financial assessment, 184-185, 184-185 (exhibits)
  health care reform, 189, 190, 192 (exhibit)
  human resources/staffing, 186
  implementation planning, 192-194
  information/outreach subsystems in, 186
  internal environmental analysis, 181-187
  mission/vision statements, 187, 188 (exhibit)
  needs/capacity assessment, 191-192, 193 (exhibit),
    195-196
  organizational culture, 181-184
  physical facilities, 186
  programs in, 189-190, 191 (exhibit), 193 (exhibit)
  public health services in, 176, 178 (exhibit)
  Q-sort method, 190, 193 (exhibit), 196-197
  situational analysis, 174-176
  stakeholder analysis, 177-178, 180-181 (exhibit)
  strategic management in, 173-174, 174-175
    (exhibits)
  success factors, 187, 189 (exhibit)
  trend/issue analysis, 180-181, 182-183 (exhibits)
Industrial Revolution, 110, 111
Infant mortality, 112 (exhibit)
  American Indians/Alaska Natives, 271 (exhibit)
  diarrheal disease and, 224-226, 225 (exhibits)
Infectious diseases, 90, 112-113 (exhibits)
  contact tracing, 120
  emergence of, 126
  individual rights and, 119-120
  involuntary testing, 120
  quarantine, 109-110, 111, 112 (exhibit), 121
  See also Meningococcal outbreak/New Mexico; West
    Nile virus
Information, 4, 6
  inferences and, 8
  mission statements, 12-13
  obtainable, 8
  public health informatics, 127
  systems of, 11
Information Network for Public Health Officials
  (INPHO), 127
Information sources:
  abstracts, 21-22
  bibliographies, 22
  computerized information services, 23
  dictionaries, 23
  directories, 24

  handbooks/guides, 24-27
  internet resources, 30-33, 127
  journals, 27-28
  on-line journals/publications, 28-30
  statistical sources, 33-34
Institute of Medicine (IOM), ix, 109, 111, 122
Insurance. See Payor categories
Interchem, 229, 231
InterMark, 221
International Classification of Diseases, 9th Revision,
  Clinical Modification (ICD-9-CM), 76
Internet resources, 30-33, 127
Issue analysis, 14-15
  core problem identification, 15-16
  narrow perspective in, 15
  problem statement stage, 16

Jefferson County, Alabama, 207-209, 208 (exhibit)
  acute care hospitals, 209, 210-211 (exhibits)
  Jefferson County Department of Health (JCDH),
    209, 212 (exhibit)
  Jefferson Health System (JHS), 201, 209-211, 213
    (exhibit), 215
  managed care organizations, 212 (exhibit)
  See also Alabama public health services; Cooper
    Green Hospital (CGH)
Judicial law, 119

Kaiser Permanente, 87

Laboratory standards, 119
Leadership programs. See Public health management/
  leadership
Learning. See Education
Legal issues, 4
  emerging concerns, 120-121
  English common law, 111
  individual rights vs. common health, 119-120
  laws, source of, 119
  public health powers, 118-119
  state police powers, 118, 119
  tobacco lawsuits, 113 (exhibit)
Leprosy, 109-110
Life expectancy, 113 (exhibit)
Life-span expansion, 87, 90
Local public health agencies (LPHAs), 116-118, 121-
  122, 124

Malathion, 253-255
Managed care organizations (MCOs), 78-80

Carolina ACCESS Program, 328-334, 333-335 (exhibits)
  development of, 87-89, 126
  trends in, 103-104, 104 (exhibit), 323
Management. *See* Public health management/leadership
Mantookan blood supply, 133-154 (case study)
  background, 136
  chronological sequence, 136, 138, 140-153, 141-150 (exhibits)
  decision meeting, 153
  problem in, 133-136, 134-135 (exhibits)
March of Dimes, 118
Marine Hospital Service, 112-113 (exhibits)
Marketing:
  strategies in, 11
  targets of, 10
Massachusetts Sanitary Commission Report, 112 (exhibit)
Maternal health activities, 112-113 (exhibits)
Medicaid. *See* Medicare/Medicaid
Medical examinations, 120
Medical supply industry, 95-96
Medicare Hospital Insurance Trust Fund, 96, 97, 99
Medicare/Medicaid, 90, 113 (exhibit)
  Carolina ACCESS Program, 328-334, 333-335 (exhibits)
  enrollment statistics, 205-207, 206 (exhibits)
  managed care arrangements and, 103
  outpatient services, 80
  prospective payment system (PPS) and, 76-77
  resource-based relative value (RBRV) reimbursement, 77-78, 78 (exhibit)
  skilled nursing facilities (SNFs), 80
MEDLINE, 127
Meningococcal outbreak/New Mexico, 307
  community characteristics/Cuba, New Mexico, 312-313 (exhibit)
  hantavirus pulmonary syndrome and, 307, 314, 316
  meningitis contact investigation, 311, 313-314
  New Mexico Department of Health, 308-310 (exhibit)
  response to, 314-316
Mental health programs, 114 (exhibit), 117
Metrolina Health Center. *See* C. W. Williams Health Center
Mission statements, 10, 12-13
Mortality, 113 (exhibit)
  American Indians/Alaska Natives, 271-272 (exhibits)
  diarrheal diseases, 224-226, 225 (exhibit)
  infant, 112 (exhibit)
Motor vehicle-related deaths, 379-382

Nassau County. *See* West Nile virus (WNV)
National Association of Local Boards of Health, 117
National Center for HIV, STD, and TB Prevention, 135
National Committee for Quality Assurance (NCQA), 382
National Consumers League, 118
National Electronic Disease Surveillance System (NEDSS), 127
National Environmental Health Association (NEHA), 124
National Immunization Program, 127
National Institutes of Health (NIH), 87 (exhibit), 112 (exhibit), 114 (exhibit), 126
National Library of Medicine (NLM), 127
National Medical Research Institute in Mantooka (MAMRI), 142, 154
National School Lunch and Child Nutrition Amendments, 113 (exhibit)
National Tuberculosis Association, 118
Native Americans. *See* Indian Health Service (IHS)
Nepal:
  AIDS, historical perspective, 156-157, 158-161 (exhibits)
  commercial sex workers (CSWs), 155-156, 157 (exhibit), 158 (exhibit), 162
  condom purchase/use, 156, 158-159 (exhibits)
  economic system, 172
  history/political system, 172
  India and, 155-156
  knowledge of AIDS, 157, 160-161 (exhibits)
  social/cultural environment, 172
  topography/climate, 170, 172
  See also AIDSCAP
New Hampshire. *See* Bioterrorism
New Mexico Department of Health, 308-310 (exhibit)
  See also Meningococcal outbreak/New Mexico
New York. *See* West Nile virus (WNV)
Nonphysician providers (NPPs), 207
Not-for-profit organizations, 55
Nuclear Regulatory Commission, 111
Nurse practitioners, 95, 207
Nursing home services, 95
Nutrition, 110, 112 (exhibit), 113 (exhibit)

Objectivity, 7
Occupational Safety and Health Act (OSHA), 113 (exhibit), 114
Oral presentations, 20, 35
  audience analysis, 36-38
  categories of, 36
  computer software and, 45
  credibility, establishment of, 47, 50

delivery styles, 49-50
emotional appeal, 37-38
ethical appeal, 37
evaluation of, 52-53
information quality, 38
logical appeal, 38
nonverbal communication in, 48
organization of, 39-43
question-and-answer period, 51-52
rehearsal of, 50-51
site logistics, 38-39
speech anxiety, 47
visual aids in, 43-46, 48
Oral rehydration salts (ORS), 224-226, 225 (exhibits)
Cadbury Schweppes, 229, 230, 231
Colgate & Palmolive, 231
costs of, 226, 227-230, 229 (exhibit)
delivery constraints, 226-228
distribution, 230-232, 231 (exhibit)
distribution alternatives, 231-232
Gamma Pharmaceuticals, 229, 230-231
General Pharmaceutical Ltd., 229
health care professionals, training of, 233, 233 (exhibit)
Interchem, 229, 231
Lyons Brooke Bond, 231
need/demand for, 226
packaging, 232-233
promotion of, 233-234, 235 (exhibit)
supply alternatives, 228-230
sustainability issue, 234, 236
UNICEF program development, 236
See also Diarrheal disease; Zambia
Organizations, 3
capacity of, 195
culture of, 4, 10-11, 18
decision context and, 4, 9-11
goals in, 1
government and, 55
information systems in, 11
marketing strategies, 11
mission statement, 10, 12-13
opportunities, decision-making, 11-12, 13 (exhibit)
resource limitations, 7, 11
See also Financial analysis
Outpatient services, 80

Payor categories, 96, 98-100 (exhibits)
government, 97-99
household payors, 96-97
non-patient revenues, 97
private business, 97
Pesticides:

biological, 252
chemical interactions and, 252, 263
malathion, 253-255
pyrethrins/pyrethroids, 252, 259-263
resmethrin, 256-258
Physicians:
active practitioners, 104-106, 105 (exhibits)
bargaining protection, 103-104
reimbursement of, 77-78, 78 (exhibit)
resource allocation and, 96
services of, expenditure growth, 93-94
Physician's assistants, 207
Point-of-service (POS) plans, 205
Police powers, 118, 119
Political issues, 4, 6
Pollution standards, 11-12
Preferred provider organizations (PPOs), 78, 205
Presentations. See Oral presentations
Preventive Medicine Residency (PMR) Program, 140
Problem-solving. See Case analysis; Issue analysis
Professional Standards Review Organizations (PSROs), 90
Prospective payment system (PPS), 76-77, 90
Prostitution. See AIDSCAP
Public Health Cigarette Smoking Act of 1970, 113 (exhibit)
Public health disciplines, 9
Public health management/leadership, ix, x
decision-making and, 3-4, 5 (exhibit)
See also Case analysis; Organizations; U. S. public health system
Public health response. See Case analysis
Public health science, 3, 6, 87
bacteriology, 112 (exhibit)
disease eradication, 113 (exhibit)
drug-resistance, 113 (exhibit), 126
infectious diseases, drug therapy for, 113 (exhibit), 121, 126
Public Health Service. See U. S. Public Health Service; U. S. public health system
Pyrethrins/pyrethroids, 259-263

Q-sort method, 190, 193 (exhibit), 196-197
Quality Health Care Coalition Act, 103
Quality issues, 125-126
Quarantine, 109-110, 111, 112 (exhibit), 121

Real-life cases, 4-6
Recommendations, 18-19, 20
Red tide:
blooms, 299-301, 300 (exhibit)
Escambia County, demographics, 304

media coverage, 301, 303, 304-305
   nutrient load and, 303
   public health impact, 301-303, 302 (exhibit), 304
Reference materials. *See* Information sources
Reform. *See* Health care reform
Regulatory philosophy, 9
Reimbursement:
   capitation, 78-80
   outpatient services, 80
   prospective payment system (PPS), 76-77
   resource-based relative value scale (RBRVS), 77-78,
      78 (exhibit)
   skilled nursing facilities, 80
   See also Payor categories
Research, 86-87, 86 (exhibit)
Resmethrin, 256-258
Resource-based relative value scale (RBRVS), 77-78,
   78 (exhibit), 90
Resource Conservation and Recovery Act (RCRA),
   111
Resources, 3
   allocation decisions, 96, 287-288
   competition for, 55
   organizational, 4, 7, 11
Risks:
   decision-making and, 3, 6
   managed care organizations and, 103
Rockefeller Sanitary Commission Hookworm
   Eradication Project, 116, 118

Safe Drinking Water Act (SDWA), 111
St. Louis Encephalitis (SLE) virus, 237-239
Sanitation, 110, 111, 112 (exhibit), 115, 116
Science. *See* Public health science
Seatbelt legislation, 381, 382
Services:
   categories of, 10
   market constituents, 10
Sexually transmitted diseases (STDs), 156, 158, 163-
   164
The Shattuck Report, 112 (exhibit)
Shepard-Towner Act of 1921, 112 (exhibit)
Situational analysis, 9
   decision context, 9-10
   organizational issues, 10-11, 14-16
   SWOT analysis and, 11-12, 13 (exhibit)
   See also Case analysis
Skilled Nursing Facilities (SNFs), 80
Smoking, 90, 113 (exhibit)
Social/cultural issues, 4, 6
Social Security Act of 1935, 113 (exhibit)
Social Security Amendments of 1965, 90, 113
   (exhibit), 206

Social welfare, 112 (exhibit)
Socioeconomic status, 112 (exhibit)
State government. *See* U. S. public health system
Strategic management. *See* Indiana State Department
   of Health (ISDH)
Strengths, weaknesses, opportunities, and threats
   (SWOT) analysis, 11-12, 13 (exhibit)
Substance Abuse and Mental Health Services
   Administration (SAMHSA), 114 (exhibit)
Superfund Amendments and Reauthorization Act
   (SARA), 111

Technology, 4, 9
Testing. *See* Medical examinations
Toxic Substance Control Act (TCSA), 114
Treatment, mandated, 120
Tribal Self-Governance Demonstration Project, 278
Tuberculosis, 113 (exhibit), 117, 119
   drug resistance in, 126
   drug therapy in, 121
   involuntary testing, 120
Typhoid, 116

U. S. health care system, 4, 9
   economic characteristics of, 91-96, 92-94 (exhibits)
   environmental trends, 101-106, 102 (exhibit), 104-
      105 (exhibits)
   government and, 100, 101 (exhibit)
   hospitals, 92-93, 96, 101-103, 102 (exhibit)
   managed care, 87-89, 103-104, 104 (exhibit)
   payor categories, 96-99, 98-100 (exhibits)
   physician workforce, 104-106, 105 (exhibits)
   scientific knowledge/research and, 86-87, 86
      (exhibit)
   significant events in, 90 (exhibit), 91
   spending growth, 87, 88-89 (exhibits), 89
   trends in, 85-86
U. S. Public Health Service (USPHS), 267, 268
U. S. public health system, 109
   environmental health, 111, 114, 120
   essential services in, 123-124
   expenditures in, 121-122
   federal government role in, 111, 114, 114 (exhibit)
   genetic diseases, 126-127
   government services in, 100, 101 (exhibit)
   historical perspective, 109-111, 112-113 (exhibit)
   infectious diseases, emergence of, 126
   informatics, 127
   information technology/internet, 127
   intergovernmental relationships, 125-126
   legal framework, 118-121
   local agencies (LPHAs), 116-118, 121-122, 124

managed care, 78-80, 87-89, 103-104, 104 (exhibit), 126, 205
mission statement, 122-123
providers in, 124
public health training, 124-125
reform in, 189, 191, 191 (exhibit), 202, 205-207
restructuring initiatives, state efforts, 115-116
state government role in, 115-116
systemic change, 126
See also Centers for Disease Control and Prevention (CDC); Medicare/Medicaid
United Nations International Children's Emergency Fund (UNICEF). *See* Oral rehydration program

Vaccination services. *See* Immunization
Veterans Administration, 97
Viral hemorrhagic fever viruses, 307
Vital statistics, 112 (exhibit), 120

Water Pollution Control Act of 1948, 113 (exhibit)
West Nile virus (WNV), 237-239
  biological pesticides, 252
  chemical insecticides, 252-263
  disease characteristics, 239
  environmental health office memo, 250-252, 263
  health department leadership team reports, 241-264
  health education office memo, 263-264
  infectious disease office memo, 241, 250

integrated pest management (IPM), 251-252, 263
Integrated Pest Management Mosquito Surveillance and Control program, 240
malathion, 253-255
Nassau County demographics, 239-241
Nassau County Mosquito Surveillance and Control Status Report, 242-250 (exhibit)
policy issues, 264
pyrethrins/pyrethroids, 259-263
resmethrin, 256-258
sentinel bird deaths, 240-241, 240 (exhibit)
spraying programs, 237-238, 239, 241, 251-252, 264
vector analysis, 251
Williams Health Center. *See* C. W. Williams Health Center
Women, Infants, and Children Program (WIC), 113 (exhibit)
Workmen's compensation, 97
World Health Organization (WHO), 113 (exhibit), 224, 230

Zambia, 221-222
  diarrhea incidence, 222, 224 (exhibit)
  health status/expenditures, 222
  medical facilities/providers, 222, 224 (exhibit)
  population statistics, 222, 223 (exhibit)
  private sector health services, 222-223
  See also Diarrheal disease; Oral rehydration salts (ORS)

About the Authors

Stuart A. Capper, DrPH, is Professor of Health Care Organization and Policy and Co-Director of the MidSouth Program for Public Health Practice, University of Alabama at Birmingham (UAB). He has served as Associate Dean of the School of Public Health and Chairman of the Department of Health Care Organization and Policy. Before coming to UAB, he served as Senior Staff to the Chancellor of the Tulane Medical Center. He has been a lead investigator on projects concerning the implementation of strategic management in state health departments. He also has received federal funding for the development of case studies in public health practice. In addition, he serves on the faculty of the Preventive Medicine Residency Program of the Centers for Disease Control and works with colleagues at CDC on case research projects. His publications in the area of public health management have appeared in *Public Health Reports, Public Productivity and Management Review, Health Services Management Review, Preventive Medicine, Academic Medicine, The European Journal of Public Health,* and the *Case Research Journal.* He is the recipient of the Phillip Cooper Award for the Outstanding Health Care Case Study and the UAB Faculty Award for Outstanding Public Health Service.

Peter M. Ginter is Professor and Chair of the Department of Health Care Organization and Policy in the School of Public Health and Professor of Management in the Graduate School of Management at the University of Alabama at Birmingham. He is the author or coauthor of eleven books, including *Strategic Management of Health Care Organizations* (3d ed., with Jack Duncan and Linda Swayne, 1998), *The Physician Strategist* (1996, with Duncan and Swayne), and *Strategic Issues in Health Care Management* (1992, with Duncan and Swayne). He is also coeditor (with Duncan and Swayne) of *The Handbook of Health Care Management* (1998). He has published more than 100 articles, papers, and cases in management journals, with his work appearing in such publications as the *California Management Review, Academy of Management Review, Academy of Management Executive, Business Horizons, Journal of Management Studies, Long Range Planning, Management International Review, Journal of Leadership Studies, Managerial Planning, Public Health Reports, Advances in Health Care Management,* and the *Journal of Case Research.*

Linda E. Swayne, PhD, is Professor and Chair of the Department of Marketing in the Belk College of Business Administration at The University of North Carolina at Charlotte. She serves as Editor of the *Case Research Journal* and has assisted public health practitioners in Alabama and New Mexico and at the Centers for Disease Control and Prevention with case research and writing. She has served on the Board of Directors of C. W. Williams Health Center and is on the Steering Committee for the Metrolina Health Initiative. Her consulting work has been with hospitals, pharmaceutical companies, the Mecklenburg County Medical Society (MCMS), Centers for Disease Control, and a variety of physician practices. She was presented the Friends of Medicine Award by MCMS in 1997. She has coauthored ten textbooks, more then twenty-five journal articles, and thirty-five case studies. She has served as president of three professional organizations. She cochairs the Strategic Thinking in Health Care Faculty Forum for AUPHA.